T0263168

PET Imaging of Thoracic Disease

Guest Editors

DREW A. TORIGIAN, MD
ABASS ALAVI, MD, PhD (Hon), DSc (Hon)

PET CLINICS

www.pet.theclinics.com

Consulting Editor
ABASS ALAVI, MD, PhD (Hon), DSc (Hon)

July 2011 • Volume 6 • Number 3

SAUNDERS an imprint of ELSEVIER, Inc.

W.B. SAUNDERS COMPANY
A Division of Elsevier Inc.

1600 John F. Kennedy Boulevard • Suite 1800 • Philadelphia, Pennsylvania 19103-2899

http://www.theclinics.com

PET CLINICS Volume 6, Number 3
July 2011 ISSN 1556-8598, ISBN-13: 978-1-4557-1049-2

Editor: Barton Dudlick
Developmental Editor: Eva Kulig

PET Clinics (ISSN 1556-8598) is published quarterly by Elsevier Inc., 360 Park Avenue South, New York, NY 10010-1710. Months of issue are January, April, July, and October. Periodicals postage paid at New York, NY, and additional mailing offices. Subscription prices per year are $199.00 (US individuals), $279.00 (US institutions), $102.00 (US students), $226.00 (Canadian individuals), $312.00 (Canadian institutions), $124.00 (Canadian students), $241.00 (foreign individuals), $312.00 (foreign institutions), and $124.00 (foreign students). To receive student and resident rate, orders must be accompanied by name of affiliated institution, date of term, and the signature of program/residency coordinator on institution letterhead. Orders will be billed at individual rate until proof of status is received. Foreign air speed delivery is included in all Clinics subscription prices. All prices are subject to change without notice. POSTMASTER: Send address changes to PET Clinics, Elsevier Health Sciences Division, Subscription Customer Service, 3251 Riverport Lane, Maryland Heights, MO 63043. **Customer Service: 1-800-654-2452 (U.S. and Canada); 314-447-8871 (outside U.S. and Canada). Fax: 314-447-8029. E-mail: journalscustomerservice-usa@elsevier.com (for print support); journalsonlinesupport-usa@elsevier.com (for online support).**

Reprints. For copies of 100 or more of articles in this publication, please contact the Commercial Reprints Department, Elsevier Inc., 360 Park Avenue South, New York, NY 10010-1710. Tel.: 212-633-3812; Fax: 212-462-1935; E-mail: reprints@elsevier.com.

Printed and bound by CPI Group (UK) Ltd, Croydon, CR0 4YY

Transferred to Digital Print 2011

Contributors

CONSULTING EDITOR

ABASS ALAVI, MD, PhD (Hon), DSc (Hon)
Professor of Radiology, Division of Nuclear
Medicine, University of Pennsylvania School
of Medicine, Philadelphia, Pennsylvania

GUEST EDITORS

DREW A. TORIGIAN, MD, MA
Assistant Professor, Department of Radiology,
Hospital of the University of Pennsylvania,
University of Pennsylvania School of
Medicine, Philadelphia, Pennsylvania

ABASS ALAVI, MD, PhD (Hon), DSc (Hon)
Professor of Radiology, Division of Nuclear
Medicine, University of Pennsylvania School
of Medicine, Philadelphia, Pennsylvania

AUTHORS

GAD ABIKHZER, MD
Resident, Nuclear Medicine, Division of
Nuclear Medicine, McGill University Health
Centre, Royal Victoria Hospital, Montreal,
Quebec, Canada

SCOTT ADAMS, MD
Department of Radiology, Louisiana State
University Health Sciences Center-Shreveport
(LSUHSC-S), Shreveport, Louisiana

ANSHUL AGARWAL, MD, PhD
Department of Nuclear Medicine,
University of Texas Southwestern
Medical Center, Dallas, Texas

ABASS ALAVI, MD, PhD (Hon), DSc (Hon)
Professor of Radiology, Division of Nuclear
Medicine, University of Pennsylvania School
of Medicine, Philadelphia, Pennsylvania

ASHU SEITH BHALLA, MD
Associate Professor of Radiology, Department
of Radio-Diagnosis, All India Institute of
Medical Sciences, New Delhi, India

HENNY S. BROEKHUIZEN-DE GAST, MD
Department of Radiology and Nuclear
Medicine, University Medical Center Utrecht,
Utrecht, The Netherlands

WICHANA CHAMROONRAT, MD
The Russell H. Morgan Department of
Radiology and Radiological Science,
The Johns Hopkins Hospital,
Baltimore, Maryland

MAARTEN L. DONSWIJK, MD
Department of Radiology and Nuclear
Medicine, University Medical Center Utrecht,
Utrecht, The Netherlands

ROSLYN J. FRANCIS, MBBS, FRACP, PhD
Associate Professor of Molecular Imaging,
School of Medicine and Pharmacology,
The University of Western Australia;
Nuclear Medicine/PET Physician,
Departments of Medical Oncology and
Nuclear Medicine, Sir Charles
Gairdner Hospital, Perth, Western
Australia, Australia

VICTOR H. GERBAUDO, PhD
Director, Division of Nuclear Medicine and Molecular Imaging Program, Department of Radiology, Harvard Medical School, Brigham and Women's Hospital, Boston, Massachusetts

MARC HICKESON, MD, FRCP
Assistant Professor of Nuclear Medicine, Division of Nuclear Medicine, McGill University Health Centre, Royal Victoria Hospital, Montreal, Quebec, Canada

MOHAMED HOUSENI, MD, PhD
Department of Radiology, National Liver Institute, Zamalek, Cairo, Egypt

ROLAND HUSTINX, MD, PhD
Professor of Nuclear Medicine, Chief, Division of Nuclear Medicine, University Hospital of Liége, Liége, Belgium

SHARYN I. KATZ, MD
Assistant Professor of Radiology, Department of Radiology, Hospital of the University of Pennsylvania, University of Pennsylvania School of Medicine, Philadelphia, Pennsylvania

ANTON KHOURI, MD
Department of Radiation Oncology, University Hospitals/Case Western Reserve University; Case Comprehensive Cancer Center, Cleveland, Ohio

RAKESH KUMAR, MD, PhD
Additional Professor, Department of Nuclear Medicine, All India Institute of Medical Sciences, New Delhi, India

THOMAS C. KWEE, MD, PhD
Department of Radiology and Nuclear Medicine, University Medical Center Utrecht, Utrecht, The Netherlands

MARNIX G.E.H. LAM, MD, PhD
Department of Radiology and Nuclear Medicine, University Medical Center Utrecht, Utrecht, The Netherlands

MITCHELL MACHTAY, MD
Department of Radiation Oncology, University Hospitals/Case Western Reserve University; Case Comprehensive Cancer Center, Cleveland, Ohio

NEHAL N. MEHTA, MD, MSCE
Instructor, Cardiovascular Institute, University of Pennsylvania School of Medicine, Philadelphia, Pennsylvania

GAUTHIER NAMUR, MD
Consulting Physician, Division of Nuclear Medicine, University Hospital of Liége, Liége, Belgium

ANNA K. NOWAK, MBBS, FRACP, PhD
Professor of Medicine, School of Medicine and Pharmacology, The University of Western Australia; Consultant Medical Oncologist, Department of Medical Oncology, Sir Charles Gairdner Hospital, Perth, Western Australia, Australia

KEVIN STEPHANS, MD
Department of Radiation Oncology, Cleveland Clinic; Case Comprehensive Cancer Center, Cleveland, Ohio

AMOL TAKALKAR, MD, MS
Medical Director, PET Imaging Center, Biomedical Research Foundation of Northwest Louisiana; Associate Professor of Clinical Radiology, Department of Radiology, Louisiana State University Health Sciences Center-Shreveport (LSUHSC-S), Shreveport, Louisiana

SANJAY THULKAR, MD
Associate Professor of Radiology, Dr B R Ambedkar Institute Rotary Cancer Hospital, All India Institute of Medical Sciences, New Delhi, India

DREW A. TORIGIAN, MD, MA
Assistant Professor, Department of Radiology, Hospital of the University of Pennsylvania, University of Pennsylvania School of Medicine, Philadelphia, Pennsylvania

YIDING YU, BA
Doris Duke Clinical Research Fellow, Cardiovascular Institute, University of Pennsylvania School of Medicine, Philadelphia, Pennsylvania

HONGMING ZHUANG, MD, PhD
Division of Nuclear Medicine, Department of Radiology, The Children's Hospital of Philadelphia, University of Pennsylvania School of Medicine, Philadelphia, Pennsylvania

Contents

A common clinical dilemma is the evaluation of pulmonary nodules detected on imaging. Differentiation between malignant and benign pulmonary nodules is a complex problem despite major advances in medical imaging. Accurate diagnosis helps to eliminate unnecessary surgical procedures in patients with benign diseases. It is important for the diagnostician to be aware of the role of multimodality imaging for characterization of pulmonary nodules.

Computed tomography (CT) is the primary noninvasive imaging modality for staging of non–small cell lung cancer. Magnetic resonance imaging compliments CT in tumor staging in specific situations. [^{18}F]Fluorodeoxyglucose positron emission tomography/CT is useful in detecting additional regional nodal and distant metastatic sites of disease, thereby reducing the number of unnecessary surgeries. However, noninvasive imaging modalities lack sufficient accuracy for nodal staging in all cases and, hence, preoperative lymph node sampling with invasive techniques such as mediastinoscopy, thoracoscopy, and fine-needle aspiration cytology guided by endobronchial ultrasound or endoscopic ultrasound is frequently required in selected patients.

PET has gained a major role in the evaluation and treatment of lung cancer over the past two decades. Over that time span PET and treatment techniques have both evolved substantially. While technical changes in PET and PET/computed tomography have improved accuracy and reliability, the evolution toward increasingly targeted and intensive treatment has increased the reliance upon imaging of radiation treatment. This article seeks to review the current role of PET in the evaluation and treatment of lung cancer with radiation.

Early diagnosis and accurate disease staging in patients with malignant pleural mesothelioma (MPM) are essential in classifying such patients into prognostic subgroups to allow delivery of stage-specific therapies. This review addresses the current status of multimodality imaging in the diagnosis and staging of MPM. Clinical, research, and future directions in computed tomography (CT), magnetic resonance imaging, and PET/CT diagnosis and staging of MPM are discussed, including the use of novel PET probes. The article concludes with important take-home messages summarized as the pearls and pitfalls of each diagnostic modality in the diagnosis and staging of patients with MPM.

A Multimodality Imaging Review of Malignant Pleural Mesothelioma Response Assessment

Anna K. Nowak, Roslyn J. Francis, Sharyn I. Katz, and Victor H. Gerbaudo

Assessment of response is important to interpret early phase clinical trial results and to guide individual patient management. In malignant pleural mesothelioma (MPM), the circumferential growth pattern of the disease, the presence of pleural effusion and atelectasis, and the common use of pleurodesis make this a challenging task for imaging specialists and clinicians. This article reviews the current evidence for radiological and positron emission tomography (PET) response assessment in MPM, and the pitfalls and challenges in its application. Current research and future directions in radiological and PET response are discussed, including the use of novel radiotracers.

Cardiac Assessment with PET

Amol Takalkar, Anshul Agarwal, Scott Adams, Abass Alavi, and Drew A. Torigian

Positron emission tomography (PET) has been very well validated for assessing myocardial viability, and emerging sophisticated hybrid imaging technologies involving PET with other imaging modalities offer tremendous promise for delivering an in-depth but noninvasive evaluation of cardiac perfusion and function in various pathologic conditions during a single imaging session. Moreover, several new PET radiotracers in the research and preclinical arena are poised to enter the clinical setting in the foreseeable future. With such exciting developments on the horizon, cardiac PET and PET/computed tomography imaging, and potentially integrated cardiac PET/magnetic resonance imaging have become the focus of the molecular imaging paradigm for comprehensive cardiovascular assessment.

The Role of PET with [18-F] Fluorodeoxyglucose in the Diagnosis and Management of Thoracic Vascular Disease

YiDing Yu, Drew A. Torigian, and Nehal N. Mehta

Investigating the functional activity of cellular inflammatory mediators is fundamental to understanding the pathophysiology and improving the treatment of numerous vascular conditions. PET with FDG allows noninvasive in vivo assessment of inflammatory vascular processes and may be coupled to CT or MRI to provide simultaneous anatomic information. These unique properties have provided additional insight into the pathophysiology, diagnosis, and management of thoracic vascular diseases. In this article, the role of FDG-PET in the assessment of thoracic vascular disease and the influence of this technique on the diagnostic and management approaches are discussed.

Review of Physiologic and Pathophysiologic Sources of Fluorodeoxyglucose Uptake in the Chest Wall on PET

Marc Hickeson and Gad Abikhzer

The chest wall can be defined as the osseous and soft tissue structures that form the outer framework of the thorax and move during breathing. Topics discussed in this article include physiologic uptake of fluorodeoxyglucose, benign diseases of the chest wall, and malignant tumors of the chest wall.

Brown fat is present and metabolically active in adults, and is involved in physiologic and pathologic processes. Brown fat activation can seriously interfere with correct [^{18}F]fluorodeoxyglucose-PET image interpretation if not recognized, although this can be overcome through identification of typical uptake patterns, pharmacological and nonpharmacological interventions to reduce brown fat uptake, and hybrid PET/ computed tomography and PET/magnetic resonance imaging technologies. Advanced quantitative PET imaging techniques may be used to quantify total brown fat volume and metabolic activity for assessment prior to and following various interventions, likely contributing to further understanding of brown fat.

PET Clinics

THE CLINICS ARE NOW AVAILABLE ONLINE!

Access your subscription at:
www.theclinics.com

GOAL STATEMENT

The goal of the *PET Clinics* is to keep practicing radiologists and radiology residents up to date with current clinical practice in positron emission tomography by providing timely articles reviewing the state of the art in patient care.

ACCREDITATION

PET Clinics is planned and implemented in accordance with the Essential Areas and Policies of the Accreditation Council for Continuing Medical Education (ACCME) through the joint sponsorship of the University of Virginia School of Medicine and Elsevier. The University of Virginia School of Medicine is accredited by the ACCME to provide continuing medical education for physicians.

The University of Virginia School of Medicine designates this educational activity for a maximum of 15 *AMA PRA Category 1 Credits*™ for each issue, 60 credits per year. Physicians should only claim credit commensurate with the extent of their participation in the activity.

The American Medical Association has determined that physicians not licensed in the US who participate in this CME activity are eligible for a maximum of 15 *AMA PRA Category 1 Credits*™ for each issue, 60 credits per year.

Category 1 credit can be earned by reading the text material, taking the CME examination online at http://www.theclinics.com/home/cme, and completing the evaluation. After taking the test, you will be required to review any and all incorrect answers. Following completion of the test and evaluation, your credit will be awarded and you may print your certificate.

FACULTY DISCLOSURE/CONFLICT OF INTEREST

The University of Virginia School of Medicine, as an ACCME accredited provider, endorses and strives to comply with the Accreditation Council for Continuing Medical Education (ACCME) Standards of Commercial Support, Commonwealth of Virginia statutes, University of Virginia policies and procedures, and associated federal and private regulations and guidelines on the need for disclosure and monitoring of proprietary and financial interests that may affect the scientific integrity and balance of content delivered in continuing medical education activities under our auspices.

The University of Virginia School of Medicine requires that all CME activities accredited through this institution be developed independently and be scientifically rigorous, balanced and objective in the presentation/discussion of its content, theories and practices.

All authors/editors participating in an accredited CME activity are expected to disclose to the readers relevant financial relationships with commercial entities occurring within the past 12 months (such as grants or research support, employee, consultant, stock holder, member of speakers bureau, etc.). The University of Virginia School of Medicine will employ appropriate mechanisms to resolve potential conflicts of interest to maintain the standards of fair and balanced education to the reader. Questions about specific strategies can be directed to the Office of Continuing Medical Education, University of Virginia School of Medicine, Charlottesville, Virginia.

The faculty and staff of the University of Virginia Office of Continuing Medical Education have no financial affiliations to disclose.

The authors/editors listed below have identified no professional or financial affiliations for themselves or their spouse/partner:
Gad Abikhzer, MD; Scott Adams, MD; Anshul Agarwal, MD, PhD; Abass Alavi, MD (Consulting Editor) (Guest Editor); Ashu Seith Bhalla, MD; Henny S. Broekhuizen-de Gast, MD; Wichana Chamroonrat, MD; Maarten L. Donswijk, MD; Barton Dudlick (Acquisitions Editor); Roslyn J. Francis, MBBS, FRACP, PhD; Victor H. Gerbaudo, PhD; Marc Hickeson, MD, FRCP; Mohamed Houseni, MD, PhD; Roland Hustinx, MD, PhD; Sharyn I. Katz, MD; Anton Khouri, MD; Rakesh Kumar, MD, PhD; Thomas C. Kwee, MD, PhD; Marnix G.E.H. Lam, MD, PhD; Mitchell Machtay, MD; Nehal N. Mehta, MD, MSCE; Gauthier Namur, MD; Patrice Rehm, MD (Test Editor); Kevin Stephans, MD; Amol Takalkar, MD, MS; Sanjay Thulkar, MD; YiDing Yu, BA; and Hongming Zhuang, MD, PhD.

The authors/editors listed below identified the following professional or financial affiliations for themselves or their spouse/partner:
Anna K. Nowak, MBBS, FRACP, PhD is an industry funded research/investigator for Roche Australia Pty Ltd and Pfizer Australia, and is on the Advisory Board for Roche Australia Pty Ltd.
Drew A. Torigian, MD (Guest Editor) is an industry funded research/investigator for Pfizer Corporation.

Disclosure of Discussion of Non-FDA Approved Uses for Pharmaceutical Products and/or Medical Devices
The University of Virginia School of Medicine, as an ACCME provider, requires that all faculty presenters identify and disclose any off-label uses for pharmaceutical and medical device products. The University of Virginia School of Medicine recommends that each physician fully review all the available data on new products or procedures prior to clinical use.

TO ENROLL

To enroll in the PET Clinics Continuing Medical Education program, call customer service at 1-800-654-2452 or visit us online at www.theclinics.com/home/cme. The CME program is available to subscribers for an additional fee of $196.00.

Preface
PET Imaging of Thoracic Disease

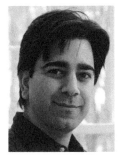
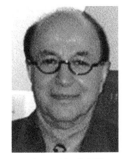

Drew A. Torigian, MD, MA   Abass Alavi, MD
Guest Editors

Thoracic disorders are common and account for a large proportion of disease-related morbidity and mortality in patients throughout the world. Multimodality imaging, predominantly with positron emission tomography (PET), computed tomography, and magnetic resonance imaging, plays a central role in the diagnosis, prognosis assessment, pretreatment planning, response assessment, and surveillance assessment of patients with such conditions. As such, in this issue of *PET Clinics*, we provide a series of state-of-the-art articles regarding the application of multimodality imaging to a wide variety of common thoracic disease conditions.

A multimodality review of lung cancer staging (based on the new 7th edition of the AJCC-UICC staging system) is provided, followed by review of lung cancer posttreatment assessment. These are particularly relevant given that lung cancer is prevalent and is the deadliest malignancy in humans. These are then followed by multimodality reviews of malignant pleural mesothelioma staging (also based on the new 7th edition AJCC-UICC staging system) and response assessment. Malignant pleural mesothelioma introduces its own set of diagnostic and therapeutic complexities given its unusual pattern of growth along the pleural surfaces. A review of multimodality imaging approaches for lung nodule assessment is then provided, which is timely given that lung nodules are prevalent and often provide a diagnostic dilemma as to their underlying etiology and clinical significance in individual patients. Reviews of the applications of PET imaging to evaluate cardiac disease and thoracic

vascular disease are included—both topics of which are important to discuss given their prevalence and high rates of associated morbidity and mortality. Last, articles on PET imaging assessment of chest wall disorders and PET imaging of brown fat are included. The former should prove useful for the diagnostician as the chest wall is not infrequently involved by pathology, and the latter is interesting as brown fat assessment may play a significant role in better understanding and treating the epidemic of obesity.

It is our hope that the readers of these articles will apply the knowledge within to help cure and ameliorate the suffering of patients worldwide who have thoracic disorders.

Drew A. Torigian, MD, MA
Department of Radiology
Hospital of the University of Pennsylvania
University of Pennsylvania School of Medicine
3400 Spruce Street
Philadelphia, PA 19104, USA

Abass Alavi, MD
Department of Radiology
Hospital of the University of Pennsylvania
University of Pennsylvania School of Medicine
3400 Spruce Street
Philadelphia, PA 19104, USA

E-mail addresses:
Drew.Torigian@uphs.upenn.edu (D.A. Torigian)
Abass.Alavi@uphs.upenn.edu (A. Alavi)

PET Clin 6 (2011) xi
doi:10.1016/j.cpet.2011.06.001
1556-8598/11/$ – see front matter © 2011 Elsevier Inc. All rights reserved.

Multimodality Imaging Assessment of Pulmonary Nodules

Mohamed Houseni, MD, PhD[a],
Wichana Chamroonrat, MD[b], Hongming Zhuang, MD, PhD[c],
Drew A. Torigian, MD, MA[d],*

KEYWORDS

• Pulmonary nodules • PET • PET/CT • MR imaging

Solitary and multiple pulmonary nodules are increasingly detected with the increased use and availability of new high quality computed tomography (CT) scans and digital radiograph machines. They are usually discovered incidentally in asymptomatic patients and pose a clinical challenge. A pulmonary nodule is defined as a discrete opacity 3 cm or less in diameter that is completely surrounded by lung parenchyma, not related to the hilum or mediastinum, and not associated with atelectasis, pleural effusion, or lymphadenopathy (whereas pulmonary masses are defined as having diameters of >3 cm).[1] The prevalence of pulmonary nodules may be as high as 69% as reported in screening studies of individuals at risk for lung cancer and as high as 75% in patients with extrapulmonary neoplasms. About 90% of newly discovered pulmonary nodules are subcentimeter in size, rendering histopathologic correlation difficult.[2–5] The differential diagnosis of pulmonary nodules spans a broad spectrum of benign and malignant causes (**Table 1**).[6–17] The most common benign causes of pulmonary nodules are granulomas and hamartomas, whereas the most common malignant causes include lung adenocarcinoma, lung squamous cell carcinoma, and metastasis. It is important for the physician to determine whether a pulmonary nodule is benign or malignant, and to decide whether further imaging investigations or tissue sampling are necessary to achieve this goal.

Based on the American College of Chest Physicians (ACCP) guidelines, the assessment of solitary pulmonary nodules should be based on the risk of cancer and the size of the nodule.[18] Patient risk stratification estimates the likelihood of malignant nature of pulmonary nodules by analyzing smoking history, patient age, history of cancer, and nodule size, morphology, and location. Several validated models based on these parameters have been generated to estimate the probability of malignancy in pulmonary nodules including the Mayo Clinic and Veterans Affairs models.[6,19–22] However, the calculations used in these models to estimate the pretest probabilities are not suitable for daily clinical practice. In addition, the accuracy of these models was similar to the accuracy of expert clinicians.[23] Some investigators have tried to stratify patients using the likelihood ratio form of the Bayes theorem and neural networks.[6,19,20,24–26] In general, the prevalence of malignancy in individuals with pulmonary nodules may range from 1.1% to 12%.[3,27–35]

[a] Department of Radiology, National Liver Institute, 1 El-Gizera El-Wousta Street, Zamalek - 11211, Cairo, Egypt
[b] The Russell H. Morgan Department of Radiology and Radiological Science, The Johns Hopkins Hospital, JHOC Building Room 3240, 601 North Caroline Street, Baltimore, MD 21287, USA
[c] Division of Nuclear Medicine, Department of Radiology, The Children's Hospital of Philadelphia, University of Pennsylvania School of Medicine, 34th Street and Civic Center Boulevard, Philadelphia, PA 19104, USA
[d] Department of Radiology, Hospital of the University of Pennsylvania, University of Pennsylvania School of Medicine, 3400 Spruce Street, Philadelphia, PA 19104, USA
* Corresponding author.
E-mail address: Drew.Torigian@uphs.upenn.edu

PET Clin 6 (2011) 231–250
doi:10.1016/j.cpet.2011.04.006
1556-8598/11/$ – see front matter © 2011 Elsevier Inc. All rights reserved.

pet.theclinics.com

Table 1
Differential diagnosis of pulmonary nodules

Malignant		Benign	
Adenocarcinoma	47%	Granuloma (healed or active)	40%
Squamous cell carcinoma	22%	Hamartoma	15%
Solitary metastasis	8%	—	
Undifferentiated non–small cell carcinoma	7%		
Small cell lung cancer	4%		
Less common causes		*Less common causes*	
Large cell carcinoma		Nonspecific inflammation/infection	
Carcinoid tumor		Abscess	
Intrapulmonary lymphoma		Round pneumonia	
Adenosquamous carcinoma		Round atelectasis	
Adenoid cystic carcinoma		Pneumoconiosis	
Malignant teratoma		Pulmonary infarction	
		Focal hemorrhage	
		Hemangioma	
		Arteriovenous malformation	

Data from Gould MK, Fletcher J, Iannettoni MD, et al. Evaluation of patients with pulmonary nodules: when is it lung cancer?: ACCP evidence-based clinical practice guidelines (2nd edition). Chest 2007;132(Suppl 3):108S–30S.

IMAGING

The value of imaging in the assessment of pulmonary nodules is to differentiate benign from malignant lesions as accurately as possible. However, up to 52% of pulmonary nodules continue to be indeterminate even after the first follow-up by radiologic evaluation.[36] Several methods have been adapted to attempt to better characterize pulmonary nodules on imaging including morphologic evaluation, growth rate assessment, perfusion analysis, and molecular imaging.

MORPHOLOGIC EVALUATION OF PULMONARY NODULES

Morphologic features of lung nodules include size, margins, attenuation, growth rate, presence and pattern of calcification, and presence of fat. Although many of these features may be typical for benignity versus malignancy, they frequently overlap, making it difficult to definitively characterize pulmonary nodules at the time of initial detection, frequently resulting in a nonspecific diagnosis requiring further evaluation.

The probability of the presence of cancer in small nodules is lower than that in large nodules, and there is a positive correlation between the risk for malignancy and the size of the nodule. The prevalence of malignancy in nodules less than 5 mm is less than 1%, is as high as 28% for nodules that are 5 to 10 mm, and ranges from 64% to 82% for nodules larger than 20 mm.[35,37–41]

The characteristics of pulmonary nodule margin can be valuable to specify the nature of the lesion. Benign nodules typically show a well-defined, smooth, and round contour, whereas malignant nodules are more likely to have an ill-defined, spiculated, and irregular contour.[19] Lobulated margins can be seen in both benign and malignant lesions, which reflects different growth rates within the nodule.[42] However, the marginal features of benign and malignant nodules may coincide. About 10% of benign nodules can be spiculated, 20% of malignant lesions have smooth margins, and most metastases are well defined.[19,43]

Pulmonary nodule attenuation can be categorized into solid, ground-glass, and mixed solid/ground-glass (**Fig. 1**). The incidence of malignancy in solid attenuation nodules ranges from 18% to 26%, whereas 59% to 73% of mixed solid/ground-glass attenuation nodules are found to be malignant.[31,35,44,45] In a CT screening study, ground-glass attenuation nodules were found to be malignant in 18% of cases.[37]

Nodule growth rate can be estimated when previous imaging is available for direct comparison, and is expressed in terms of volumetric doubling time, which is equivalent to a 26% increase in nodule diameter.[46] It can be calculated by the following formula:

Volumetric doubling time = (time in days × log2) / (3 × [log (diameter of nodule on current study/diameter on previous study)])

Malignant nodules typically have a volumetric doubling time range of 20 to 300 days,[47,48]

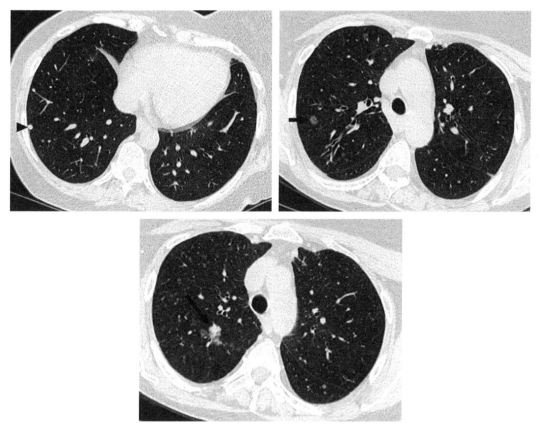

Fig. 1. Axial CT images show solid (*arrowhead*), ground-glass (*short arrow*), and mixed (*long arrow*) attenuation nodules in right lung. The ground-glass attenuation nodule is caused by bronchioloalveolar cell lung carcinoma (BAC), and the mixed attenuation nodule is caused by transformation of BAC into lung adenocarcinoma.

although most malignant nodules in clinical practice have a volumetric doubling time less than 100 days.[49] According to these findings, a 2-year stability in the size of a nodule should suggest a benign cause. However, some investigators suggest a longer follow-up for subcentimeter nodules because they may require a longer volumetric doubling time.[37,50] A longer follow-up is also suggested for ground-glass attenuation nodules when bronchioloalveolar lung carcinoma is suspected, because they frequently have longer volumetric doubling times.[51]

The presence of calcification in a pulmonary nodule increases the probability of a benign cause. However, differential diagnostic considerations of a calcified nodule include granuloma, hamartoma, carcinoid, metastasis, and bronchogenic carcinoma. Four patterns of nodule calcification are characteristic for benign causes, including the diffuse (**Fig. 2**), central, laminated, and popcorn calcification patterns. However, stippled, eccentric (**Fig. 3**), amorphous, punctuate, and reticular patterns are not specific for benignity, and may

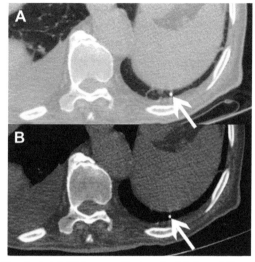

Fig. 2. Axial CT images displayed with lung (*A*) and soft tissue (*B*) window and level settings show diffuse calcification of lung nodule (*arrow*), indicating benignity.

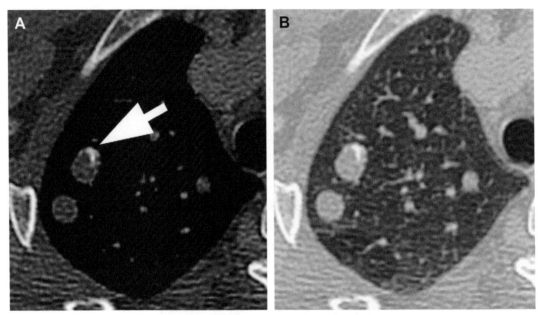

Fig. 3. Axial CT images displayed with lung (*A*) and soft tissue (*B*) window and level settings reveal eccentric calcification (*arrow*) in lung nodule caused by metastasis from osteogenic sarcoma.

be seen in malignant nodules. Sometimes, diffuse calcification can be seen in nodules caused by metastases, although this is uncommon.[18,52,53] Presence of macroscopic fat in a nodule is diagnostic for a pulmonary hamartoma.[54]

CHEST RADIOGRAPHY

Pulmonary nodules are typically evaluated with frontal and lateral chest radiographs. Normal structures such as nipples, articular surfaces of the anterior ribs, and skin lesions should be distinguished from abnormal lung lesions. Oblique chest radiographs may be useful to distinguish true pulmonary nodules from apparent nodular densities caused by superimposition of vascular and/or osseous structures. Metallic nipple markers can also be useful to reliably identify the nipple shadows. Location, shape, density, and size of the lesions affect their detectability on radiograph (**Fig. 4**). Although chest radiographs can sometimes detect nodules as small as 5 mm, many subcentimeter nodules are frequently missed.[55]

Location is another factor that influences nodules detection. Lesions located in the lung apex or in a peripheral location are the most

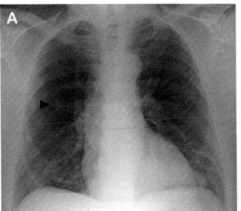
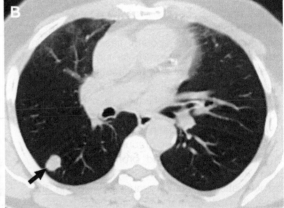

Fig. 4. Frontal chest radiograph (*A*) shows 1.4-cm nodule (*arrowhead*) in right midlung zone. Axial CT image (*B*) shows corresponding lobulated nodule (*arrow*) in right lower lobe, in keeping with squamous cell lung carcinoma.

frequently missed than nodules located elsewhere in the lung.[56,57] Nodules that are superimposed on the heart, hila, or diaphragms are also more difficult to visualize.

Dual-energy subtraction digital radiography and dual-energy subtraction digital tomosynthesis significantly improve the sensitivity of chest radiography for pulmonary nodule detection including noncalcified nodules and lesions behind the heart or near the diaphragm. Dual-energy digital subtraction radiography is based on low-voltage (60 kVp) and high-voltage (120 kVp) exposure, associated with soft tissue or bone subtraction. Tomograms of the desired layer thickness can be reconstructed from a single tomographic scan using a three-dimensional (3D) filtered back-projection algorithm.[58,59]

CT

CT is significantly more sensitive and specific than chest radiography in the assessment of pulmonary nodules. Multislice scanners have the ability of volumetric acquisition of whole chest in a few seconds with multiplanar reconstruction capability. Several software models can be used to generate a pulmonary nodule analysis report. CT evaluation includes size and/or volume measurement, growth rate assessment, morphologic assessment, attenuation measurement, lobar and segmental localization, and assessment of the 3D relationship to the bronchi without intravenous contrast material (Fig. 5). Furthermore, CT can be used to evaluate lymph node status, mediastinal, pleural, and chest wall involvement by disease, the presence of a pleural effusion, and associated pulmonary parenchymal abnormalities.[18,60,61] Intravenous contrast material is useful for evaluation of the nonpulmonary structures of the thorax, and also enables assessment of the degree and pattern of enhancement of lung nodules. CT is typically used to further characterize nodules that are detected on other imaging tests such as chest radiography, and is also frequently used in

patients at high risk for pulmonary malignancy. Unenhanced CT with a low-dose technique may be useful to minimize the risks of radiation exposure and contrast exposure in patients undergoing follow-up for pulmonary nodules.[62]

Benign features of pulmonary nodules on CT images include small size, smooth margins, stability or interval decrease in size more than time, a benign calcification pattern, and presence of macroscopic fat. Arteriovenous malformations, which are benign lesions that can mimic pulmonary nodules on chest radiography, are identified by their tubular configuration, presence of 1 or more feeding arteries and draining veins, and enhancement characteristics similar to other vessels (Fig. 6). Pulmonary infarction appears as a peripheral wedge-shaped opacity, which may have air bronchograms, often in association with a visualized central hypoattenuating filling defect caused by acute pulmonary embolism in an associated pulmonary arterial branch (Fig. 7). Round atelectasis typically shows a subpleural nodular opacity adjacent to an area of pleural thickening or pleural effusion, and a curvilinear swirling appearance of adjacent vessels and bronchi on and around the opacity (also known as the comet tail sign) (Fig. 8). Malignant features of pulmonary nodules on CT include large size, interval increase in size over time, spiculated or lobulated margins (Figs. 9 and 10), cavitation with thick or irregular walls, mixed attenuation, endobronchial location, or stippled, eccentric, punctuate, amorphous calcification patterns.[39,40,63–65]

Application of postprocessing techniques including maximal intensity projection (MIP) has been shown to improve the detection rate of pulmonary nodules. Small pulmonary nodules are significantly better detected on MIP images, especially when less than 5 mm in diameter (Fig. 11). In a study included 103 patients, MIP images were found to detect 37.5% more pulmonary nodules than standard axial images.[66] This study proposed MIP at 5-mm slice thickness and found it to be

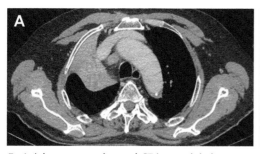
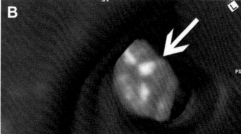

Fig. 5. Axial contrast-enhanced CT image (A) shows complete right upper lobe atelectasis. Virtual CT bronchoscopy image (B) reveals central lobulated endobronchial nodule in right upper lobe bronchus caused by bronchogenic carcinoma (arrow).

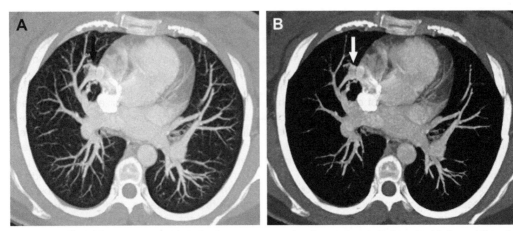

Fig. 6. Axial contrast-enhanced maximal intensity projection (MIP) CT images displayed with lung (*A*) and soft tissue (*B*) window and level settings show tubular configuration of 2-cm nodule in medial right middle lobe with enhancement similar to other vessels. Also note feeding pulmonary artery and draining pulmonary vein. These findings are diagnostic for pulmonary arteriovenous malformation in this patient with history of hereditary hemorrhagic telangiectasia.

superior to axial standard reconstructions. However, another study examined different slab thicknesses and reported that MIP images with a slab thickness of 8 mm are superior to those with other thicknesses in the detection of pulmonary nodules.[67]

Dynamic contrast-enhanced (DCE) CT imaging (also known as CT densitometry) has been used

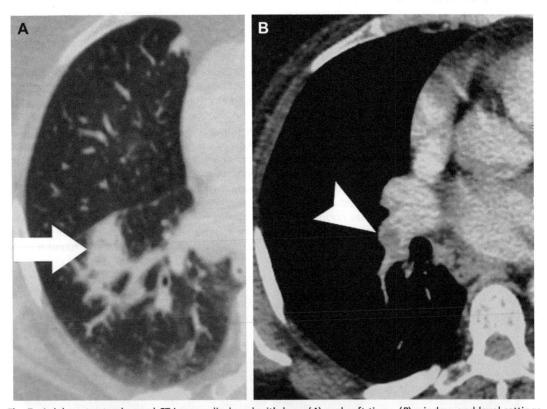

Fig. 7. Axial contrast-enhanced CT images displayed with lung (*A*) and soft tissue (*B*) window and level settings show peripheral nodular opacity in right lower lobe (*arrow*) consistent with pulmonary infarction (*A*). Associated hypoattenuating central filling defect in right interlobar pulmonary artery is caused by acute pulmonary embolus (*arrowhead*).

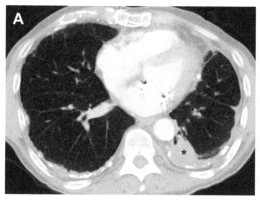 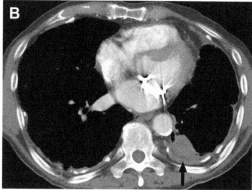

Fig. 8. Axial contrast-enhanced CT images displayed with lung (*A*) and soft tissue (*B*) window and level settings reveal subpleural 2.9-cm round nodular opacity in medial left lower lobe (*) adjacent to area of pleural thickening (*arrow*) along with curvilinear swirling appearance of adjacent vessels and bronchi on and around opacity, in keeping with round atelectasis.

by some investigators to identify malignant nodules. It is performed by first acquiring unenhanced CT images, followed by a series of CT images after intravenous injection of contrast medium. The degree of enhancement is estimated by measuring the attenuation at various time points after the start of intravenous contrast injection. A specificity of 93% has been associated with enhancement equal to or more than 25 HU,[68] whereas the most sensitive results have been reported for enhancement of more than 15 HU. In addition, absence of enhancement strongly suggests a benign cause, with a 96.5% negative predictive value. The enhancement features have been reported to reflect the number of small vessels and the distribution of elastic fibers within the nodule.[69–72]

The availability of multislice CT facilitates dynamic sequential imaging in a short time with high resolution, while maintaining adequate coverage, thus overcoming the limitations of single-slice scanners. Moreover, temporal and spatial analysis of wash in and wash out characteristics of pulmonary nodules may further improve the specificity of this technique. For example, malignant nodules have been associated with a wash in of 25 HU or greater and a wash out of 5 to 31 HU, whereas benign nodules have been associated with a wash in of less than 25 HU, a wash in of 25 HU or greater combined with a wash out of greater than 31 HU, or a wash in of 25 HU or greater with persistent enhancement.[73,74] Major disadvantages of this technique that have prevented widespread use of this approach in the community include an increased complexity of image acquisition and image analysis, nonstandardization of the optimal image acquisition and image analysis approaches, and an increased radiation dose exposure.

Dual-energy CT is another technique that facilitates material decomposition of substances based on attenuation differences at different energy

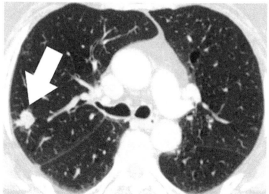 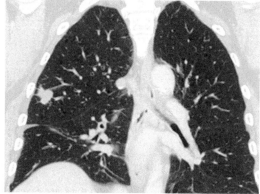

Fig. 9. Axial (*upper*) and coronal (*lower*) CT images show spiculated lung nodule with pleural tail (*arrow*) in peripheral right upper lobe caused by lung carcinoma. Note subcentimeter foci of lucency within lung parenchyma indicating centrilobular emphysema caused by tobacco use.

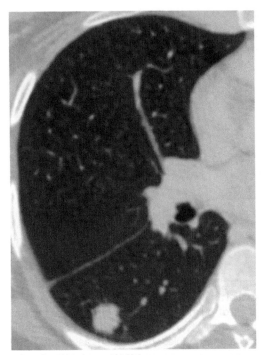

Fig. 10. Axial CT image shows lobulated nodule in superior segment of right lower lobe caused by lung adenocarcinoma.

levels. To study pulmonary nodules, dual-energy CT is typically performed by scanning the chest at 140-kVp and at 80-kVp settings. This technique can detect different calcium or iodine concentrations on an experimental basis and can be potentially useful in clinical practice to better

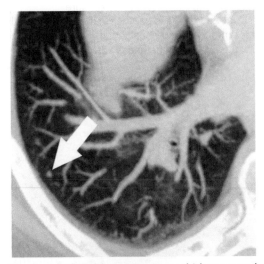

Fig. 11. Axial MIP CT image at 8-mm thickness reveals peripheral 3-mm nodule in the right lower lobe, unchanged on follow-up CT imaging (not shown), likely benign in nature.

characterize pulmonary nodules.[75,76] This approach also adjusts for inaccuracies in the measurement of attenuation values caused by the nonuniformity of thoracic structures, and also limits the incorrect characterization of calcification that may occur with dense fibrous tissues.[77] The major limitations of this technique include an increased radiation dose exposure as well as non-standardization of image analysis techniques.

CT volumetric measurements can now be performed on thin-section CT datasets through automated computer software programs.[78,79] These programs provide a quantitative volumetric measurement of nodule volume (**Fig. 12**) and allow for comparisons to be made with previous CT studies for assessment of volumetric doubling time. However, volumetric measurement of ground-glass attenuation nodules is difficult because of the low nodule-to-lung parenchyma contrast. Other factors that may challenge the volumetric measurements include motion artifacts, presence of adjacent normal structures such as the pleural surface or pulmonary vessels, and the underlying cardiac phase.[80]

POSITRON EMISSION TOMOGRAPHY AND PET/CT

Positron emission tomography (PET) is a molecular imaging technology that uses positron-emitting radiotracers to assess various metabolic characteristics of lesions in a noninvasive and quantitative approach. Its role in oncology is well established by its ability to evaluate and characterize the metabolic and functional parameters of cancerous growth.[81,82] PET/CT synergistically combines molecular and structural information provided by PET and CT, improving its diagnostic performance in a wide variety of clinical settings.[83]

Fluorodeoxyglucose (FDG) is a glucose analog that enters the glucose metabolic pathway in healthy and diseased tissues.[84] Malignant cells are characterized by enhanced glucose consumption, resulting in increased accumulation of FDG within tumor cells,[85,86] and therefore FDG-PET imaging allows for the identification and characterization of cancer based on the presence and degree of FDG uptake.

In the lungs, focal increased FDG uptake greater than the mediastinal blood pool is considered abnormal. FDG-PET may characterize pulmonary nodules with a sensitivity range from 80% to 100% and a specificity range from 40% to 100%,[8,9,11,13,15,16,87–89] with pooled sensitivity and specificity measures 87% and 83%, respectively.[41] If malignancy is suggested, FDG-PET/CT plays a critical role in staging, treatment

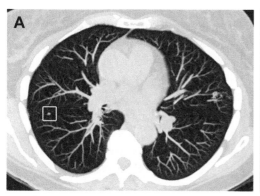
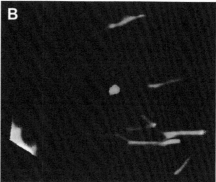

Fig. 12. Axial MIP CT image (A) shows 4-mm nodule in right lung, which is likely benign in nature. Coronal 3D volume-rendered image reveals segmented nodule with volumetric measurement of 25.09 mm³.

planning, response assessment, and restaging. FDG-PET or PET/CT is typically performed to evaluate intermediate-risk or high-risk patients with lung nodules when CT findings are indeterminate.[90] Although negative PET results in these patients may not always exclude the presence of malignancy, these tumors tend to have a more favorable prognosis because they are generally more well differentiated.[91] Patients in this clinical setting may be followed with CT imaging for 2 years, or may undergo needle biopsy when the probability of malignancy is high.[18]

Bronchioloalveolar cell lung carcinoma, carcinoid, mucinous adenocarcinoma, low-grade lymphoma, and metastasis from primary bone tumors (Fig. 13) may give false-negative results because these tumors are differentiated and characterized by low glycolytic activity. False-negative results on FDG-PET have been reported to occur in about 5% of lung cancers less than 3 cm in diameter.[92] In addition, lesions located adjacent to sites of physiologic FDG uptake as well as small nodules may be difficult to assess, and may lead to false-negative results as well. Infectious diseases (Fig. 14), sarcoidosis, radiation pneumonitis, and postoperative changes with active fibrosis have been described to take up FDG on PET imaging, and can be a source of false-positive results. This situation is because inflammatory cells including neutrophils and activated macrophages have increased glycolysis.[93]

A distinctive feature of PET imaging is its quantitative nature. Semiquantitative analysis can be performed by measuring the standardized uptake value (SUV) of a tissue of interest, which is a measurement of radiotracer concentration in the tissue of interest that is normalized to the injected dose of radiotracer and a feature of body habitus such as body weight. Many investigators have suggested the use of a cutoff value to differentiate benign from malignant lesions.[94,95] However, SUV measurement depends on several factors that can adversely affect its reliability, such that there is much overlap in the SUV of benign and malignant lung nodules.[96,97] Several methods have been proposed to allow the optimal use of SUV, including partial volume correction for FDG uptake in small lesions, correction for motion (respiration), dual-time-point imaging technique, and global metabolic assessment. These methods are among the tools that can improve the role and reliability of SUV measurements for clinical and research purposes.[98]

The partial volume effect is mainly related to limitations in scanner resolution and image sampling, resulting in significant underestimation of the amount of radiotracer uptake within a lesion, particularly when small in size. It is well established that in lesions smaller than 3 cm in diameter, SUV measurements are substantially lower than the true values (Fig. 15). Partial volume correction techniques may be useful to compensate for this phenomenon, and can improve the differentiation

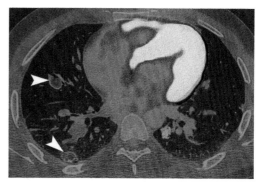

Fig. 13. FDG-PET/CT image shows mild FDG uptake within multiple right lung nodules caused by metastases from osteogenic sarcoma.

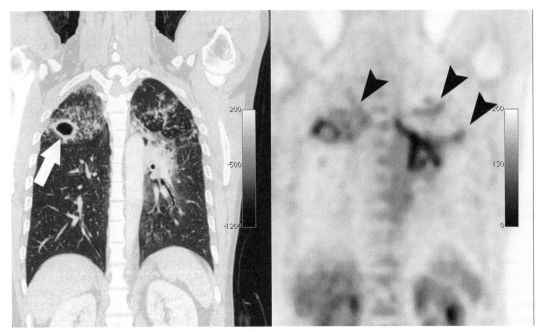

Fig. 14. Coronal CT image (*left*) and FDG-PET image (*right*) reveal cavitary nodule in right upper lobe with thickened wall (*arrow*) and increased FDG uptake as well as fibronodular opacities in upper lobes with faint FDG uptake (*arrowheads*), in keeping with reactivation mycobacterium tuberculous infection.

between benign and malignant lung nodules.[99] Several methods have been implemented for partial volume correction such as recovery coefficient curves as well as reconstruction-based and image-based correction methods. A significant difference has been reported in the SUV measurement of small lung lesions by use of partial volume correction. Studies have shown that partial volume correction can increase the SUV measurement by 5% to 80% according to lesion size.[100,101]

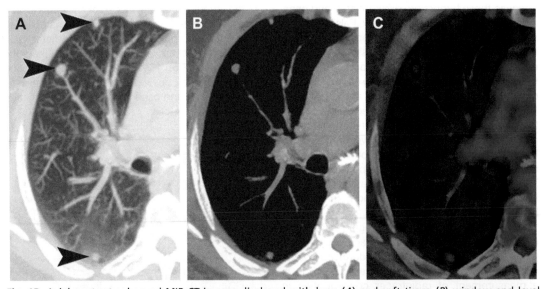

Fig. 15. Axial contrast-enhanced MIP CT images displayed with lung (*A*) and soft tissue (*B*) window and level settings and FDG-PET/CT image show multiple subcentimeter noncalcified nodules in right lung caused by colon cancer metastases with only mild apparent FDG uptake. This latter observation is caused by the partial volume effect in relation to small nodule size, leading to significant underestimation of true radiotracer uptake in these lesions.

In an effort to maximize the use of SUV measurements, dual-time-point imaging has been introduced. Dual-time-point FDG-PET imaging includes early (approximately 60 minutes after FDG administration) and delayed (approximately 90 minutes after FDG administration) PET image acquisitions, allowing for calculation of the percentage change in SUV of a lesion from early to delayed time points, reflecting the dynamics of lesional glucose metabolism. This approach is useful because malignant cells continue to concentrate FDG for several hours, whereas most benign lesions reach the maximum level of FDG accumulation within the first hour. This is believed to be caused by decreased amounts of glucose-6-phosphatase, an enzyme that breaks down FDG-6-phosphate to FDG, in malignant tissues but with abundant amounts of enzyme in normal tissues. The use of dual-time-point FDG-PET imaging has been shown to be useful to distinguish malignant from benign lung nodules (**Fig. 16**).[102] Furthermore, it shows prognostic value in patients with lung cancer.[103] In a study of 265 patients with pulmonary nodules, an increase in SUV over time was reported to have the highest specificity and accuracy among parameters that were evaluated.[104] In another study, pulmonary nodules that showed mild metabolic activity with SUV less than 2.5 were

selectively analyzed, and it was reported that the finding of an increase in SUV of more than 10% over time had an accuracy of 84.8% for the characterization of lung nodules as malignant.[105]

FDG-PET is also useful for planning the most appropriate site of biopsy by identification of metabolically active lung nodules and delineation of the most metabolically active portions of a particular nodule of interest to decrease sampling error.[106] This strategy may be especially useful when biopsy is difficult, unsuccessful, or indeterminate (**Fig. 17**).

Use of a diagnostic quality CT in conjunction with PET/CT imaging may further enhance the diagnostic yield of the study. Semiquantitative parameters from PET together with morphologic, volumetric, and densitometric parameters from CT can be analyzed in a single study. This approach may improve the accuracy for differentiation of malignant from benign nodules even further, although some investigators do not believe that the addition of diagnostic quality CT significantly adds to the diagnostic capability already provided by FDG-PET/CT. Through use of this approach, 1 group of investigators reported that they were able to correctly identify all malignant nodules in a study of 56 patients.[107] However, the main disadvantages of this approach are the increased radiation dose exposure and increased costs.

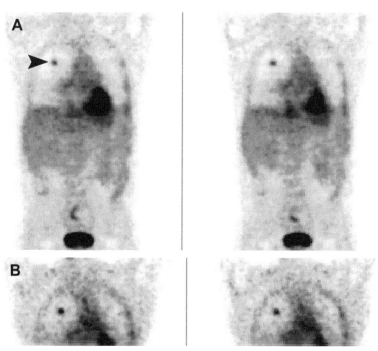

Fig. 16. Coronal early (*A*) and delayed (*B*) dual-time-point FDG-PET images show focally increased FDG uptake in subcentimeter right upper lobe pulmonary nodule with maximum SUV of 2.2 and 3.0 on early and delayed images, respectively, for a 36.4% increase in FDG accumulation over time, in keeping with lung carcinoma.

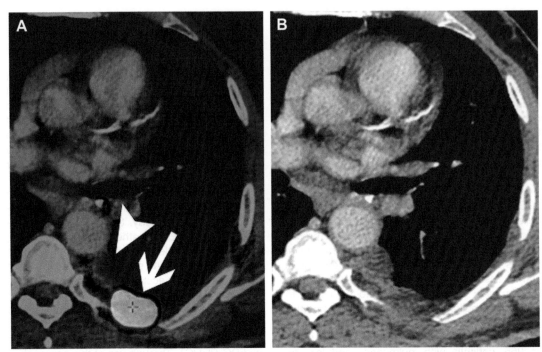

Fig. 17. Axial contrast-enhanced FDG-PET/CT (*A*) and CT (*B*) images reveal FDG avid soft tissue mass (*arrow*) involving posterior left chest wall and more medially located nonmetabolically active postsurgical fluid collection (*arrowhead*) in patient with recurrent squamous cell lung carcinoma after surgical resection. The FDG-PET image data were useful to guide biopsy.

Introduction of new positron-emitting radiotracers has helped PET imaging to gain more diagnostic prominence. Several imaging strategies with these radiotracers have recently been described to measure selected properties of tumors such as cell proliferation, overexpression of receptors such as epidermal growth factor receptor, angiogenesis, hypoxia, apoptosis, and invasive and metastatic potential, potentially improving diagnostic confidence for evaluation of lung nodules.[108–114] For example, [18F]fluorothymidine can be used to improve on the sensitivity and specificity of FDG-PET imaging to differentiate benign from malignant pulmonary nodules by revealing differences in cell proliferation.[115] [68Ga]-tetraazacyclododecane tetraacetic acid (DOTA) is a PET radiotracer that directly binds to somatostatin receptors, which has been shown to be useful for detection and characterization of lung nodules as neuroendocrine tumors.[116] It is beyond the scope of this article to provide a comprehensive review of the novel PET radiotracers that are available for this purpose.

MAGNETIC RESONANCE IMAGING

Magnetic resonance (MR) imaging for assessment of the lung is still evolving. MR imaging is characterized by the lack of ionizing radiation, and may be advantageous for the evaluation of certain lung pathologies in children and in patients who are undergoing frequent follow-up imaging tests. Furthermore, MR imaging provides superior soft tissue contrast compared with CT for assessment of certain parts of the thorax such as the chest wall.[117] Some studies have shown that 90% of 3-mm lung nodules and all nodules larger than 5 mm can be detected with common MR image sequences, including heavily T2-weighted fast spin echo and T1-weighted gradient-recalled echo images. Grossly calcified nodules may appear dark on all MR imaging sequences, and are suboptimally evaluated on MR imaging.[118,119] Overall, the diagnostic performance of MR imaging for the assessment of lung nodules is inferior to that of CT, particularly when lung nodules are small, because of susceptibility artifacts related to multiple gas-tissue interfaces, respiratory and cardiac motion artifacts, and the slightly superior spatial resolution of CT compared with MR imaging.[120]

Contrast-enhanced MR imaging improves the diagnostic yield of pulmonary nodules (**Fig. 18**). A nodular enhancement pattern has been described for malignant nodules, whereas peripheral enhancement is more often associated with

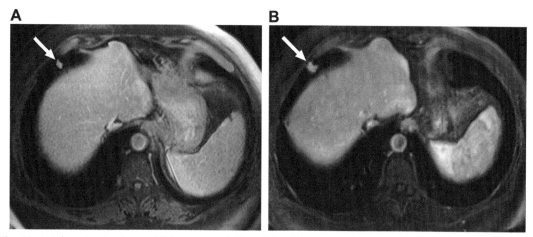

Fig. 18. Axial contrast-enhanced fat-suppressed T1-weighted images at baseline (*A*) and 1 year later (*B*) show lobulated enhancing nodule in right middle lobe (*arrows*) with interval growth over time, in keeping with metastasis from hepatocellular carcinoma.

benign nodules.[121] DCE lung MR imaging can be obtained after intravenous contrast administration by obtaining multiple MR images over time through a nodule of interest. Subsequently, the signal intensity of a lung nodule at different time points after intravenous contrast administration can be measured to generate a time-intensity curve. Several quantitative parameters such as transit time, blood volume, and blood flow can then be derived from the time-intensity curve. The enhancement ratio has been reported to be high in both malignant and active inflammatory nodules, although significant washout has been observed in malignant nodules. A study of 68 patients with lung nodules showed progressive enhancement dynamics, up to 4 minutes, for 12 nodules with active inflammation, whereas 40 malignant nodules showed about 35% wash out at the 4-minute time point.[122] In another study of 51 patients with lung nodules, a significant decrease of signal intensity over time was noted in 52% of malignant nodules with a specificity of 100%.[121] MR imaging parameters of enhancement have previously been correlated with the degree of angiogenesis in malignant tumors, and have also been used to evaluate responses to anti-angiogenic therapy.[123] Major disadvantages of this technique that have prevented widespread use of this approach in the community include an increased complexity of image acquisition and image analysis, and nonstandardization of the optimal image acquisition and image analysis approaches.

Some recent studies have shown a promising role for diffusion-weighted (DW) MR imaging to differentiate benign from malignant lung lesions.[124,125] A nodule signal intensity greater than or equal to that of the spinal cord on DW imaging has been reported to correctly identify malignant pulmonary nodules in 79.6% of cases. However, when the nodule size is less than 2 cm, no significant difference between malignant and benign lesions on DW imaging was observed.[126] A recent study by Tondo and colleagues[127] reported that use of an apparent diffusion coefficient threshold value of 1.25×10^{-3} mm^2/s can differentiate malignant from benign nodules in 91% of cases.

BAYESIAN ANALYSIS

Bayesian analysis has been used to define the weight of different clinical and imaging risk factors based on the available literature.[19] The incorporation of advanced imaging techniques such as FDG-PET and DCE CT in Bayesian models is suggested for more precise evaluation of pulmonary nodules.[128,129] Clinical parameters may include the presence of hemoptysis, a history of malignancy, a history of tobacco use, and patient age. Imaging-based parameters may include morphologic features, growth rate, location, enhancement features, and SUV measurements of lung nodules. A hierarchy of likelihood ratios for various risk factors of malignancy in lung nodules is presented in **Table 2**.

The main purpose of Bayesian analysis is to incorporate both clinical and imaging-based characteristics to derive an estimate of the probability of malignancy in pulmonary nodules. Through the Bayes theorem, the probabilities of different risk factors can be combined into an overall estimate to calculate the risk of malignancy of pulmonary nodules.[20] In more sophisticated work, artificial neural networks have been used. They are

Table 2
Risk factors and likelihood ratios of malignancy

Characteristics Suggest Malignancy	Likelihood Ratio of Malignancy	Characteristics Support Benign Nature	Likelihood Ratio of Malignancy
Cavity wall thickness >16 mm	38.0	Benign growth rate	0.01
PET SUV >2.5	7.1	Benign calcification	0.01
Spiculated margin	5.54	CT enhancement <15 HU	0.04
Size >3.0 cm	5.23	Age 20–29 y	0.05
Hemoptysis	5.08	PET SUV <2.5	0.06
History of malignancy	4.95	Size <4 mm	0.07
Smoking >40 packs/y	3.7	Nonsmoker	0.15
Size 2.1–3.0 cm	3.67	Age 30–39 y	0.24
Malignant growth rate	3.4	Smooth margin	0.3
Age 60–69 y	2.64	Size 0–1 cm	0.52
CT enhancement >15 HU	2.32	Lower lobe location	0.66
Noncalcified nodule	2.2	Size 5–15 mm	0.72
Smoking 30–39 packs/y	2.0	Smoking <30 packs/y	0.74
Age 50–59 y	1.9	Size 1.1–2.0 cm	0.74
Upper/middle lobe location	1.22	Lobulated outline	0.74
		Age 40–49 y	0.94
		No hemoptysis	1.0
		No previous malignancy	1.0

Data from Refs.[9,19,20,22]

designed to adapt training and adjust their patterns based on the presented objectives. Some investigators[26] have reported a potential value of neural networks to accurately classify lung nodules as malignant.

NEEDLE ASPIRATION/BIOPSY

Image-guided transthoracic needle aspiration or biopsy may help to obtain the correct diagnosis for indeterminate pulmonary nodules in high-risk patients,[130] and has been shown to affect the management of indeterminate nodules ~50% of the time.[131] Image guidance can be achieved with CT, fluoroscopy, or ultrasonography. Endobronchial ultrasound-guided transbronchial needle aspiration (EBUS-TBNA) is considered as a minimally invasive staging and diagnostic procedure usually performed for central and hilar lung lesions. It has been reported to have ~81% sensitivity and up to 100% specificity. In addition, it allows for real-time sampling with improved performance compared with mediastinoscopy.[132] The effectiveness of EBUS-TBNA depends on multiple factors including the size and location of the lesion undergoing sampling, and whether the lesion is visible by ultrasonography.[133] Transthoracic needle aspiration is generally more sensitive than bronchoscopy and EBUS-TBNA in the

assessment of peripheral lung lesions.[134] With a transthoracic approach, it is almost always possible to reach visible nodules, although a high apical location and a location near the diaphragm tend to increase the difficulty of the approach. Although nodule aspiration/biopsy can identify benign and malignant lesions, the definitive diagnosis of benignity and the differentiation between different cell types of cancer are still evolving.[73]

The diagnostic accuracy of transthoracic needle aspiration/biopsy depends on the size of the lesion. Nodules less than 15 mm in size may require a high level of experience and more than a single attempt to obtain enough sample tissue. If an adequate technique is performed, the accuracy of transthoracic needle biopsy can be as high as 96%.[135] Complications such as pneumothorax and hemorrhage may occur in about 5% to 30% of cases of transthoracic needle biopsy. The risk of pneumothorax can be limited with the use of postbiopsy positional restrictions, although the risk is increased when emphysema is present. Hemorrhage is self-limited in most cases.[130]

GENERAL GUIDELINES FOR THE MANAGEMENT FOR LUNG NODULES

Together with imaging, clinical evaluation should be incorporated in the assessment of patients

Table 3
Fleischner Society guidelines for follow-up of incidental pulmonary nodules

Nodule size[a]	≤4 mm	>4–6 mm	>6–8 mm	>8 mm
Low risk[b]	No follow-up needed	Follow-up CT at 12 mo; if no change, no further follow-up[c]	Initial follow-up CT at 6–12 then at 18–24 mo if no change	Follow-up CT at around 3, 9, and 24 mo, PET, DCE CT, and/or biopsy
High risk[b]	Follow-up CT at 12 mo; if no change, no further follow-up[c]	Initial follow-up CT at 6–12 then at 18–24 mo if no change[c]	Initial follow-up CT at 3–6 then at 9–12 and 24 mo if no change	

These guidelines apply only to patients 35 years of age or older with nodules that are incidental (ie, unrelated to known underlying disease). For patients less than 35 years of age, 1 follow-up CT at 6–12 months is suggested. Comparison studies should be obtained whenever possible to assess for interval change. Low-dose thin-section unenhanced CT technique is suggested for follow-up CT examination when lung nodule follow-up is the only clinical indication for imaging.
[a] Average of nodule length and width.
[b] Risk is based on history of smoking or of other known risk factors.
[c] Ground-glass attenuation or mixed attenuation nodules may require longer follow-up.
Data from MacMahon H, Austin JH, Gamsu G, et al. Guidelines for management of small pulmonary nodules detected on CT scans: a statement from the Fleischner Society. Radiology 2005;237(2):395–400.

with pulmonary nodules. According to the probability of malignancy, management options for pulmonary nodules include surgical resection, tissue biopsy, or watchful waiting with clinical and imaging follow-up. Biopsy and surgery are invasive techniques that are typically performed in patients with lung nodules that have an intermediate or high probability of malignancy, respectively. Clinical and imaging follow-up is favored for patients with a low probability of malignancy. Observation may extend for a period of 1 to 2 years depending on nodule morphologic features and other risk factors, preferably with CT. More frequent imaging may be obtained for patients at higher risk of malignancy, whereas a longer follow-up period is advised for ground-glass attenuation nodules. General follow-up guidelines for incidental pulmonary nodules are presented in **Table 3**.

SUMMARY

Advances in imaging have led to increased detection of pulmonary nodules. CT continues to be the modality of choice for the detection and characterization of pulmonary nodules. In addition, molecular imaging, mainly with PET imaging, provides indispensable information that significantly affects the diagnosis and management of patients with pulmonary nodules. The ongoing development and refinement of more advanced techniques to improve the diagnostic performance of MR imaging for lung nodule evaluation may make MR imaging an attractive radiation-free alternative in selected patient populations.

REFERENCES

1. Hansell DM, Bankier AA, MacMahon H, et al. Fleischner Society: glossary of terms for thoracic imaging. Radiology 2008;246(3):697–722.
2. Gohagan JK, Marcus PM, Fagerstrom RM, et al. Final results of the Lung Screening Study, a randomized feasibility study of spiral CT versus chest X-ray screening for lung cancer. Lung Cancer 2005;47(1):9–15.
3. Swensen SJ, Jett JR, Hartman TE, et al. Lung cancer screening with CT: Mayo Clinic experience. Radiology 2003;226(3):756–61.
4. Veronesi G, Bellomi M, Mulshine JL, et al. Lung cancer screening with low-dose computed tomography: a non-invasive diagnostic protocol for baseline lung nodules. Lung Cancer 2008;61(3):340–9.
5. Hanamiya M, Aoki T, Yamashita Y, et al. Frequency and significance of pulmonary nodules on thin-section CT in patients with extrapulmonary malignant neoplasms. Eur J Radiol 2011. [Epub ahead of print].
6. Cummings SR, Lillington GA, Richard RJ. Estimating the probability of malignancy in solitary pulmonary nodules. A Bayesian approach. Am Rev Respir Dis 1986;134(3):449–52.
7. Dewan NA, Gupta NC, Redepenning LS, et al. Diagnostic efficacy of PET-FDG imaging in solitary pulmonary nodules. Potential role in evaluation and management. Chest 1993;104(4):997–1002.

8. Dewan NA, Reeb SD, Gupta NC, et al. PET-FDG imaging and transthoracic needle lung aspiration biopsy in evaluation of pulmonary lesions. A comparative risk-benefit analysis. Chest 1995; 108(2):441–6.

9. Dewan NA, Shehan CJ, Reeb SD, et al. Likelihood of malignancy in a solitary pulmonary nodule: comparison of Bayesian analysis and results of FDG-PET scan. Chest 1997;112(2):416–22.

10. Gupta NC, Frank AR, Dewan NA, et al. Solitary pulmonary nodules: detection of malignancy with PET with 2-[F-18]-fluoro-2-deoxy-D-glucose. Radiology 1992;184(2):441–4.

11. Gupta NC, Maloof J, Gunel E. Probability of malignancy in solitary pulmonary nodules using fluorine-18-FDG and PET. J Nucl Med 1996;37(6):943–8.

12. Lowe VJ, Duhaylongsod FG, Patz EF, et al. Pulmonary abnormalities and PET data analysis: a retrospective study. Radiology 1997;202(2):435–9.

13. Lowe VJ, Fletcher JW, Gobar L, et al. Prospective investigation of positron emission tomography in lung nodules. J Clin Oncol 1998;16(3):1075–84.

14. Orino K, Kawamura M, Hatazawa J, et al. Efficacy of F-18 fluorodeoxyglucose positron emission tomography (FDG-PET) scans in diagnosis of pulmonary nodules. Jpn J Thorac Cardiovasc Surg 1998;46(12):1267–74 [in Japanese].

15. Patz EF Jr, Lowe VJ, Hoffman JM, et al. Focal pulmonary abnormalities: evaluation with F-18 fluorodeoxyglucose PET scanning. Radiology 1993; 188(2):487–90.

16. Prauer HW, Weber WA, Romer W, et al. Controlled prospective study of positron emission tomography using the glucose analogue [18f]fluorodeoxyglucose in the evaluation of pulmonary nodules. Br J Surg 1998;85(11):1506–11.

17. Seely JM, Mayo JR, Miller RR, et al. T1 lung cancer: prevalence of mediastinal nodal metastases and diagnostic accuracy of CT. Radiology 1993; 186(1):129–32.

18. Gould MK, Fletcher J, Iannettoni MD, et al. Evaluation of patients with pulmonary nodules: when is it lung cancer?: ACCP evidence-based clinical practice guidelines (2nd edition). Chest 2007;132(Suppl 3): 108S–30S.

19. Gurney JW. Determining the likelihood of malignancy in solitary pulmonary nodules with Bayesian analysis. Part I. Theory. Radiology 1993;186(2): 405–13.

20. Gurney JW, Lyddon DM, McKay JA. Determining the likelihood of malignancy in solitary pulmonary nodules with Bayesian analysis. Part II. Application. Radiology 1993;186(2):415–22.

21. Gurney JW, Swensen SJ. Solitary pulmonary nodules: determining the likelihood of malignancy with neural network analysis. Radiology 1995; 196(3):823–9.

22. Swensen SJ, Silverstein MD, Ilstrup DM, et al. The probability of malignancy in solitary pulmonary nodules. Application to small radiologically indeterminate nodules. Arch Intern Med 1997;157(8): 849–55.

23. Swensen SJ, Silverstein MD, Edell ES, et al. Solitary pulmonary nodules: clinical prediction model versus physicians. Mayo Clin Proc 1999;74(4): 319–29.

24. Henschke CI, Yankelevitz DF, Mateescu I, et al. Neural networks for the analysis of small pulmonary nodules. Clin Imaging 1997;21(6):390–9.

25. Matsuki Y, Nakamura K, Watanabe H, et al. Usefulness of an artificial neural network for differentiating benign from malignant pulmonary nodules on high-resolution CT: evaluation with receiver operating characteristic analysis. AJR Am J Roentgenol 2002;178(3):657–63.

26. Nakamura K, Yoshida H, Engelmann R, et al. Computerized analysis of the likelihood of malignancy in solitary pulmonary nodules with use of artificial neural networks. Radiology 2000;214(3): 823–30.

27. Diederich S, Thomas M, Semik M, et al. Screening for early lung cancer with low-dose spiral computed tomography: results of annual follow-up examinations in asymptomatic smokers. Eur Radiol 2004; 14(4):691–702.

28. Gohagan J, Marcus P, Fagerstrom R, et al. Baseline findings of a randomized feasibility trial of lung cancer screening with spiral CT scan vs chest radiograph: the Lung Screening Study of the National Cancer Institute. Chest 2004;126(1):114–21.

29. Henschke CI, Yankelevitz DF, Libby DM, et al. Early lung cancer action project: annual screening using single-slice helical CT. Ann N Y Acad Sci 2001;952: 124–34.

30. Li F, Sone S, Abe H, et al. Lung cancers missed at low-dose helical CT screening in a general population: comparison of clinical, histopathologic, and imaging findings. Radiology 2002;225(3):673–83.

31. Li F, Sone S, Abe H, et al. Malignant versus benign nodules at CT screening for lung cancer: comparison of thin-section CT findings. Radiology 2004; 233(3):793–8.

32. Nawa T, Nakagawa T, Kusano S, et al. Lung cancer screening using low-dose spiral CT: results of baseline and 1-year follow-up studies. Chest 2002;122(1):15–20.

33. Sone S, Li F, Yang ZG, et al. Results of three-year mass screening programme for lung cancer using mobile low-dose spiral computed tomography scanner. Br J Cancer 2001;84(1):25–32.

34. Swensen SJ, Jett JR, Sloan JA, et al. Screening for lung cancer with low-dose spiral computed tomography. Am J Respir Crit Care Med 2002;165(4): 508–13.

35. Takashima S, Sone S, Li F, et al. Small solitary pulmonary nodules (< or =1 cm) detected at population-based CT screening for lung cancer: reliable high-resolution CT features of benign lesions. AJR Am J Roentgenol 2003;180(4):955–64.

36. Takashima S, Sone S, Li F, et al. Indeterminate solitary pulmonary nodules revealed at population-based CT screening of the lung: using first follow-up diagnostic CT to differentiate benign and malignant lesions. AJR Am J Roentgenol 2003;180(5):1255–63.

37. Henschke CI, Yankelevitz DF, Mirtcheva R, et al. CT screening for lung cancer: frequency and significance of part-solid and nonsolid nodules. AJR Am J Roentgenol 2002;178(5):1053–7.

38. Henschke CI, Yankelevitz DF, Naidich DP, et al. CT screening for lung cancer: suspiciousness of nodules according to size on baseline scans. Radiology 2004;231(1):164–8.

39. Siegelman SS, Khouri NF, Leo FP, et al. Solitary pulmonary nodules: CT assessment. Radiology 1986;160(2):307–12.

40. Zerhouni EA, Stitik FP, Siegelman SS, et al. CT of the pulmonary nodule: a cooperative study. Radiology 1986;160(2):319–27.

41. Wahidi MM, Govert JA, Goudar RK, et al. Evidence for the treatment of patients with pulmonary nodules: when is it lung cancer?: ACCP evidence-based clinical practice guidelines (2nd edition). Chest 2007;132(Suppl 3):94S–107S.

42. Heitzman ER, Markarian B, Raasch BN, et al. Pathways of tumor spread through the lung: radiologic correlations with anatomy and pathology. Radiology 1982;144(1):3–14.

43. Winer-Muram HT. The solitary pulmonary nodule. Radiology 2006;239(1):34–49.

44. Asamura H, Suzuki K, Watanabe S, et al. A clinicopathological study of resected subcentimeter lung cancers: a favorable prognosis for ground glass opacity lesions. Ann Thorac Surg 2003;76(4):1016–22.

45. Diederich S, Wormanns D, Lenzen H, et al. Screening for asymptomatic early bronchogenic carcinoma with low dose CT of the chest. Cancer 2000;89(Suppl 11):2483–4.

46. Geddes DM. The natural history of lung cancer: a review based on rates of tumour growth. Br J Dis Chest 1979;73(1):1–17.

47. Albert RH, Russell JJ. Evaluation of the solitary pulmonary nodule. Am Fam Physician 2009;80(8):827–31.

48. Revel MP, Merlin A, Peyrard S, et al. Software volumetric evaluation of doubling times for differentiating benign versus malignant pulmonary nodules. AJR Am J Roentgenol 2006;187(1):135–42.

49. Bach PB, Silvestri GA, Hanger M, et al. Screening for lung cancer: ACCP evidence-based clinical practice guidelines (2nd edition). Chest 2007;132(Suppl 3):69S–77S.

50. Hasegawa M, Sone S, Takashima S, et al. Growth rate of small lung cancers detected on mass CT screening. Br J Radiol 2000;73(876):1252–9.

51. Aoki T, Nakata H, Watanabe H, et al. Evolution of peripheral lung adenocarcinomas: CT findings correlated with histology and tumor doubling time. AJR Am J Roentgenol 2000;174(3):763–8.

52. Khan AN, Al-Jahdali HH, Allen CM, et al. The calcified lung nodule: what does it mean? Ann Thorac Med 2010;5(2):67–79.

53. Soubani AO. The evaluation and management of the solitary pulmonary nodule. Postgrad Med J 2008;84(995):459–66.

54. Siegelman SS, Khouri NF, Scott WW Jr, et al. Pulmonary hamartoma: CT findings. Radiology 1986;160(2):313–7.

55. Muhm JR, Miller WE, Fontana RS, et al. Lung cancer detected during a screening program using four-month chest radiographs. Radiology 1983;148(3):609–15.

56. Quekel L, Kessels AG, Goei R, et al. Miss rate of lung cancer on the chest radiograph in clinical practice. Chest 1999;115(3):720.

57. Shah PK, Austin JH, White CS, et al. Missed non-small cell lung cancer: radiographic findings of potentially resectable lesions evident only in retrospect. Radiology 2003;226(1):235–41.

58. Gomi T, Nakajima M, Fujiwara H, et al. Comparison of chest dual-energy subtraction digital tomosynthesis imaging and dual-energy subtraction radiography to detect simulated pulmonary nodules with and without calcifications a phantom study. Acad Radiol 2011;18(2):191–6.

59. Oda S, Awai K, Funama Y, et al. Detection of small pulmonary nodules on chest radiographs: efficacy of dual-energy subtraction technique using flat-panel detector chest radiography. Clin Radiol 2010;65(8):609–15.

60. Picozzi G, Paci E, Lopez Pegna A, et al. Screening of lung cancer with low dose spiral CT: results of a three year pilot study and design of the randomised controlled trial 'Italung-CT'. Radiol Med 2005;109(1–2):17–26 [in English, Italian].

61. Volterrani L, Mazzei MA, Scialpi M, et al. Three-dimensional analysis of pulmonary nodules by MSCT with Advanced Lung Analysis (ALA1) software. Radiol Med 2006;111(3):343–54 [in English, Italian].

62. Mayo JR, Aldrich J, Muller NL. Radiation exposure at chest CT: a statement of the Fleischner Society. Radiology 2003;228(1):15–21.

63. Kishi K, Homma S, Kurosaki A, et al. Small lung tumors with the size of 1cm or less in diameter: clinical, radiological, and histopathological characteristics. Lung Cancer 2004;44(1):43–51.

64. Seemann MD, Seemann O, Luboldt W, et al. Differentiation of malignant from benign solitary pulmonary lesions using chest radiography, spiral CT and HRCT. Lung Cancer 2000;29(2):105–24.

65. Woodring JH, Fried AM. Significance of wall thickness in solitary cavities of the lung: a follow-up study. AJR Am J Roentgenol 1983;140(3):473–4.

66. Eibel R, Turk TR, Kulinna C, et al. Multidetector-row CT of the lungs: multiplanar reconstructions and maximum intensity projections for the detection of pulmonary nodules. Rofo 2001;173(9):815–21 [in German].

67. Kawel N, Seifert B, Luetolf M, et al. Effect of slab thickness on the CT detection of pulmonary nodules: use of sliding thin-slab maximum intensity projection and volume rendering. AJR Am J Roentgenol 2009;192(5):1324–9.

68. Yi CA, Lee KS, Kim BT, et al. Tissue characterization of solitary pulmonary nodule: comparative study between helical dynamic CT and integrated PET/CT. J Nucl Med 2006;47(3):443–50.

69. Swensen SJ, Viggiano RW, Midthun DE, et al. Lung nodule enhancement at CT: multicenter study. Radiology 2000;214(1):73–80.

70. Yamashita K, Matsunobe S, Tsuda T, et al. Solitary pulmonary nodule: preliminary study of evaluation with incremental dynamic CT. Radiology 1995; 194(2):399–405.

71. Yi CA, Lee KS, Kim EA, et al. Solitary pulmonary nodules: dynamic enhanced multi-detector row CT study and comparison with vascular endothelial growth factor and microvessel density. Radiology 2004;233(1):191–9.

72. Zhang M, Kono M. Solitary pulmonary nodules: evaluation of blood flow patterns with dynamic CT. Radiology 1997;205(2):471–8.

73. Jeong YJ, Lee KS, Jeong SY, et al. Solitary pulmonary nodule: characterization with combined wash-in and washout features at dynamic multi-detector row CT. Radiology 2005;237(2):675–83.

74. Lee KS, Yi CA, Jeong SY, et al. Solid or partly solid solitary pulmonary nodules: their characterization using contrast wash-in and morphologic features at helical CT. Chest 2007;131(5):1516–25.

75. Bhalla M, Shepard JA, Nakamura K, et al. Dual kV CT to detect calcification in solitary pulmonary nodule. J Comput Assist Tomogr 1995;19(1):44–7.

76. Sieren JC, Ohno Y, Koyama H, et al. Recent technological and application developments in computed tomography and magnetic resonance imaging for improved pulmonary nodule detection and lung cancer staging. J Magn Reson Imaging 2010;32(6):1353–69.

77. Cann CE, Gamsu G, Birnberg FA, et al. Quantification of calcium in solitary pulmonary nodules using single- and dual-energy CT. Radiology 1982; 145(2):493–6.

78. Yankelevitz DF, Reeves AP, Kostis WJ, et al. Small pulmonary nodules: volumetrically determined growth rates based on CT evaluation. Radiology 2000;217(1):251–6.

79. Wormanns D, Kohl G, Klotz E, et al. Volumetric measurements of pulmonary nodules at multi-row detector CT: in vivo reproducibility. Eur Radiol 2004;14(1):86–92.

80. Ko JP, Rusinek H, Jacobs EL, et al. Small pulmonary nodules: volume measurement at chest CT–phantom study. Radiology 2003;228(3):864–70.

81. Basu S, Alavi A. Unparalleled contribution of 18F-FDG PET to medicine over 3 decades. J Nucl Med 2008;49(10):17N–21N, 37N.

82. Facey K, Bradbury I, Laking G, et al. Overview of the clinical effectiveness of positron emission tomography imaging in selected cancers. Health Technol Assess 2007;11(44):iii–iiv, xi–267.

83. Torigian DA, Huang SS, Houseni M, et al. Functional imaging of cancer with emphasis on molecular techniques. CA Cancer J Clin 2007;57(4):206–24.

84. Alavi A, Reivich M. Guest editorial: the conception of FDG-PET imaging. Semin Nucl Med 2002;32(1):2–5.

85. Warburg O, Posener K, Negelein E. The metabolism of the carcinoma cell. The metabolism of tumors. New York: Richard R Smith; 1931. p. 129–69.

86. Kostakoglu L, Agress H Jr, Goldsmith SJ. Clinical role of FDG PET in evaluation of cancer patients. Radiographics 2003;23(2):315–40 [quiz: 533].

87. Duhaylongsod FG, Lowe VJ, Patz EF Jr, et al. Lung tumor growth correlates with glucose metabolism measured by fluoride-18 fluorodeoxyglucose positron emission tomography. Ann Thorac Surg 1995; 60(5):1348–52.

88. Herder GJ, Golding RP, Hoekstra OS, et al. The performance of(18)F-fluorodeoxyglucose positron emission tomography in small solitary pulmonary nodules. Eur J Nucl Med Mol Imaging 2004;31(9): 1231–6.

89. Hung GU, Shiau YC, Tsai SC, et al. Differentiation of radiographically indeterminate solitary pulmonary nodules with [18F]fluoro-2-deoxyglucose positron emission tomography. Jpn J Clin Oncol 2001; 31(2):51–4.

90. Gould MK, Sanders GD, Barnett PG, et al. Cost-effectiveness of alternative management strategies for patients with solitary pulmonary nodules. Ann Intern Med 2003;138(9):724–35.

91. Cheran SK, Nielsen ND, Patz EF Jr. False-negative findings for primary lung tumors on FDG positron emission tomography: staging and prognostic implications. AJR Am J Roentgenol 2004;182(5): 1129–32.

92. Lee KS, Jeong YJ, Han J, et al. T1 non-small cell lung cancer: imaging and histopathologic findings and their prognostic implications. Radiographics 2004;24(6):1617–36 [discussion: 32–6].

93. Alavi A, Gupta N, Alberini JL, et al. Positron emission tomography imaging in nonmalignant thoracic disorders. Semin Nucl Med 2002;32(4):293–321.

94. Khalaf M, Abdel-Nabi H, Baker J, et al. Relation between nodule size and 18F-FDG-PET SUV for malignant and benign pulmonary nodules. J Hematol Oncol 2008;1:13.

95. Lowe VJ, Hoffman JM, DeLong DM, et al. Semiquantitative and visual analysis of FDG-PET images in pulmonary abnormalities. J Nucl Med 1994;35(11):1771–6.

96. Keyes JW Jr. SUV: standard uptake or silly useless value? J Nucl Med 1995;36(10):1836–9.

97. Huang SC. Anatomy of SUV. Standardized uptake value. Nucl Med Biol 2000;27(7):643–6.

98. Basu S, Zaidi H, Houseni M, et al. Novel quantitative techniques for assessing regional and global function and structure based on modern imaging modalities: implications for normal variation, aging and diseased states. Semin Nucl Med 2007; 37(3):223–39.

99. Bural G, Torigian DA, Houseni M, et al. Tumor metabolism measured by partial volume corrected standardized uptake value varies considerably in primary and metastatic sites in patients with lung cancer. A new observation. Hell J Nucl Med 2009;12(3):218–22.

100. Hoetjes NJ, van Velden FH, Hoekstra OS, et al. Partial volume correction strategies for quantitative FDG PET in oncology. Eur J Nucl Med Mol Imaging 2010;37(9):1679–87.

101. Srinivas SM, Dhurairaj T, Basu S, et al. A recovery coefficient method for partial volume correction of PET images. Ann Nucl Med 2009;23(4):341–8.

102. Matthies A, Hickeson M, Cuchiara A, et al. Dual time point 18F-FDG PET for the evaluation of pulmonary nodules. J Nucl Med 2002;43(7):871–5.

103. Houseni M, Chamroonrat W, Zhuang J, et al. Prognostic implication of dual-phase PET in adenocarcinoma of the lung. J Nucl Med 2010; 51(4):535–42.

104. Alkhawaldeh K, Bural G, Kumar R, et al. Impact of dual-time-point (18)F-FDG PET imaging and partial volume correction in the assessment of solitary pulmonary nodules. Eur J Nucl Med Mol Imaging 2008;35(2):246–52.

105. Xiu Y, Bhutani C, Dhurairaj T, et al. Dual-time point FDG PET imaging in the evaluation of pulmonary nodules with minimally increased metabolic activity. Clin Nucl Med 2007;32(2):101–5.

106. Rankin S. [(18)F]2-fluoro-2-deoxy-D-glucose PET/CT in mediastinal masses. Cancer Imaging 2010; 10(Spec no A):S156–60.

107. Orlacchio A, Schillaci O, Antonelli L, et al. Solitary pulmonary nodules: morphological and metabolic characterisation by FDG-PET-MDCT. Radiol Med 2007;112(2):157–73 [in English, Italian].

108. Bading JR, Shields AF. Imaging of cell proliferation: status and prospects. J Nucl Med 2008;49(Suppl 2): 64S–80S.

109. Cai W, Niu G, Chen X. Multimodality imaging of the HER-kinase axis in cancer. Eur J Nucl Med Mol Imaging 2008;35(1):186–208.

110. Dass K, Ahmad A, Azmi AS, et al. Evolving role of uPA/uPAR system in human cancers. Cancer Treat Rev 2008;34(2):122–36.

111. Jacobson O, Weiss ID, Szajek L, et al. 64Cu-AMD3100–a novel imaging agent for targeting chemokine receptor CXCR4. Bioorg Med Chem 2009; 17(4):1486–93.

112. Kenny LM, Coombes RC, Oulie I, et al. Phase I trial of the positron-emitting Arg-Gly-Asp (RGD) peptide radioligand 18F-AH111585 in breast cancer patients. J Nucl Med 2008;49(6):879–86.

113. Li ZB, Niu G, Wang H, et al. Imaging of urokinase-type plasminogen activator receptor expression using a 64Cu-labeled linear peptide antagonist by microPET. Clin Cancer Res 2008;14(15):4758–66.

114. Zannetti A, Del Vecchio S, Iommelli F, et al. Imaging of alpha(v)beta(3) expression by a bifunctional chimeric RGD peptide not cross-reacting with alpha(v)beta(5). Clin Cancer Res 2009;15(16): 5224–33.

115. Tian J, Yang X, Yu L, et al. A multicenter clinical trial on the diagnostic value of dual-tracer PET/CT in pulmonary lesions using 3'-deoxy-3'-18F-fluorothymidine and 18F-FDG. J Nucl Med 2008;49(2):186–94.

116. Ambrosini V, Castellucci P, Rubello D, et al. 68Ga-DOTA-NOC: a new PET tracer for evaluating patients with bronchial carcinoid. Nucl Med Commun 2009;30(4):281–6.

117. Biederer J, Hintze C, Fabel M. MRI of pulmonary nodules: technique and diagnostic value. Cancer Imaging 2008;8:125–30.

118. Both M, Schultze J, Reuter M, et al. Fast T1- and T2-weighted pulmonary MR-imaging in patients with bronchial carcinoma. Eur J Radiol 2005; 53(3):478–88.

119. Bruegel M, Gaa J, Woertler K, et al. MRI of the lung: value of different turbo spin-echo, single-shot turbo spin-echo, and 3D gradient-echo pulse sequences for the detection of pulmonary metastases. J Magn Reson Imaging 2007;25(1):73–81.

120. Girvin F, Ko JP. Pulmonary nodules: detection, assessment, and CAD. AJR Am J Roentgenol 2008;191(4):1057–69.

121. Schaefer JF, Vollmar J, Schick F, et al. Solitary pulmonary nodules: dynamic contrast-enhanced MR imaging–perfusion differences in malignant and benign lesions. Radiology 2004;232(2):544–53.

122. Zou Y, Zhang M, Wang Q, et al. Quantitative investigation of solitary pulmonary nodules: dynamic contrast-enhanced MRI and histopathologic analysis. AJR Am J Roentgenol 2008;191(1):252–9.

123. Matsuoka S, Hunsaker AR, Gill RR, et al. Functional MR imaging of the lung. Magn Reson Imaging Clin N Am 2008;16(2):275–89, ix.

124. Karabulut N. Accuracy of diffusion-weighted MR imaging for differentiation of pulmonary lesions. Radiology 2009;253(3):899 [author reply: 899–900].

125. Liu H, Liu Y, Yu T, et al. Usefulness of diffusion-weighted MR imaging in the evaluation of pulmonary lesions. Eur Radiol 2010;20(4):807–15.

126. Satoh S, Kitazume Y, Ohdama S, et al. Can malignant and benign pulmonary nodules be differentiated with diffusion-weighted MRI? AJR Am J Roentgenol 2008;191(2):464–70.

127. Tondo F, Saponaro A, Stecco A, et al. Role of diffusion-weighted imaging in the differential diagnosis of benign and malignant lesions of the chest-mediastinum. Radiol Med 2011. [Epub ahead of print].

128. Meert AP. Pulmonary nodule: a Bayesian approach. Rev Med Brux 2010;31(2):117–21 [in French].

129. Menzel C, Hamer OW. Characterization and management of incidentally detected solitary pulmonary nodules. Radiologe 2010;50(1):53–60 [in German].

130. Cham MD, Lane ME, Henschke CI, et al. Lung biopsy: special techniques. Semin Respir Crit Care Med 2008;29(4):335–49.

131. Yankelevitz DF, Vazquez M, Henschke CI. Special techniques in transthoracic needle biopsy of pulmonary nodules. Radiol Clin North Am 2000; 38(2):267–79.

132. Medford AR. Endobronchial ultrasound-guided transbronchial needle aspiration. Pol Arch Med Wewn 2010;120(11):459–66.

133. Yung RC. Tissue diagnosis of suspected lung cancer: selecting between bronchoscopy, transthoracic needle aspiration, and resectional biopsy. Respir Care Clin N Am 2003;9(1):51–76.

134. Rivera MP, Mehta AC. Initial diagnosis of lung cancer: ACCP evidence-based clinical practice guidelines (2nd edition). Chest 2007;132(Suppl 3): 131S–48S.

135. Li H, Boiselle PM, Shepard JO, et al. Diagnostic accuracy and safety of CT-guided percutaneous needle aspiration biopsy of the lung: comparison of small and large pulmonary nodules. AJR Am J Roentgenol 1996;167(1):105–9.

Multimodality Staging of Lung Cancer

Sanjay Thulkar, MD[a],*, Gauthier Namur, MD[b],
Roland Hustinx, MD, PhD[b], Ashu Seith Bhalla, MD[c],
Rakesh Kumar, MD, PhD[d]

KEYWORDS

• Lung cancer • Staging • Lymph nodes • Metastases

Lung cancer is among the most common and lethal cancers around the world. Most lung cancers are directly attributed to smoking.[1] Common histologic subtypes of lung carcinomas are squamous cell carcinoma, adenocarcinoma, and large cell carcinoma. These carcinomas have similar presentations and are primarily treated surgically. Hence, these are usually classified as non–small cell lung carcinoma (NSCLC). Small cell lung carcinoma (SCLC) is an aggressive neuroendocrine tumor with a generally poor prognosis.[2] It usually presents with massive mediastinal lymphadenopathy and widespread metastases at initial diagnosis, and is usually treated with chemotherapy and radiotherapy; surgery has little role.

Cough, dyspnea, and hemoptysis are the consistent clinical features of most lung cancers. Advanced tumors with pleural, chest wall, or mediastinal invasion produce a variety of additional clinical features such as chest pain, brachial plexus neuropathy, Horner syndrome, phrenic or recurrent laryngeal nerve palsy, dysphagia, or superior vena cava syndrome. Some of the lung cancers are detected as small pulmonary nodules in asymptomatic individuals.

DIAGNOSIS OF LUNG CANCER

Chest radiography is the primary modality for the detection of lung cancer. Typically, lung cancer is seen as a solitary pulmonary nodule or mass.

Although large tumors are readily shown, those smaller than 2 cm or located centrally near the hilum are frequently missed on chest radiographs.[3] Other lung cancers may present with atypical (or indirect) signs on chest radiographs, such as nonresolving or recurring pneumonia, atelectasis, mediastinal lymphadenopathy, or pleural effusion.

Computed tomography (CT) imaging is frequently used in patients suspected to have lung cancer. It is more accurate for detection and characterization of lung cancers compared with chest radiography. Most lung cancers are readily shown as nodules ($\leq$3 cm) or masses (>3 cm) on CT. Some central tumors may not be visible, and, in this situation, the diagnosis is based on other modalities such as bronchoscopy and biopsy.

METHODS TO ESTABLISH TISSUE DIAGNOSIS

Pathologic diagnosis of lung cancer is normally obtained with bronchoscopic or CT-guided biopsy. Bronchoscopy is most useful for central tumors and diagnostic yield exceeds 90% for visible tumors.[1] Nonvisible lesions can also be sampled using indirect bronchoscopic methods such as lavage, brushing, or biopsy forceps. CT-guided transthoracic fine-needle aspiration cytology (FNAC) or core biopsy is accurate for tumors not amenable to bronchoscopic visualization. If there is a strong clinical or radiological suspicion for presence of a lung cancer, nondiagnostic or nonspecific

Financial support: not applicable.
[a] Dr B R Ambedkar Institute Rotary Cancer Hospital, All India Institute of Medical Sciences, New Delhi 110029, India
[b] Division of Nuclear Medicine, University Hospital of Liège, B-4000 Liège, Belgium
[c] Department of Radio-diagnosis, All India Institute of Medical Sciences, New Delhi 110029, India
[d] Department of Nuclear Medicine, All India Institute of Medical Sciences, New Delhi 110029, India
* Corresponding author.
E-mail address: thulkar@hotmail.com

PET Clin 6 (2011) 251–263
doi:10.1016/j.cpet.2011.05.001
1556-8598/11/$ – see front matter © 2011 Published by Elsevier Inc.

benign results are not reliable and repeat biopsy should generally be performed in these situations.[4]

STAGING OF LUNG CANCER

After the diagnosis of lung cancer, accurate staging is required to determine the treatment options and prognosis. The most important issue is to determine whether the tumor is resectable and, if so, the type and extent of the surgery that may be required. NSCLC is staged according to the new seventh edition of American Joint Committee on Cancer (AJCC)/Union Internationale Contre le Cancer (UICC) staging system, which is based on the recommendations of the International Association for Study of Lung cancer (IASLC), published in 2009 (**Tables 1** and **2**).[5]

Traditionally, SCLC is staged into 2 stages depending on whether or not the disease can be included in a single radiation field. There is limited disease stage (disease in ipsilateral lung with unilateral or bilateral mediastinal lymph nodes) and extensive disease stage (involvement of contralateral lung and/or distant metastases). However, the new seventh edition of TNM-based lung cancer staging system is also recommended for staging of SCLC.

Table 2
Seventh edition of AJCC-UICC Staging of Lung Cancer: stage groups

T/M	Subgroups	N0	N1	N2	N3
T1	T1a T1b	IA	IIA	IIIA	IIIB
T2	T2a T2b	IB IIA	IIA IIB	IIIA	IIIB
T3		IIB	IIIA	IIIA	IIIB
T4		IIIA	IIIA	IIIB	IIIB
M1	M1a M2b	IV	IV	IV	IV

Data from Detterbeck FC, Boffa DJ, Tanoue LT. The new lung cancer staging system. Chest 2009;136:260–71.

WORK-UP FOR THE STAGING OF LUNG CANCER

Chest radiographs are useful for diagnosis of the lung cancer but generally not for staging. Although presence of lung metastases, bone marrow metastases, or phrenic nerve involvement, as suggested by increase of the diaphragm on chest radiography, makes the lung cancer unresectable, these are of limited usefulness for staging

Table 1
Seventh edition of AJCC-UICC Staging of Lung Cancer: tumor-node-metastasis (TNM) descriptors

Descriptors	Definitions
T1	Up to 3 cm diameter, surrounded by lung or visceral pleura, not more proximal than lobar bronchus T1a up to 2 cm, T1b>2–3 cm
T2	>3–7 cm diameter or any tumor up to 7 cm that invades visceral pleura, involves main bronchus ≥2 cm distal to carina, atelectasis/pneumonia extending to hilum but not involving entire lung T2a>3–5 cm; T2b>5–7 cm
T3	>7 cm diameter, main bronchus involvement <2 cm distal to carina, involvement of chest wall, diaphragm, phrenic nerve, mediastinal pleura, pericardium, atelectasis/pneumonia of entire lung, separate nodule(s) in same lobe
T4	Any size tumor with involvement of mediastinum, heart, great vessels, carina, trachea, esophagus, vertebral body, recurrent laryngeal nerve, separate nodule(s) in different ipsilateral lobe
N0	No lymph nodes metastases
N1	Ipsilateral intrapulmonary/peribronchial/hilar lymph nodes, including direct extension
N2	Ipsilateral mediastinal/subcarinal lymph nodes
N3	Contralateral mediastinal/hilar, any scalene or supraclavicular lymph nodes
M0	No distant metastases
M1	Distant metastases M1a: separate tumor nodule in contralateral lung, malignant pleural/pericardial effusion M1b: presence of distant metastases

Data from Detterbeck FC, Boffa DJ, Tanoue LT. The new lung cancer staging system. Chest 2009;136:260–71.

purposes. Contrast-enhanced CT (CECT) of the thorax and upper abdomen including liver and adrenals is the primary imaging modality for staging of the lung cancer. Based on the CT findings, 1 or more of the complimentary modalities are also used in the staging work-up. These include mediastinoscopy, video-assisted thoracoscopic surgery (VATS), endoscopic ultrasonography (EUS), transbronchial ultrasonography (TBUS), pleural fluid cytology, and FNAC or biopsy of suspected distant metastases. Magnetic resonance (MR) imaging is not a standard lung cancer staging modality; however, it is occasionally used in specific situations. [^{18}F]Fluorodeoxyglucose (FDG) positron emission tomography (PET)/CT is the most important upcoming modality for lung cancer staging, especially for regional nodal and distant metastatic staging.

Depending on the clinical findings, tumor stage, and histology of the lung cancer, other imaging techniques for the metastatic work-up may also be required. These techniques include CECT of abdomen and pelvis, CT or MR imaging of the brain, and bone scintigraphy. Protocols to use different imaging studies for staging of lung cancer also vary according to local institutional protocols. A useful guideline for the rational use of various imaging modalities has been published by American College of Radiology (ACR; Appropriateness Criteria for Staging of Bronchogenic Carcinoma).[6]

TUMOR STAGING

The primary goal of the tumor staging (T staging) in lung cancer is to assess surgical resectability by assessment of the size and extent of the primary tumor. T1 and T2 tumors are localized within the lung and visceral pleura (**Fig. 1**). On CT, location

and size of the tumor should be defined. It is also important to determine the relationship of the tumor with the lobar or mainstem bronchus, and whether or not tumor has involved the fissure, major pulmonary artery, or major pulmonary veins (**Fig. 2**). This information is taken into consideration to determine the type of surgery to be implemented (ie, lobectomy, sleeve lobectomy, or pneumonectomy).[7] T3 tumors may have chest wall or early mediastinal involvement, or are located within 2 cm of the carina (**Fig. 3** A–C). T4 tumors involve the carina or other major mediastinal structures (**Fig. 4**). It is important to distinguish T3 from T4 tumors, because the latter are not resectable.

On CECT, most centrally located lung cancers are seen as minimally enhancing, soft tissue masses, whereas obstructive atelectasis shows significant enhancement. However, some tumors cannot be separately defined from obstructive atelectasis and/or pneumonia on CT. Although this limitation normally does not affect the assessment of surgical resectability, accurate tumor delineation is an important requirement for radiotherapy. Such distinction is readily made with FDG-PET, because atelectasis usually shows mild to moderate uptake compared with the tumor (**Fig. 5**). MR imaging may also be helpful in these situations. Atelectatic lung may be hyperintense compared with tumor on T2-weighted images, and contrast-enhanced T1-weighted images may also be useful in tumor delineation.[8]

MEDIASTINAL INVASION

Tumor extension deeper to the mediastinal pleura or pericardium precludes surgical resection. On CT, visualization of tumor merely abutting the

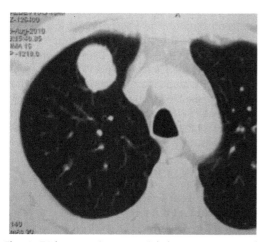

Fig. 1. T1 lung carcinoma. Axial chest CT image with lung windowing shows small, well-defined lung mass in right upper lobe, surrounded by lung parenchyma only.

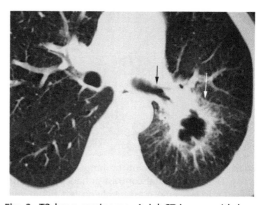

Fig. 2. T2 lung carcinoma. Axial CT image with lung windowing shows cavitary left lower lobe lung mass. Left main bronchus is not involved by tumor (*black arrow*), whereas major fissure is involved and retracted by tumor (*white arrow*).

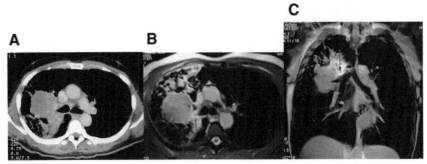

Fig. 3. T3 lung carcinoma. (*A*) Axial contrast-enhanced CT image shows right central pulmonary/hilar mass that is involving right main bronchus within 2 cm of carina. Tumor abuts mediastinum on anterior aspect of right main bronchus, although depth of mediastinal invasion is not well defined. (*B*) Axial T2-weighted and (*C*) coronal post-contrast T1-weighted MR images of chest show separation of tumor mass from mediastinum by hyperintense and enhancing inflammatory tissue (*black arrows*). No mediastinal invasion was found at surgery.

mediastinum is insufficient to establish presence of mediastinal invasion. Preservation of mediastinal fat planes, tumor contact with the mediastinum of less than 3 cm, and tumor contact with the aorta of less than 90 degrees exclude mediastinal invasion.[9] However, loss of mediastinal fat planes, tumor contact with the mediastinum of greater than 3 cm, or tumor contact with the aorta of greater than 90 degrees do not necessarily indicate unresectable tumor. Deep penetration of the tumor within mediastinum, involvement of major vessels, heart, carina, trachea, esophagus, or vertebra are the only reliable signs of deep mediastinal invasion (ie, T4 tumor; see **Fig. 4**). The accuracy of MR imaging for mediastinal invasion is similar to CT, although it may sometimes be useful to better define bronchial encasement (see

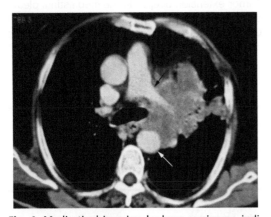

Fig. 4. Mediastinal invasion by lung carcinoma indicating T4 disease. Axial contrast-enhanced CT image shows large left lung mass involving left hilum with deep extension into mediastinum. Left main pulmonary artery is encased and narrowed by tumor (*black arrow*). Descending aorta is also involved, as suggested by wide angle of contact with tumor and contour deformity (*white arrow*).

Fig. 3) or intrapericardial extension of tumor along the pulmonary veins.[7] Endobronchial ultrasound (EBUS) is also useful to differentiate between compression and infiltration of bronchi by tumor.[10]

CHEST WALL INVASION

Invasion of the chest wall or diaphragm does not necessarily make lung cancer unresectable, but does adversely affect prognosis. Surgical treatment may be extensive, and resection of the chest wall, sometimes with reconstruction, is required. Early chest wall invasion may be difficult to confirm or exclude on CT. Various signs that suggest invasion of the parietal pleura by lung cancer include an obtuse angle of contact between tumor and chest wall, obliteration of the extrapleural fat plane, pleural thickening, and presence of an extrapleural soft tissue component. Presence of 1 or more of these signs indicates a high likelihood of chest wall invasion.[11] Extrathoracic tumor extension through the intercostal space and rib destruction are the only definitive signs of chest wall invasion on CT (**Fig. 6**). Clinically, presence of local chest pain is highly specific for chest wall invasion. Thoracoscopy is more accurate than imaging for excluding chest wall invasion in equivocal cases.[12] The accuracy of MR imaging is similar or slightly superior to CT in the diagnosis of chest wall invasion.[13,14]

PANCOAST TUMOR

Pancoast or superior sulcus tumors are apical lung cancers that can be of any histologic type. These tumors arise in the superior part of the lung and have a propensity to invade the adjacent chest wall, brachial plexus, subclavian vessels, ribs, scapula, vertebrae, and base of the neck. Horner syndrome, caused by involvement of the sympathetic chain, is

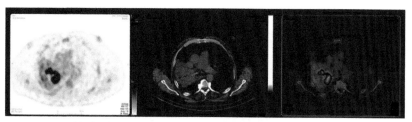

Fig. 5. Transverse PET, CT, and hybrid PET/CT images from FDG-PET/CT study show right pulmonary/hilar squamous cell lung carcinoma. Note clear differentiation between central highly metabolic tumor and peripheral nonhypermetabolic obstructive atelectasis.

the characteristic clinical feature of superior sulcus tumors.

On chest radiography, a superior sulcus tumor appears as an apical lung mass or asymmetric pleural thickening. CT shows the full extent of the lung mass to a better extent. Bone involvement and invasions of vessels have important surgical implications, and are well shown on CT. Multiplanar reconstructions (MPR) of CT images are particularly important (**Fig. 7**). In equivocal cases, MR imaging is more useful to diagnose invasion of the chest wall, brachial plexus, neural foramina, and subclavian vessels.[14] Because of the close and complex relationships among the anatomic structures at the thoracic inlet, the combination of both CT and MR imaging may be useful for the accurate assessment of resectability of superior sulcus tumors.[15]

ADDITIONAL LUNG NODULES

Lung cancer can metastasize to the lungs. A tumor nodule in the same lobe as the primary tumor is considered as T3 disease, and a tumor nodule in a different ipsilateral lobe is considered as T4

disease, whereas a tumor nodule in the contralateral lung is considered to be an intrathoracic metastasis (M1a disease) (**Fig. 8**). However, the significance of additional small noncalcified pulmonary nodules detected at CT is difficult to determine, because about 75% of such nodules may be benign.[16,17]

REGIONAL LYMPH NODE STAGING

Presence or absence of lymph node metastases has important implications for the resectability of lung cancer. In patients treated with surgery, presence or absence of mediastinal lymph node involvement on pathology is the most important predictor of the treatment outcome and survival.[18] Tumors of more than 3 cm and adenocarcinoma histology have greater chances of mediastinal lymph node involvement.

In the new staging system, lymph nodes have been grouped into 7 nodal zones. These zones are supraclavicular, upper zone (paratracheal, retrotracheal, and prevascular), aorticopulmonary (aorticopulmonary window and para-aortic), lower zone (paraesophageal and pulmonary ligament),

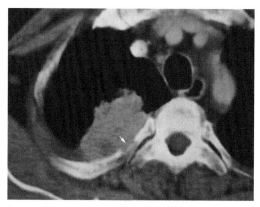

Fig. 6. Chest wall invasion by lung carcinoma indicating T3 disease. Axial CT image with bone windowing shows right upper lobe lung mass with large area of contact with chest wall and erosion of posterior rib (*arrow*).

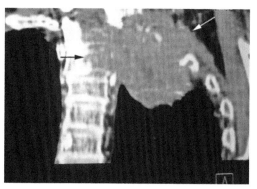

Fig. 7. Superior sulcus tumor caused by lung carcinoma. Coronal reconstructed contrast-enhanced CT image shows left apical lung mass with destruction of ribs by tumor with extrathoracic tumor extension (*white arrow*) and destruction of vertebra (*black arrow*) indicating T4 disease.

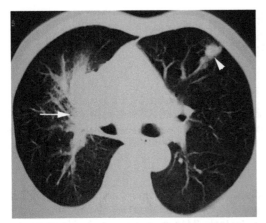

Fig. 8. Axial CT image with lung windowing shows right hilar mass caused by lung carcinoma. There is an additional lung nodule seen in contralateral lung (*arrowhead*) in keeping with metastasis (M1a disease).

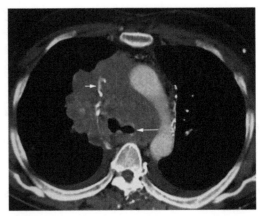

Fig. 10. Bilateral mediastinal lymphadenopathy caused by SCLC indicating N3 disease. Axial contrast-enhanced CT image shows extensive and conglomerate bilateral lymph node enlargement with encasement of superior vena cava (*small arrow*) and carina (*large arrow*).

subcarinal, hilar-interlobar, and peripheral groups (lobar, segmental, subsegmental); the last 2 groups are the N1 nodes.[19] Hilar (N1) lymph nodes are extramediastinal and can be removed within the pneumonectomy. Ipsilateral mediastinal lymph nodes, as well as midline nodes such as central prevascular or subcarinal lymph nodes, are N2 lymph nodes (**Fig. 9**). Contralateral mediastinal, contralateral hilar, and any scalene or supraclavicular lymph nodes are N3 nodes (**Fig. 10**). Patients with gross ipsilateral (N2) or any contralateral (N3) mediastinal lymph nodal involvement are not candidates for curative surgery. If mediastinal lymph nodes are contiguous with primary tumor and not separately defined, they are considered as part of the tumor and staged as such. Lymph node involvement at any other site outside the

thorax is considered as distant metastatic disease (M1b).

On CT, enlarged lymph nodes (short-axis diameter of 10 mm or more) are generally considered to be lymph node metastases. The attenuation pattern of lymph nodes is not helpful to diagnose lymph node metastases in lung cancer.[7] Size criteria for the diagnosis of lymph node metastases has obvious limitations. Substantial interobserver variation in designation of lymph node location and measurement of size further complicates the problem.[20] A meta-analysis has found that the overall sensitivity and specificity of CT for the diagnosis of lymph node metastases in lung cancer is 57% and 82%, respectively.[21] False-positive lymph node enlargement on CT can be caused by postobstructive pneumonia and atelectasis, and is more common with central and large primary tumors.[7] False-negative CT results are especially common with central adenocarcinomas.[22] MR imaging also relies on size criteria for lymph node involvement in lung cancer, and hence its accuracy is similar to CT.[7,13] Morphology of lymph nodes may be better evaluated on MR imaging but does not improve the sensitivity.[23] Diffusion-weighted MR imaging techniques may be more accurate, although there is limited evidence at present.[24]

The added value of metabolic imaging in the mediastinal staging is well established. A meta-analysis reviewed 39 studies, including a total of 1959 patients evaluated with FDG-PET.[25] Median sensitivity and specificity were 61% and 79%, respectively, which are similar to the figures reported by Toloza and colleagues[21] in the same year. For FDG-PET, these values were 85% and

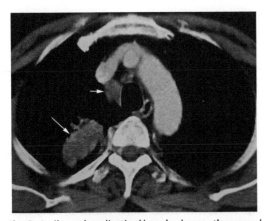

Fig. 9. Ipsilateral mediastinal lymphadenopathy caused by lung carcinoma indicating N2 disease. Axial contrast-enhanced CT image shows right upper lobe lung mass (*large arrow*) with ipsilateral paratracheal lymph node enlargement (*small arrow*).

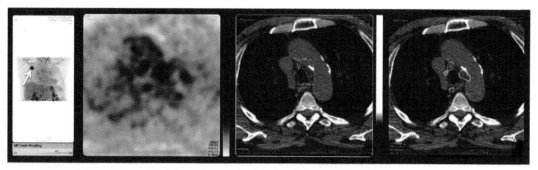

Fig. 11. Coronal FDG-PET maximal intensity projection (MIP) image shows hypermetabolic right upper lobe nodule caused by NSCLC (*arrow*). Transverse FDG-PET, unenhanced CT, and hybrid FDG-PET/CT images show hypermetabolic mediastinal lymph nodes suspicious for involvement by tumor, although smaller than 10 mm in short axis. EBUS-FNAC confirmed malignant involvement of the pretracheal node.

90%, respectively. FDG-PET was significantly more accurate than CT and it was particularly sensitive, but less specific, when CT depicted enlarged lymph nodes. Integrated FDG-PET/CT has also proved superior to stand-alone CT for mediastinal staging.[26,27] As always with FDG-PET imaging, false-positive nodal accumulation of FDG may occur in cases of inflammatory or infectious diseases. It is thus important to recognize patterns of uptake that are suggestive of benign involvement.[28,29] In regions with high prevalence of tuberculosis, it is possible to maintain a reasonable accuracy and a high specificity for PET/CT by considering CT features such as calcification as negative for cancer, but at the cost of decreased sensitivity.[30,31] Low sensitivity has also been reported in other circumstances, such as early-stage disease. For example, the sensitivity was only 42% in a series of 150 patients with stage T1 disease at CT.[32] Nonetheless, small lymph nodes (10–15 mm) without FDG uptake are associated with a low posttest probability of malignant involvement (5%).[33] Typical examples are provided in **Figs. 11** and **12**.

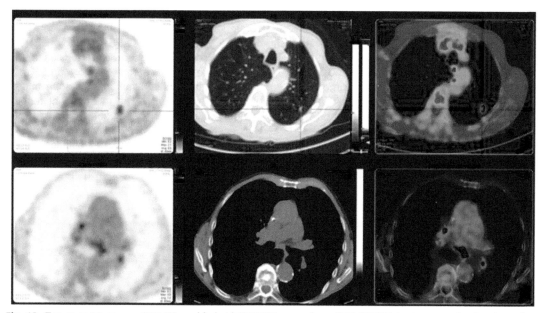

Fig. 12. Top row: transverse PET, CT, and hybrid PET/CT images from FDG-PET/CT staging examination in patient with lung carcinoma show small, highly metabolic pulmonary epidermoid carcinoma in left upper lobe (*crosshair*). Bottom row: transverse PET, CT, and hybrid PET/CT images from FDG-PET/CT examination in the same patient show mildly hypermetabolic small mediastinal and bilateral hilar nodes, which are nonspecific in this patient with a long history of tobacco use. Negative EBUS-FNAC and follow-up assessments at 5 months suggest that they are benign and likely inflammatory in nature.

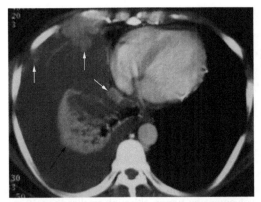

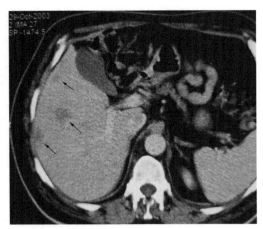

Fig. 13. Malignant pleural effusion caused by lung carcinoma. Axial contrast-enhanced CT image in patient with right hilar lung cancer shows atelectasis of right lung (*black arrow*) surrounded by large right pleural effusion and multiple nodular pleural deposits of tumor (*white arrows*), indicating M1a disease.

Fig. 15. Liver metastases caused by lung carcinoma indicating M1b disease. Axial contrast-enhanced CT image shows multiple hypoattenuating nodules in liver (*arrows*).

Because noninvasive imaging techniques are not sufficiently reliable, several invasive techniques are used with the aim of establishing pathologically accurate lymph nodal stage before curative surgery. Mediastinoscopy and lymph node biopsy is a reliable and widely used invasive technique for nodal staging of NSCLC. However, protocols for mediastinoscopic lymph node sampling are variable. Most surgeons do it only with positive lymph nodes on CT or PET, because this decreases the number of unnecessary mediastinoscopies, whereas others do it in all patients.[34] VATS is sometimes used but permits lymph node sampling of only 1 side of the mediastinum, although it also permits assessment of mediastinal or chest wall invasion by the primary tumor at the same time. EUS with transesophageal FNAC is also useful to diagnose mediastinal lymph node metastases.[35] It is especially suitable for the paratracheal and subcarinal lymph nodes. EBUS with transbronchial needle aspiration (EBUS-TBNA) is a new technique that is also useful for this purpose.[36] The combination of EBUS and

FDG-PET/CT is probably the most powerful for mediastinal staging. It should improve the overall specificity, although the negative predictive value may be as low as 60% because of sampling errors.[37] It may also enhance the sensitivity, particularly for adenocarcinomas.[38] Squamous cell carcinomas consistently display high FDG uptake, and few false-negative results are found in this tumor type.

In 2007, the European Society of Thoracic Surgeons recommended omitting invasive procedures in patients with peripheral tumors and negative mediastinal FDG-PET findings, whereas central tumors, PET-based hilar N1 disease, low FDG uptake of the primary tumor, and lymph nodes greater than 15 mm on CT scan should be surgically staged.[39] The most recent recommendations from the National Comprehensive Cancer Network (NCCN) indicate that positive FDG-PET findings should be clarified using EBUS-TBNA whenever possible, or pathologically confirmed by mediastinoscopy when the EBUS is negative.

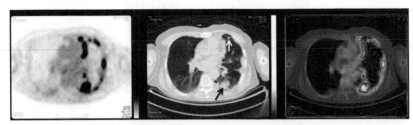

Fig. 14. Transverse PET, CT, and hybrid PET/CT images from FDG-PET/CT staging examination show hypermetabolic NSCLC of superior segment of left lower lobe (*black arrow*). Note subpleural metastasis in left upper lobe (*white arrow*) indicating T4 disease as well as multiple hypermetabolic pleural metastases indicating M1a disease. Bilateral metastatic mediastinal nodes were also present (not shown), indicating N3 disease.

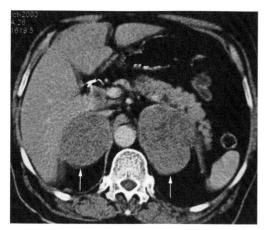

Fig. 16. Adrenal metastases caused by lung carcinoma indicating M1b disease. Axial contrast-enhanced CT image shows bilateral large adrenal masses (*arrows*).

PLEURAL EFFUSION

Malignant pleural effusion significantly worsens the prognosis of lung cancer, and for this reason it has been changed from T4 disease in the previous staging system to distant metastatic disease (M1a) in the new staging system. Pleura can be involved by direct invasion or by metastatic tumor deposits. Pleural effusion is generally considered as malignant unless the patient has other reasons for pleural effusion or if the effusion has been shown to be nonmalignant by multiple cytologic examinations. However, large pleural effusions associated with lung cancer, whether or not cytologically proven, almost always indicate a poor prognosis.[40] Among patients with T4 NSCLC, high FDG uptake in malignancy involving the pleural space is associated with a significantly worse prognosis than in those with a lower degree of uptake.[41] Benign and malignant pleural effusions cannot be differentiated on structural imaging unless pleural masses are seen (**Fig. 13**). Large pleural deposits of tumor are well shown on CT, but small pleural deposits may be missed.[42] FDG-

PET is helpful in this situation, because it shows a high sensitivity for detection of both primary pleural tumors and secondary lesions (**Fig. 14**).[43] On ultrasonography, presence of debris, septations, or pleural thickening does not necessarily mean that the pleural effusion is malignant, because these findings can be seen in benign pleural effusions as well.[44] Pleural effusion can occur with any lung cancer, although it is most common with adenocarcinomas. Sometimes, pleural involvement by adenocarcinoma of the lung produces diffuse nodular pleural thickening that mimics malignant pleural mesothelioma.[45]

DISTANT METASTASES

Liver, bone marrow, brain, and adrenal glands are the common sites of metastasis from lung cancer, although any organ in the body can be affected by metastatic lung cancer.[1] CT imaging performed for evaluation of patients with NSCLC should always include upper abdomen for the assessment of the adrenal glands. Liver metastases can be reliably detected on CT, and biopsy for confirmation is generally not required (**Fig. 15**). Adrenal metastases are seen in up to 20% of patients with NSCLC at presentation. Incidental nonfunctional adrenal adenomas are also common, and hence a small solitary adrenal nodule in a patient with NSCLC is more likely to be benign than caused by a metastasis.[46] Adrenal nodules less than 12 HU in attenuation on unenhanced CT are likely caused by adrenal adenomas. However, adrenal masses of more than 2 cm are usually caused by metastases (**Fig. 16**). The combination of CT criteria (size and attenuation) with metabolic features (standardized uptake value [SUV] or SUV ratio relative to normal liver) effectively characterizes adrenal involvement in most patients (**Fig. 17**).[47] In infrequent equivocal cases, MR imaging characterization or biopsy is recommended, especially if this is the only finding that may make the disease inoperable.[48] Lung cancer is a common cause of brain metastases, and these

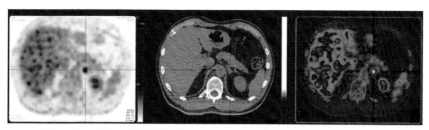

Fig. 17. Transverse PET, CT, and hybrid PET/CT images from FDG-PET/CT staging examination in patient with NSCLC. Although only minimally enlarged, left adrenal gland is highly hypermetabolic, in keeping with metastasis, indicating M1b disease.

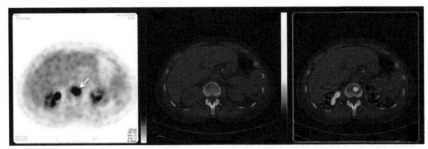

Fig. 18. Transverse PET, CT, and hybrid PET/CT images from FDG-PET/CT staging examination in patient with lung adenocarcinoma. Note hypermetabolic bone marrow metastasis in L2 vertebral body (*arrow*) that is not visible on corresponding CT image because no lytic destruction is present, indicating M1b disease. Because no sclerosis is present, this would also not be visible on bone scintigraphy.

are more commonly seen with poorly differentiated tumors or adenocarcinomas. MR imaging is more accurate than CT in their diagnosis.[49] MR imaging of brain is recommended in symptomatic patients as well as patients suspected to have stage III and IV NSCLC.[1] Bone marrow metastases are common in lung cancer, and bone scintigraphy may be used for their detection, although this imaging modality has limitations to its diagnostic performance. Because FDG-PET is both more sensitive and specific in this setting,[50] bone scintigraphy is no longer recommended, at least whenever FDG-PET/CT is performed (**Fig. 18**).

FDG-PET/CT is the most important single imaging modality for the overall metastatic work-up of patients with lung cancer. In a randomized controlled trial in 2002, van Tinteren and colleagues[51] showed that performing FDG-PET in patients who were operable according to the conventional work-up decreased the number of unnecessary thoracotomies by a factor 2, from 41% to 21%. More recently, 2 additional randomized trials further established the role of FDG-PET/CT in reducing the proportion of futile surgeries.[52,53] FDG-PET/CT is highly sensitive for detecting bone marrow, adrenal gland, and liver

metastases, as well as metastases in other unusual locations (**Fig. 19**) except for the brain, given the normal avid FDG uptake in the gray matter, so that dedicated brain imaging, preferably with MR imaging, remains necessary. Whole-body MR imaging with diffusion-weighted imaging may also have comparable accuracy for this purpose,[54] although this technique is currently in the early stages of the validation process. However, several studies have shown the cost-effectiveness of PET[55,56] and PET/CT.[57,58] The evidence regarding the clinical usefulness of metabolic imaging in the preoperative evaluation of NSCLC has reached levels rarely achieved for any other imaging technique in any other clinical situation.

SUMMARY

CT is the primary noninvasive imaging modality for staging of NSCLC. MR imaging compliments CT in tumor staging in specific situations. FDG-PET/CT is useful in detecting additional regional nodal and distant metastatic sites of disease, thereby reducing the number of unnecessary surgeries. However, noninvasive imaging modalities lack sufficient accuracy for nodal staging in all cases

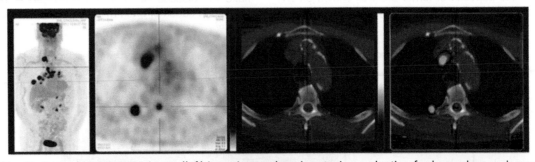

Fig. 19. Coronal FDG-PET MIP image (*left*) in patient undergoing staging evaluation for lung adenocarcinoma indicates presence of disseminated metastatic disease, which generally implies that chemotherapy is the only therapeutic option. Transverse FDG-PET, unenhanced CT, and hybrid FDG-PET/CT images show hypermetabolic intrathecal metastatic lesion at T5 level (*crosshair*), which is amenable to external radiotherapy treatment.

and, hence, preoperative lymph node sampling with invasive techniques such as mediastinoscopy, thoracoscopy, and FNAC guided by EBUS or EUS is frequently required in selected patients.

REFERENCES

1. Schrump D, Giaccone G, Kelsey C. Non small cell lung cancer. In: DeVita VT, Lawrence TS, Rosenberg SA, editors. Cancer: principles and practice of oncology. 8th edition. Philadelphia: Lippincott Williams & Wilkins; 2008. p. 896.

2. Munden RF, Bragg DG. Primary malignancies of the thorax. In: Bragg DG, Rubin P, Hricack H, editors. Oncologic imaging. 2nd edition. Philadelphia: WB Saunders; 2002. p. 313.

3. Hayashi H, Ashizawa K, Uetani M, et al. Detectability of peripheral lung cancer on chest radiographs: effect of the size, location and extent of ground-glass opacity. Br J Radiol 2009;82:272.

4. Quint LE, Kretschmer M, Chang A, et al. CT-guided thoracic core biopsies: value of a negative result. Cancer Imaging 2006;6:163.

5. Detterbeck FC, Boffa DJ, Tanoue LT. The new lung cancer staging system. Chest 2009;136:260.

6. American College of Radiology. Available at: http://www.acr.org/SecondaryMainMenuCategories/quality_safety/app_criteria/pdf/ExpertPanelonThoracicImaging/StagingofBronchogenicCarcinomaDoc11.aspx. Accessed March 7, 2011.

7. Hansell DM, Armstrong P, Lynch DA, et al. Neoplasms of the lungs, airway and pleura. In: Hansell DM, Armstrong P, Lynch DA, editors. Imaging of diseases of the chest. 4th edition. Philadelphia: Elsevier Mosby; 2005. p. 785.

8. Stiglbauer R, Schurawitzki H, Klepetko W, et al. Contrast-enhanced MRI for the staging of bronchogenic carcinoma: comparison with CT and histopathologic staging–preliminary results. Clin Radiol 1991;44:293.

9. Glazer HS, Kaiser LR, Anderson DJ, et al. Indeterminate mediastinal invasion in bronchogenic carcinoma: CT evaluation. Radiology 1989;173:37.

10. Herth F, Ernst A, Schulz M, et al. Endobronchial ultrasound reliably differentiates between airway infiltration and compression by tumor. Chest 2003;123:458.

11. Ratto GB, Piacenza G, Frola C, et al. Chest wall involvement by lung cancer: computed tomographic detection and results of operation. Ann Thorac Surg 1991;51:182.

12. Roberts JR, Blum MG, Arildsen R, et al. Prospective comparison of radiologic, thoracoscopic, and pathologic staging in patients with early non-small cell lung cancer. Ann Thorac Surg 1999;68:1154.

13. Webb WR, Gatsonis C, Zerhouni EA, et al. CT and MR imaging in staging non-small cell bronchogenic carcinoma: report of the Radiologic Diagnostic Oncology Group. Radiology 1991;178:705.

14. Freundlich IM, Chasen MH, Varma DG. Magnetic resonance imaging of pulmonary apical tumors. J Thorac Imaging 1996;11:210.

15. Bruzzi JF, Komaki R, Walsh GL, et al. Imaging of non-small cell lung cancer of the superior sulcus: part 2: initial staging and assessment of resectability and therapeutic response. Radiographics 2008;28:561.

16. Keogan MT, Tung KT, Kaplan DK, et al. The significance of pulmonary nodules detected on CT staging for lung cancer. Clin Radiol 1993;48:94.

17. Yuan Y, Matsumoto T, Hiyama A, et al. The probability of malignancy in small pulmonary nodules coexisting with potentially operable lung cancer detected by CT. Eur Radiol 2003;13:2447.

18. Myrdal G, Lambe M, Gustafsson G, et al. Survival in primary lung cancer potentially cured by operation: influence of tumor stage and clinical characteristics. Ann Thorac Surg 2003;75:356.

19. Rusch VW, Asamura H, Watanabe H, et al. The IASLC lung cancer staging project: a proposal for a new international lymph node map in the forthcoming seventh edition of the TNM classification for lung cancer. J Thorac Oncol 2009;4:568.

20. Guyatt GH, Lefcoe M, Walter S, et al. Interobserver variation in the computed tomographic evaluation of mediastinal lymph node size in patients with potentially resectable lung cancer. Canadian Lung Oncology Group. Chest 1995;107:116.

21. Toloza EM, Harpole L, McCrory DC. Noninvasive staging of non-small cell lung cancer: a review of the current evidence. Chest 2003;123:137S.

22. Daly BD Jr, Faling LJ, Bite G, et al. Mediastinal lymph node evaluation by computed tomography in lung cancer. An analysis of 345 patients grouped by TNM staging, tumor size, and tumor location. J Thorac Cardiovasc Surg 1987;94:664.

23. Kim HY, Yi CA, Lee KS, et al. Nodal metastasis in non-small cell lung cancer: accuracy of 3.0-T MR imaging. Radiology 2008;246:596.

24. Hasegawa I, Boiselle PM, Kuwabara K, et al. Mediastinal lymph nodes in patients with non-small cell lung cancer: preliminary experience with diffusion-weighted MR imaging. J Thorac Imaging 2008;23:157.

25. Gould MK, Kuschner WG, Rydzak CE, et al. Test performance of positron emission tomography and computed tomography for mediastinal staging in patients with non-small-cell lung cancer: a meta-analysis. Ann Intern Med 2003;139:879.

26. Shim SS, Lee KS, Kim BT, et al. Non-small cell lung cancer: prospective comparison of integrated FDG PET/CT and CT alone for preoperative staging. Radiology 2005;236:1011.

27. Tournoy KG, Maddens S, Gosselin R, et al. Integrated FDG-PET/CT does not make invasive staging of the intrathoracic lymph nodes in non-small cell

lung cancer redundant: a prospective study. Thorax 2007;62:696.

28. Karam M, Roberts-Klein S, Shet N, et al. Bilateral hilar foci on 18F-FDG PET scan in patients without lung cancer: variables associated with benign and malignant etiology. J Nucl Med 2008;49:1429.

29. Chowdhury FU, Sheerin F, Bradley KM, et al. Sarcoid-like reaction to malignancy on whole-body integrated (18)F-FDG PET/CT: prevalence and disease pattern. Clin Radiol 2009;64:675.

30. Kim YK, Lee KS, Kim BT, et al. Mediastinal nodal staging of nonsmall cell lung cancer using integrated 18F-FDG PET/CT in a tuberculosis-endemic country: diagnostic efficacy in 674 patients. Cancer 2007;109:1068.

31. Lee JW, Kim BS, Lee DS, et al. 18F-FDG PET/CT in mediastinal lymph node staging of non-small-cell lung cancer in a tuberculosis-endemic country: consideration of lymph node calcification and distribution pattern to improve specificity. Eur J Nucl Med Mol Imaging 2009;36:1794.

32. Kim BT, Lee KS, Shim SS, et al. Stage T1 non-small cell lung cancer: preoperative mediastinal nodal staging with integrated FDG PET/CT–a prospective study. Radiology 2006;241:501.

33. de Langen AJ, Raijmakers P, Riphagen I, et al. The size of mediastinal lymph nodes and its relation with metastatic involvement: a meta-analysis. Eur J Cardiothorac Surg 2006;29:26.

34. Choi YS, Shim YM, Kim J, et al. Mediastinoscopy in patients with clinical stage I non-small cell lung cancer. Ann Thorac Surg 2003;75:364.

35. Fritscher-Ravens A, Bohuslavizki KH, Brandt L, et al. Mediastinal lymph node involvement in potentially resectable lung cancer: comparison of CT, positron emission tomography, and endoscopic ultrasonography with and without fine-needle aspiration. Chest 2003;123:442.

36. Herth FJ, Krasnik M, Vilmann P. EBUS-TBNA for the diagnosis and staging of lung cancer. Endoscopy 2006;38(Suppl 1):S101.

37. Rintoul RC, Tournoy KG, El Daly H, et al. EBUS-TBNA for the clarification of PET positive intrathoracic lymph nodes-an international multi-centre experience. J Thorac Oncol 2009;4:44.

38. Hwangbo B, Kim SK, Lee HS, et al. Application of endobronchial ultrasound-guided transbronchial needle aspiration following integrated PET/CT in mediastinal staging of potentially operable non-small cell lung cancer. Chest 2009;135:1280.

39. De Leyn P, Lardinois D, Van Schil PE, et al. ESTS guidelines for preoperative lymph node staging for non-small cell lung cancer. Eur J Cardiothorac Surg 2007;32:1.

40. Decker DA, Dines DE, Payne WS, et al. The significance of a cytologically negative pleural effusion in bronchogenic carcinoma. Chest 1978;74:640.

41. Duysinx B, Corhay JL, Larock MP, et al. Prognostic value of metabolic imaging in non-small cell lung cancers with neoplasic pleural effusion. Nucl Med Commun 2008;29:982.

42. Arenas-Jimenez J, Alonso-Charterina S, Sanchez-Paya J, et al. Evaluation of CT findings for diagnosis of pleural effusions. Eur Radiol 2000;10:681.

43. Duysinx B, Nguyen D, Louis R, et al. Evaluation of pleural disease with 18-fluorodeoxyglucose positron emission tomography imaging. Chest 2004;125:489.

44. Gorg C, Restrepo I, Schwerk WB. Sonography of malignant pleural effusion. Eur Radiol 1997;7:1195.

45. Woodring JH, Stelling CB. Adenocarcinoma of the lung: a tumor with a changing pleomorphic character. AJR Am J Roentgenol 1983;140:657.

46. Oliver TW Jr, Bernardino ME, Miller JI, et al. Isolated adrenal masses in nonsmall-cell bronchogenic carcinoma. Radiology 1984;153:217.

47. Brady MJ, Thomas J, Wong TZ, et al. Adrenal nodules at FDG PET/CT in patients known to have or suspected of having lung cancer: a proposal for an efficient diagnostic algorithm. Radiology 2009;250:523.

48. Kim HK, Choi YS, Kim K, et al. Preoperative evaluation of adrenal lesions based on imaging studies and laparoscopic adrenalectomy in patients with otherwise operable lung cancer. Lung Cancer 2007;58:342.

49. Yokoi K, Kamiya N, Matsuguma H, et al. Detection of brain metastasis in potentially operable non-small cell lung cancer: a comparison of CT and MRI. Chest 1999;115:714.

50. Cheran SK, Herndon JE 2nd, Patz EF Jr. Comparison of whole-body FDG-PET to bone scan for detection of bone metastases in patients with a new diagnosis of lung cancer. Lung Cancer 2004;44:317.

51. van Tinteren H, Hoekstra OS, Smit EF, et al. Effectiveness of positron emission tomography in the preoperative assessment of patients with suspected non-small-cell lung cancer: the PLUS multicentre randomised trial. Lancet 2002;359:1388.

52. Maziak DE, Darling GE, Inculet RI, et al. Positron emission tomography in staging early lung cancer: a randomized trial. Ann Intern Med 2009;151:221.

53. Fischer B, Lassen U, Mortensen J, et al. Preoperative staging of lung cancer with combined PET-CT. N Engl J Med 2009;361:32.

54. Ohno Y, Koyama H, Onishi Y, et al. Non-small cell lung cancer: whole-body MR examination for M-stage assessment–utility for whole-body diffusion-weighted imaging compared with integrated FDG PET/CT. Radiology 2008;248:643.

55. Dietlein M, Weber K, Gandjour A, et al. Cost-effectiveness of FDG-PET for the management of solitary pulmonary nodules: a decision analysis based on cost reimbursement in Germany. Eur J Nucl Med 2000;27:1441.

56. Farjah F, Flum DR, Ramsey SD, et al. Multi-modality mediastinal staging for lung cancer among Medicare beneficiaries. J Thorac Oncol 2009;4:355.

57. Sogaard R, Fischer BM, Mortensen J, et al. Preoperative staging of lung cancer with PET/CT: cost-effectiveness evaluation alongside a randomized controlled trial. Eur J Nucl Med Mol Imaging 2011; 38(5):802.

58. Schreyogg J, Weller J, Stargardt T, et al. Cost-effectiveness of hybrid PET/CT for staging of non-small cell lung cancer. J Nucl Med 2010;51: 1668.

The Role of PET in the Evaluation, Treatment, and Ongoing Management of Lung Cancer

Kevin Stephans, MD[a,c],*, Anton Khouri, MD[b,c], Mitchell Machtay, MD[a,b]

KEYWORDS

- PET • Radiation • Lung cancer • Staging
- Response assessment

[18F]-fluorodeoxyglucose positron emission tomography (FDG-PET) has gained a major role in the evaluation and treatment of lung cancer over the past two decades. Over that time span PET and treatment techniques have both evolved substantially. While technical changes in PET and PET/computed tomography (CT) have improved accuracy and reliability, the evolution toward increasingly targeted and intensive treatment has increased the reliance upon imaging for radiation treatment. This article seeks to review the current role of PET in the evaluation and treatment of lung cancer with radiation.

DIAGNOSIS

The FDG PET imaging has attained a central role in both the evaluation of new pulmonary lesions and the staging of lung cancer. A meta-analysis of 40 prospective studies suggested a sensitivity of 96.8% and specificity of 77.8%[1] for FDG-PET in the evaluation of a new lung nodule. This finding makes PET an excellent frontline study, even prior to pathologic diagnosis of lung cancer. FDG-PET is extremely useful in guiding the need for biopsy, given that PET-negative lesions are rarely malignant and therefore can typically be followed clinically. Most PET false-negative lung cancers are bronchioloalveolar cell lung carcinomas. These lesions have unique CT characteristics and are typically low grade with a slow-growth pattern demonstrating progression over only long intervals, therefore the urgency of diagnosis may be less. As the specificity of FDG-PET is only 77.8%,[1] biopsy confirmation of malignancy remains vital. Biopsy offers confirmation of malignancy justifying treatment, as well as histology, which is critical. For example, small cell lung cancer (SCLC) and non–small cell lung cancer (NSCLC) may be treated very differently despite otherwise identical presentation.

Combining PET with CT allows the potential for integrated imaging, which should improve sensitivity by eliminating from consideration areas of increased standardized uptake value (SUV) with no associated CT changes. The specificity of PET/CT might be greater than the 77.8% reported for PET alone in the aforementioned meta-analysis,

This work was done independently of any grant or research funding.

[a] Department of Radiation Oncology, Cleveland Clinic, 9500 Euclid Avenue, T28, Cleveland, OH 44195, USA
[b] Department of Radiation Oncology, University Hospitals/Case Western Reserve University, 11100 Euclid Avenue, Cleveland, OH 44106, USA
[c] Case Comprehensive Cancer Center, Wearn 152, 11100 Euclid Avenue, Cleveland, OH, USA
* Corresponding author. Department of Radiation Oncology, Cleveland Clinic, 9500 Euclid Avenue, T28, Cleveland, OH 44195.
E-mail address: stephak@ccf.org

PET Clin 6 (2011) 265–274
doi:10.1016/j.cpet.2011.05.003
1556-8598/11/$ – see front matter © 2011 Elsevier Inc. All rights reserved.

pet.theclinics.com

though comparative data at this point are limited. Some investigators have even suggested that combining CT and PET features may even give some insight into tumor histology[2]; this may take on further interest with the future availability of additional PET radio tracers.

An important exception to the requirement for tissue diagnosis comes in medically inoperable patients with highly suspected NSCLC. Biopsy may be high risk in patients with extremely poor lung function or in those with history of contralateral pneumonectomy, and otherwise unreliable in patients with small but PET-positive lesions located in areas where access is technically challenging. Such patients are typically treated based on radiographic criteria, which may vary by institution. To consider empiric treatment, a lesion is required to be both increasing in size on serial CT over a 6-week to 3-month interval, and positive on FDG-PET with an SUV of greater than 3.0. The numbers of patients treated in this manner are small and the population is heterogeneous, making reliable analysis of these criteria difficult. However, the fact that the rate of future distant metastasis is comparable in a series of stage I patients treated with histologic versus radiographic characteristics suggests these criteria are reasonable.[3]

STAGING

Once a biopsy diagnosis is reached, FDG-PET/CT is the gold standard for noninvasive staging. PET offers substantial improvements in both mediastinal and distant staging over CT criteria alone, and is the standard of care for all patients with newly diagnosed NSCLC.

Mediastinal Staging

According to a recent meta-analysis the addition of PET to standard CT increases the sensitivity for the detection of mediastinal nodal involvement from 61% to 85%, while specificity is improved from 79% to 90%.[4] Of interest, when CT demonstrated enlarged mediastinal lymph nodes PET was more sensitive (100%), but less specific than at baseline (78%). Conversely, when CT showed no nodal enlargement, sensitivity was near baseline at 82% and specificity 93%. This finding has important treatment planning implications: enlarged but PET-negative nodes therefore are unlikely to contain disease (as PET was 100% sensitive in this series), whereas small but PET-positive nodes are very likely to be malignant. Given the association of target size and PET SUV measurement, both of these conclusions are logical, and have important implications for both staging and treatment planning.

Even after PET, patients who are surgical candidates frequently proceed to additional staging by mediastinoscopy prior to the final selection of treatment modality. The ACOSOG Z0050 trial[5] investigated the correlation of CT, PET, and mediastinoscopy in 303 potentially resectable patients with NSCLC. PET detected microscopic N2 nodal disease in 58% of patients. However, as sensitivity was only 61% and negative predictive value 87%, the ability of PET to detect microscopic N2 disease appears to be modest. In addition, a Cleveland Clinic review[6] of 87 patients with pathologic stage IIIA NSCLC by mediastinoscopy reported that 38% of pN2+ patients had no previous abnormal PET findings in the mediastinum. Other reports suggest higher accuracy of PET, including a recent Korean report[7] of 750 NSCLC patients who were mediastinal node negative by CT and PET criteria and who underwent mediastinoscopy. Only 6.8% of these patients were found to have N2 disease on mediastinoscopy, though an additional 8.5% were later found to have N2 disease on final surgical dissection after completion of neoadjuvant therapy. A similar Japanese study[8] suggested an 11% (24 out of 224) incidence of mediastinoscopy-detected microscopic N2 disease present in NSCLC patients who were node negative by PET. Of note, most metastases were small, with two-thirds being less than 4 mm. Multivariate analysis identified adenocarcinoma, tumors located in upper or middle lobe, tumor size larger than 3 cm, and maximum SUV of primary tumor greater than 4.0 g/mL as significant risk factors for microscopic nodal metastasis. An Irish review by Al-Sarraf and colleagues[9] demonstrated a 16% incidence of microscopic N2 disease in PET-negative patients, and identified central tumors, right upper lobe tumors, and PET-positive uptake in hilar (N1) nodes as significant risk factors for undetected microscopic N2 disease. Based on the aforementioned studies the incidence of PET false-negative mediastinal nodes ranges substantially, from 10% to as much as 40%. For this reason mediastinoscopy remains clinically indicated for most patients undergoing surgical resection. Conversely, for patients with locally advanced NSCLC undergoing chemoradiation (as well as medically inoperable stage I NSCLC) mediastinoscopy, an invasive procedure that would delay the start of radiotherapy is not typically performed. The standard staging system for these patients is based on PET. Additional mediastinal staging tools such as endobronchial ultrasound sampling, magnetic resonance (MR) imaging, or MR spectroscopy are currently under investigation as a supplement to PET in these patients. Despite the high sensitivity and specificity of PET, findings which do not fit clinical context or expectations should be investigated further (**Fig. 1**).

Despite some limitations in the detection of microscopic disease, PET remains an important supplement to mediastinoscopy. Limitations to mediastinoscopy include variation in the number of nodes sampled by individual surgeons as well as access only to a limited number of mediastinal nodal stations. This is illustrated in a Danish randomized trial[10] of 189 patients to mediastinoscopy with or without preceding PET/CT. The accuracy of nodal staging was improved from 85% to 95% with the addition of PET/CT.

For locally advanced NSCLC patients treated with chemoradiation, as well as stage I medically inoperable NSCLC, mediastinoscopy has not been part of the standard staging with target volumes primarily based on CT, PET, and clinical judgment. The accuracy of staging in this population has been less well studied, with no large cooperative group trials, and is inherently more challenging because of the absence of pathologic confirmation accompanying resection in surgical series. Data assessing the accuracy of staging for nonsurgical patients is therefore based primarily on outcomes, that is, patterns of failure.

The overall limited prognosis of many of these patients, due to comorbidities in the medically inoperable stage I population, and progressive disease in the locally advanced chemoradiation population, makes accurate assessment of staging difficult in these settings. Preradiation PET staging alone appears to be justified in stage I NSCLC because isolated nodal failure is less than 5% despite treatment to the primary site alone.[3,11,12] In the locally advanced population, precise staging of the mediastinum has been historically less important because of the widespread use of comprehensive elective nodal radiation. However, mediastinal staging is becoming a topic of greater interest, with modernly tailored fields and selective dose escalation. This trend is discussed in greater detail in the section on treatment planning. The difference between PET and mediastinoscopy staging is important to consider when comparing outcomes of surgical and nonoperative series.

Distant Staging

In addition to improvements in mediastinal nodal staging, PET has substantial impact on treatment choices by improving systemic staging. In the ACOSOG Z0050 trial,[5] 6.3% of patients were

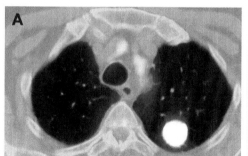
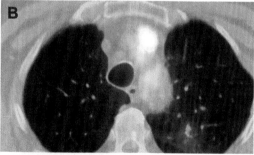
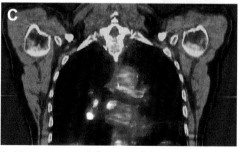

Fig. 1. A 84 year old male with biopsy proven left upper lobe adenocarcinoma with SUV 9.1 (*A*). PET shows increased uptake throughout mediastinum (*B, C*), and bilateral hilum (*C*) with SUV at all stations between 4.5 and 6.1, highest uptake in R10. Because of clinically unusual picture of small primary with diffuse mediastinal and even contralateral hilar uptake pathological verification was sought by endobronchial ultrasound guided sampling revealing benign lymphatic tissue and calcified granulomas at all stations. Patient was treated with stereotactic radiation to left upper lobe primary for presumed stage IB NSCLC (48 Gy in 4 fractions) and is disease free at 18 months. While PET SUV >5 is highly specific clinically atypical results should be verified pathologically.

found to have extracranial distant metastasis not seen on previous CT staging at the time of PET scan. A meta-analysis of more than 1000 patients[13] suggested a sensitivity of 94% and specificity of 97% in the detection of distant metastasis. Overall there was a 12% rate of detection of distant metastasis, and a change in the therapeutic plan for 18% of patients (in some cases CT-diagnosed metastasis were excluded) through the use of PET rather than conventional imaging. PET is excellent at detecting metastasis in otherwise normal-appearing soft tissue (liver, adrenals, omentum, and upper abdominal nodes) as well as in the evaluation of otherwise benign enlargements such as adrenal adenomas and bone islands (Fig. 2). The detection of metastasis also increases with increasing stage. MacManus and colleagues[14] found a 7.5% incidence of metastasis in stage I NSCLC, increasing to 18% in stage II and 24% in stage III. As PET is poor at

detecting brain metastasis because of high background metabolism in the gray matter, dedicated brain imaging (contrast-enhanced CT or magnetic resonance imaging (MRI)) is recommended as a supplement to PET by National Comprehensive Cancer Center guidelines for asymptomatic stage II and higher NSCLC, and is optional for patients with asymptomatic stage I disease (recommended for all patients with central nervous system symptoms). PET is also more accurate than bone scintigraphy in evaluation for bone marrow metastasis.[15,16] The only setting where bone scintigraphy may be preferred (in combination with serum alkaline phosphatase) is in previously established stage IV disease where PET is not otherwise needed and bone scintigraphy may be more cost effective. The same seems to be true for SCLC, where PET appears to be equally accurate as CT plus bone scintigraphy and bone marrow analysis, though with more limited data.[17,18]

In summary, FDG-PET is recommended for the staging of all patients with a new diagnosis of lung cancer, and has been shown to be cost effective because of its ability to more appropriately select therapeutic choices,[19] which is particularly true in the age of dose-escalated radiotherapy with elimination of elective nodal radiation. This aspect will increase the importance of the staging PET scan, discussed in greater detail below. For patients under evaluation for surgical therapy, mediastinoscopy should supplement PET findings prior to thoracotomy, as microscopic nodal metastasis may be missed by PET in 10% to 40% of cases.

PROGNOSIS

In a systematic review[20] of 13 studies comprising 1474 patients with NSCLC, increasing maximum SUV on FDG-PET was found to be prognostic as a continuous variable for lower overall survival, though no clear cutoff was identified. This result has been confirmed individually in patients undergoing surgical resection for a range of NSCLCs,[21,22] stage I NSCLC,[23] and chemoradiation for locally advanced NSCLC.[24,25] Of note, the only two studies looking at stereotactic radiation for stage I NSCLC did not find a correlation between maximum pretreatment SUV and local control, distant failure, or overall survival.[26,27] A third study including a large number of stage I NSCLC patients was also inconclusive.[28] The critical unanswered question is whether the mechanism for the relationship of maximal pretreatment SUV to affect overall survival is through the inability to control local disease, or rather a higher potential for distant metastasis (or perhaps both). Insight into this would

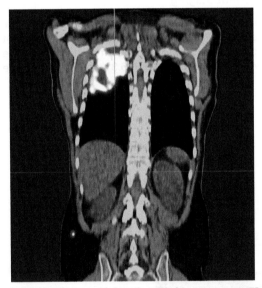

Fig. 2. A 46 year old female with biopsy proven T3 right upper lobe adenocarcinoma with chest wall invasion. PET demonstrated no hilar or mediastinal uptake but did show right flank 1.1 cm PET avid soft tissue nodule not seen on previous CT but on ultrasound guided biopsy demonstrated to be metastatic adenocarcinoma. Given excellent performance and limited metastasis was treated with induction chemoradiation (45 Gy with concurrent cisplatin and etoposide) and right upper lobectomy/limited chest wall resection + needle localization abdominal wall excision. Final pathology demonstrated complete response to neoadjuvant treatment. She was treated with consolidation carboplatin and alimta and remains disease free at 15 months. Unusual plan of care, however PET allowed for management of very early oligometastatic disease.

allow for appropriate escalation of therapy, with either additional local therapy or the addition of systemic therapies in appropriately selected patients.

One major limiting confounding factor in answering this question is that because of respiratory motion and other measurement factors, larger tumors will have higher maximum SUV values than similarly active smaller tumors. Tumor size is a known risk factor for both nodal and distant metastasis, and this association between size and SUV may not always be controlled for adequately. For example, in the analysis by Ikushima and colleagues[24] from M.D. Anderson, tumor SUV strongly predicted for local control, distant metastasis, and overall survival in a series of 149 patients with locally advanced NSCLC treated with chemoradiation. When tumor size alone was corrected, this association weakened substantially. On multivariate analysis of patients receiving integrated PET/CT, SUV was not significant for any outcome measure.

The lack of correlation of pretreatment tumor SUV to outcomes after stereotactic radiation[26–28] is also of interest given its frequent correlation for other treatment modalities; this may simply be due to limited numbers of patients and follow-up in this series. Other potential explanations include the possibility that the extremely dose-escalated treatment overcomes radioresistance. In addition, perhaps the inclusion of low-grade, poorly margined tumors (which may be more challenging to target), particularly in series including patients without biopsy confirmation, introduces the possibility of bimodal distribution of SUV-related outcomes.

Overall it is well established that, in general, tumors with high pretreatment maximum SUV on FDG-PET have inferior prognosis; however, the mechanisms for this are not well established, and there may be differences among disease stages and treatment modalities.

TREATMENT PLANNING

FDG-PET imaging has significant implications for treatment volumes, particularly in the setting of locally advanced NSCLC. The impact of improved disease targeting should continue to increase in the newer era of dose-escalated, image-guided radiation to smaller, more precise treatment fields, as this will emphasize the importance of accuracy in field design.

For medically inoperable stage I NSCLC, PET will rarely change treatment fields, outside of the impact on initial staging, as most lesions are well defined given the clear boundary between an isolated pulmonary nodule and surrounding air. Aside

from occasional demonstration of clear invasion into the mediastinum, the boundary between tumor and either mediastinum or chest wall is typically more clearly seen on CT or MR imaging. The primary role of PET in delineation of target volumes for stage I NSCLC is in the differentiation of tumor from occasional downstream atelectasis, particularly with larger lesions.

Medically inoperable stage II NSCLC is a relatively uncommon and poorly defined entity. As such, a standard of care does not truly exist and the concept of elective nodal radiation is poorly defined in this context. The primary lesion and ipsilateral hilar nodal regions clearly will be targeted. The use of at least some elective mediastinal nodal radiation is relatively common, given the association of PET-positive hilar nodes to mediastinal micrometastasis. Other previously identified risk factors are tumor size larger than 3 cm, upper or middle lobe tumors, central tumors, primary tumor SUV greater than 4, and adenocarcinoma histology.[8,9] The final decision on field size and mediastinal radiation in these patients is frequently a compromise, weighing the risk factors for mediastinal disease against the patient's overall performance as well as medical comorbidities that prohibited surgery in the first place. Consideration should be given to mediastinoscopy or endobronchial ultrasound sampling in appropriate patients.

In stage III NSCLC, evidence for improved overall survival with dose escalation is mounting. An analysis of data from 7 randomized Radiation Therapy Oncology Group (RTOG) trials demonstrated total radiation dose to be strongly correlated with both local control and overall survival.[29] Each 1-Gy increase in biological equivalent dose was associated with a 4% relative improvement in survival and 3% improvement in local control. Furthermore, a randomized Chinese trial of standard dose radiation with elective nodal coverage versus escalated radiation dose to involved disease alone demonstrated an improvement in 2-year overall survival from 26% to 39% in favor of escalated dose to the involved target volume only.[30] At the same time, toxicity-related breaks in treatment have been shown to have a deleterious effect on survival.[31] As clinical recurrence in areas of omitted elective nodal radiation has been documented to be rare,[30,32–34] there is a strong movement to dose-escalated radiation to involved nodes only, with consideration of elective coverage only to the highest risk mediastinal nodes, to maximize dose while minimizing toxicity. PET is thus a critical tool in identification of the true involved target volume, and has been demonstrated to affect treatment volumes in many stage III patients, changing the electively targeted volume from CT alone along with the corresponding volume of normal lung and esophagus irradiated in the majority of patients (**Fig. 3**).[32–35] RTOG 0515,[32] a recent prospective multicenter cooperative group phase 2 trial, demonstrated a 10% reduction in treatment volumes when adding PET information to CT contours with a corresponding trend to decrease in median lung dose, without significant change in the number of involved nodes or median esophageal dose. Only one patient (2%) had developed an out-of-field elective nodal failure with 12.9-month median follow-up.

PET-guided selective nodal radiation with consideration of escalation of radiation dose is the current standard of care for locally advanced NSCLC based on the aforementioned results.

ADAPTIVE TREATMENT

The concept of adaptive replanning during treatment to adjust for changes in tumor size is most common in head and neck cancer. This concept has gained popularity for this site for two reasons: the observed rapid treatment response of some large neck lymph nodes involved with squamous cell carcinoma; and the resultant change in dosimetry to both normal structures and tumor, due to treatment to a small area of the body with changing surface dimensions and close association of critical tissue. The importance of this concept may be slightly less in lung cancer because of the far lesser extent of changes in

surface anatomy during therapy. Nevertheless, with local control rates not much more than 50% even with dose-escalated therapy, there may be room for further escalation and volume reduction. Two studies[36,37] of volume changes with mid-treatment PET scan after 5 to 6 weeks of radiation, with the goal of reduced volume high-dose boost, have demonstrated modest reductions in full-dose radiation target volume by 20% to 44%, though the expected benefit in normal tissue complications averaged only 2%. This is a novel and interesting concept, which at this point remains experimental and requires further study.

RESPONSE ASSESSMENT

The significance of posttreatment imaging changes in NSCLC can be extremely complicated because of the common presence of postradiation fibrosis, atelectasis, and inflammatory changes during the standard follow-up interval. Furthermore, the modest rate of local control, even with modern dose-escalated radiation, provides rationale for consideration of further intensification of therapy if local failure, or at least poor response, can be identified early (**Fig. 4**). This concept has led to interest in the role of PET in response assessment. A prospective Australian study by MacManus and colleagues[38] suggested a much more powerful correlation of outcome to PET metabolic response versus CT response. At a median of 70 days post treatment 2-year overall survivals of 61%, 34%,

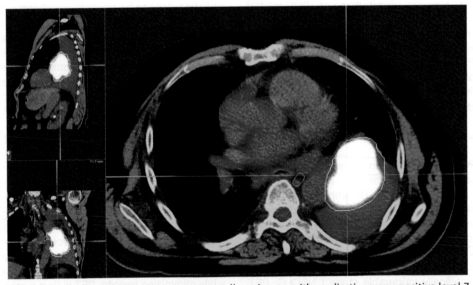

Fig. 3. A 58 year old male with stage IIIa squamous cell carcinoma with mediastinoscopy positive level 7 and 4L nodes. Treated with definitive chemotherapy and radiation to 70 Gy with weekly carboplatinum and paclitaxel followed by consolidation chemotherapy. PET scan was critical in defining target volume for high-dose radiation given surrounding lung collapse. Internal target volume in yellow created from PET + 4D CT scan then expanded to planning target volume (not shown).

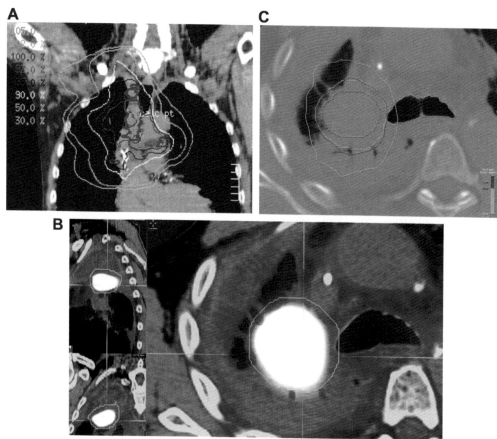

Fig. 4. A 78 year old male with stage IIIB NSCLC of the right upper lobe s/p combined chemoRT (*A*). 20 months post treatment possible enlargement in post-treatment effect on CT noted, PET verified increased metabolic activity and biopsy demonstrated recurrent NSCLC without evidence of distant metastasis. Treated with salvage sterotactic radiation to 50 Gy in 5 fractions after creating ITV from PET and 4DCT which was expanded by 5 mm to create PTV in blue (*B*). Stereotactic treatment plan, ITV in purple, PTV in blue, dose as per table (*C*).

20%, and 18% were noted respectively for patients with a metabolic complete response, versus partial response, stable disease, or progressive disease. Furthermore, metabolic complete response was much more common than CT complete response (47% vs 14%), with poor concordance between PET and CT responses. Inflammatory changes were also noted in normal tissue, and appeared to correlate positively with the degree of metabolic tumor response, suggesting linkage between normal tissue radiosensitivity and tumor response.[39] Rosenzweig and colleagues[40] likewise demonstrated improvement in local control of 83% compared with 23% for patients with 4-month postradiation tumor SUV of less than 3.5 versus SUV greater than 3.5. Decreases in maximum SUV during and just after treatment have also been shown to correlate with improved survival for both induction chemotherapy[41] and chemoradiation.[25] A large prospective multi-institutional trial of PET response to chemoradiation

(ACRIN 6668/RTOG 0235) has recently been completed, with results pending.[42] These data will help further establish the role of PET in the early posttreatment response assessment, and likely will serve as a springboard for further attempts to improve outcome.

Although the field of stereotactic radiation (SBRT) for NSCLC is relatively new, early data are available regarding PET response to treatment. These data are of increased interest to SBRT given the high incidence of posttreatment inflammatory changes, which can be very intense, prolonged, and easily mistaken for tumor progression. As part of a prospective pilot study,[43] 14 patients treated to 60 Gy in 3 fractions underwent repeat PET at 2, 26, and 52 weeks after SBRT. While maximum SUVs generally decreased over time, the median was higher at 52 weeks than at 26 weeks. Six patients with maximum SUV remaining above 3.5 had no evidence of local progression with further follow-up (the only patient with a persistently rising SUV had repeat biopsy negative for disease, but died shortly thereafter of infection, limiting further follow-up data). A similar study from Georgetown[44] evaluating 20 patients demonstrated some mild individual elevations in maximum SUV, though the average decreased from 6.2 to 2.3. At 18 to 24 months, however, controlled tumors showed a narrow range of SUVs (1.5 to 2.8), whereas a single confirmed local failure exhibited an SUV of 8.4. Additional data will be derived from RTOG 0618, which is a prospective multi-institutional trial of stereotactic body radiation therapy (SBRT) in medically operable patients and includes post-treatment PET evaluation for identification of patients for surgical salvage.[45] Further investigation is needed, although early results suggest occasional early reactive increase in SUV but long-term declines in controlled patients. Thus any patient with a persistently elevated or increasing SUV should be evaluated and given the potential for salvage therapy. Elevated SUV alone, however, should not be automatically assumed to represent recurrence/progression, and repeat biopsy is strongly recommended. Assessment of post-SBRT PET response will gain increasing importance as a trigger for biopsy and/or surgical salvage with increasing use of SBRT in medically operable early-stage NSCLC.

NOVEL DIRECTIONS

FDG-PET is well established. However, a host of other PET radiotracers that are analogues to thymidine, methionine, choline, annexin V, as well as proliferative and hypoxic markers, plus a variety of other cellular activity markers are under further investigation. These agents may help clarify the biological blueprint of tumors to identify prognosis, give insight into tumor histology, predict toxicity and, more significantly, lead to novel methods of treatment selection and targeted therapies. Along with mapping of tumor DNA and protein, as well as MR spectroscopy, novel PET analogues represent the horizon of individualized tumor therapy, though substantial prospective assessment is required before the clinical impact can be confirmed and realized.

SUMMARY

PET is central to the diagnosis and staging of lung cancer. The transition to dose-escalate radiation with increasingly selective nodal radiation has made the accurate characterization of nodal status critical to successful treatment. Although mediastinoscopy increases the detection of microscopic

nodal metastasis to a greater extent than PET alone, treatment failure in omitted elective nodal areas is rare with PET-guided modern chemoradiation. New horizons for PET scanning include the ability to potentially allow for early detection of salvageable poor treatment responses or local recurrence, as well as to improve the molecular blueprint of tumors with novel tracers to assist with treatment selection and delivery of targeted therapy. The role of PET imaging in the management of lung cancer is likely to continue to increase in the future.

REFERENCES

1. Gould MK, Maclean CC, Kuschner WG, et al. Accuracy of positron emission tomography for diagnosis of pulmonary nodules and mass lesions: a meta-analysis. JAMA 2001;285(7):914–24.
2. Sun JS, Park KJ, Sheen SS, et al. Clinical usefulness of the fluorodeoxyglucose (FDG)-PET maximal standardized uptake value (SUV) in combination with CT features for the differentiation of adenocarcinoma with a bronchioloalveolar carcinoma from other subtypes of non-small cell lung cancers. Lung Cancer 2009;66(2):205–10.
3. Stephans KL, Djemil T, Reddy CA, et al. A comparison of two stereotactic body radiation fractionation schedules for medically inoperable stage I non-small cell lung cancer: the Cleveland Clinic experience. J Thorac Oncol 2009;4(8): 976–82.
4. Gould MK, Kuschner WG, Rydzak CE, et al. Test performance of positron emission tomography and computed tomography for mediastinal staging in patients with non-small-cell lung cancer: a meta-analysis. Ann Intern Med 2003;139(11):879–92.
5. Reed CE, Harpole DH, Posther KE, et al. Results of the American College of Surgeons Oncology Group Z0050 trial: the utility of positron emission tomography in staging potentially operable non-small cell lung cancer. J Thorac Cardiovasc Surg 2003; 126(6):1943–51.
6. Videtic GM, Rice TW, Murthy S, et al. Utility of positron emission tomography compared with mediastinoscopy for delineating involved lymph nodes in stage III lung cancer: insights for radiotherapy planning from a surgical cohort. Int J Radiat Oncol Biol Phys 2008;72(3):702–6.
7. Kim HK, Choi YS, Kim K, et al. Outcomes of mediastinoscopy and surgery with or without neoadjuvant therapy in patients with non-small cell lung cancer who are N2 negative on positron emission tomography and computed tomography. J Thorac Oncol 2011;6(2):336–42.
8. Kanzaki R, Higashiyama M, Fujiwara A, et al. Occult mediastinal lymph node metastasis in NSCLC

patients diagnosed as clinical N0-1 by preoperative integrated FDG-PET/CT and CT: risk factors, pattern, and histopathological study. Lung Cancer 2011; 71(3):333–7.

9. Al-Sarraf N, Aziz R, Gately K, et al. Pattern and predictors of occult mediastinal lymph node involvement in non-small cell lung cancer patients with negative mediastinal uptake on positron emission tomography. Eur J Cardiothorac Surg 2008;33(1): 104–9.

10. Fischer BM, Mortensen J, Hansen H, et al. Multimodality approach to mediastinal staging in non-small cell lung cancer. Faults and benefits of PET-CT: a randomised trial. Thorax 2010. [Epub ahead of print].

11. Bradley JD, El Naqa I, Drzymala RE, et al. Stereotactic body radiation therapy for early-stage non-small-cell lung cancer: the pattern of failure is distant. Int J Radiat Oncol Biol Phys 2010;77(4): 1146–50.

12. Timmerman R, Paulus R, Galvin J, et al. Stereotactic body radiation therapy for inoperable early stage lung cancer. JAMA 2010;303(11):1070–6.

13. Hellwig D, Ukena D, Paulsen F, et al. Meta-analysis of the efficacy of positron emission tomography with F-18-fluorodeoxyglucose in lung tumors. Basis for discussion of the German Consensus Conference on PET in Oncology 2000. Pneumologie 2001;55(8):367–77.

14. MacManus MP, Hicks RJ, Matthews JP, et al. High rate of detection of unsuspected distant metastases by PET in apparent stage III non-small-cell lung cancer: implications for radical radiation therapy. Int J Radiat Oncol Biol Phys 2001;50(2): 287–93.

15. Ak I, Sivrikoz MC, Entok E, et al. Discordant findings in patients with non-small-cell lung cancer: absolutely normal bone scans versus disseminated bone metastases on positron-emission tomography/computed tomography. Eur J Cardiothorac Surg 2010;37(4): 792–6.

16. Song JW, Oh YM, Shim TS, et al. Efficacy comparison between (18)F-FDG PET/CT and bone scintigraphy in detecting bony metastases of non-small-cell lung cancer. Lung Cancer 2009;65(3):333–8.

17. Bradley JD, Dehdashti F, Mintun MA, et al. Positron emission tomography in limited-stage small-cell lung cancer: a prospective study. J Clin Oncol 2004;22(16):3248–54.

18. Fischer BM, Mortensen J, Langer SW, et al. A prospective study of PET/CT in initial staging of small-cell lung cancer: comparison with CT, bone scintigraphy and bone marrow analysis. Ann Oncol 2007;18(2):338–45.

19. Schreyogg J, Weller J, Stargardt T, et al. Cost-effectiveness of hybrid PET/CT for staging of non-small cell lung cancer. J Nucl Med 2010; 51(11):1668–75.

20. Paesmans M, Berghmans T, Dusart M, et al. Primary tumor standardized uptake value measured on fluorodeoxyglucose positron emission tomography is of prognostic value for survival in non-small cell lung cancer: update of a systematic review and meta-analysis by the European Lung Cancer Working Party for the International Association for the Study of Lung Cancer Staging Project. J Thorac Oncol 2010;5(5):612–9.

21. Downey RJ, Akhurst T, Gonen M, et al. Preoperative F-18 fluorodeoxyglucose-positron emission tomography maximal standardized uptake value predicts survival after lung cancer resection. J Clin Oncol 2004;22(16):3255–60.

22. Okereke IC, Gangadharan SP, Kent MS, et al. Standard uptake value predicts survival in non-small cell lung cancer. Ann Thorac Surg 2009;88(3):911–5 [discussion: 915–6].

23. Nair VS, Barnett PG, Ananth L, et al. PET scan ^{18}F-fluorodeoxyglucose uptake and prognosis in patients with resected clinical stage IA non-small cell lung cancer. Chest 2010;137(5):1150–6.

24. Ikushima H, Dong L, Erasmus J, et al. Predictive value of ^{18}F-fluorodeoxyglucose uptake by positron emission tomography for non-small cell lung cancer patients treated with radical radiotherapy. J Radiat Res (Tokyo) 2010;51(4):465–71.

25. Zhang HQ, Yu JM, Meng X, et al. Prognostic value of serial [(18)F]fluorodeoxyglucose PET-CT uptake in stage III patients with non-small cell lung cancer treated by concurrent chemoradiotherapy. Eur J Radiol 2011;77(1):92–6.

26. Burdick MJ, Stephans KL, Reddy CA, et al. Maximum standardized uptake value from staging FDG-PET/CT does not predict treatment outcome for early-stage non-small-cell lung cancer treated with stereotactic body radiotherapy. Int J Radiat Oncol Biol Phys 2010;78(4):1033–9.

27. Hoopes DJ, Tann M, Fletcher JW, et al. FDG-PET and stereotactic body radiotherapy (SBRT) for stage I non-small-cell lung cancer. Lung Cancer 2007; 56(2):229–34.

28. Coon D, Gokhale AS, Burton SA, et al. Fractionated stereotactic body radiation therapy in the treatment of primary, recurrent, and metastatic lung tumors: the role of positron emission tomography/computed tomography-based treatment planning. Clin Lung Cancer 2008;9(4):217–21.

29. Machtay M, Bae K, Movsas B, et al. Higher biologically effective dose of radiotherapy is associated with improved outcomes for locally advanced non-small cell lung carcinoma treated with chemoradiation: an analysis of the Radiation Therapy Oncology Group. Int J Radiat Oncol Biol Phys 2010. [Epub ahead of print].

30. Yuan S, Sun X, Li M, et al. A randomized study of involved-field irradiation versus elective nodal

irradiation in combination with concurrent chemotherapy for inoperable stage III nonsmall cell lung cancer. Am J Clin Oncol 2007;30(3):239–44.

31. Machtay M, Hsu C, Komaki R, et al. Effect of overall treatment time on outcomes after concurrent chemoradiation for locally advanced non-small-cell lung carcinoma: analysis of the Radiation Therapy Oncology Group (RTOG) experience. Int J Radiat Oncol Biol Phys 2005;63(3):667–71.

32. Bradley J, Bae K, Choi N, et al. A phase II comparative study of gross tumor volume definition with or without PET/CT fusion in dosimetric planning for non-small-cell lung cancer (NSCLC): primary analysis of Radiation Therapy Oncology Group (RTOG) 0515. Int J Radiat Oncol Biol Phys 2010. [Epub ahead of print].

33. Fernandes AT, Shen J, Finlay J, et al. Elective nodal irradiation (ENI) vs. involved field radiotherapy (IFRT) for locally advanced non-small cell lung cancer (NSCLC): a comparative analysis of toxicities and clinical outcomes. Radiother Oncol 2010;95(2): 178–84.

34. Sulman EP, Komaki R, Klopp AH, et al. Exclusion of elective nodal irradiation is associated with minimal elective nodal failure in non-small cell lung cancer. Radiat Oncol 2009;4:5.

35. Bradley J, Thorstad WL, Mutic S, et al. Impact of FDG-PET on radiation therapy volume delineation in non-small-cell lung cancer. Int J Radiat Oncol Biol Phys 2004;59(1):78–86.

36. Feng M, Kong FM, Gross M, et al. Using fluorodeoxyglucose positron emission tomography to assess tumor volume during radiotherapy for non-small-cell lung cancer and its potential impact on adaptive dose escalation and normal tissue sparing. Int J Radiat Oncol Biol Phys 2009;73(4): 1228–34.

37. Gillham C, Zips D, Ponisch F, et al. Additional PET/CT in week 5-6 of radiotherapy for patients with stage III non-small cell lung cancer as a means of dose escalation planning? Radiother Oncol 2008; 88(3):335–41.

38. MacManus MP, Hicks RJ, Matthews JP, et al. Positron emission tomography is superior to computed tomography scanning for response-assessment after radical radiotherapy or chemoradiotherapy in patients with non-small-cell lung cancer. J Clin Oncol 2003;21(7):1285–92.

39. Hicks RJ, MacManus MP, Matthews JP, et al. Early FDG-PET imaging after radical radiotherapy for non-small-cell lung cancer: inflammatory changes in normal tissues correlate with tumor response and do not confound therapeutic response evaluation. Int J Radiat Oncol Biol Phys 2004;60(2): 412–8.

40. Rosenzweig KE, Fox JL, Giraud P. Response to radiation. Semin Radiat Oncol 2004;14(4):322–5.

41. Eschmann SM, Friedel G, Paulsen F, et al. Repeat ^{18}F-FDG PET for monitoring neoadjuvant chemotherapy in patients with stage III non-small cell lung cancer. Lung Cancer 2007;55(2):165–71.

42. ACRIN 6668/RTOG 0235. Available at: http://www.acrin.org/TabID/155/Default.aspx. Accessed January 31, 2011.

43. Henderson MA, Hoopes DJ, Fletcher JW, et al. A pilot trial of serial ^{18}F-fluorodeoxyglucose positron emission tomography in patients with medically inoperable stage I non-small-cell lung cancer treated with hypofractionated stereotactic body radiotherapy. Int J Radiat Oncol Biol Phys 2010;76(3):789–95.

44. Vahdat S, Oermann EK, Collins SP, et al. CyberKnife radiosurgery for inoperable stage IA non-small cell lung cancer: ^{18}F-fluorodeoxyglucose positron emission tomography/computed tomography serial tumor response assessment. J Hematol Oncol 2010;3:6.

45. RTOG 0618. Available at: http://www.rtog.org/members/protocols/0618/0618.pdf. Accessed January 31, 2011.

Multimodality Imaging Review of Malignant Pleural Mesothelioma Diagnosis and Staging

Victor H. Gerbaudo, PhD[a],*, Sharyn I. Katz, MD[b],
Anna K. Nowak, MBBS, FRACP, PhD[c],
Roslyn J. Francis, MBBS, FRACP, PhD[c,d]

KEYWORDS

- Mesothelioma • Fluorodeoxyglucose • PET/CT
- Computed tomography • Magnetic resonance imaging
- Fluorothymidine • Fluoromisonidazole

Malignant pleural mesothelioma (MPM) is a highly aggressive tumor of mesothelial cells with an annual incidence of approximately 15 patients per million, a male to female ratio of approximately 4:1, and a projected number of 68,000 deaths between 2008 and 2042 in the United States.[1,2] Its worldwide incidence is expected to increase in the next 20 years. The disease manifests clinically 30 to 40 years (range 15–60 years) after exposure to asbestos fibers, with approximately 65% of the patients developing the disease at an average age of 60 years.[3–5] Other causes and/or cofactors for MPM include exposure to nonasbestos mineral fibers such as erionite and tremolite, therapeutic radiation, and diethylstilbestrol. Exposure to the Simian Virus 40 (SV40) in contaminated polio vaccines as an additional etiologic factor for MPM has been contested by recent reports.[6,7]

According to the 2004 World Health Organization (WHO) histologic classification of MPM, there are 3 main histologic subtypes: epithelioid (50%– 60%), sarcomatoid (10%), and a combination of both consisting of at least 10% of each, called biphasic or mixed subtype (30%–40%). Some sarcomatoid tumors may contain a significant desmoplastic component that, when found in more than 50% of the tumor, is categorized as desmoplastic MPM.[8]

Differentiating MPM from other malignancies or benign pleural processes is a significant diagnostic challenge.[9] It is important to be able to differentiate among mesothelioma subtypes (epithelioid, sarcomatoid, and mixed), because they have different biological behaviors. Better survival rates have been reported for patients with the epithelial subtype than for those with sarcomatoid and mixed histologies. In a good number of cases, epithelioid MPM may resemble a metastatic lesion to the pleura such as from lung, breast, or ovarian carcinomas. Moreover, a benign inflammatory or reactive pleural lesion consisting of atypical mesothelial hyperplasia may resemble early-stage

[a] Division of Nuclear Medicine and Molecular Imaging, Department of Radiology, Harvard Medical School, Brigham & Women's Hospital, 75 Francis Street, Boston, MA 02115, USA
[b] Department of Radiology, Hospital of the University of Pennsylvania, University of Pennsylvania School of Medicine, 1 Silverstein Building, 3400 Spruce Street, Philadelphia, PA 19104, USA
[c] Department of Medical Oncology, School of Medicine and Pharmacology, University of Western Australia, Sir Charles Gairdner Hospital, Hospital Avenue, Nedlands 6009, Western Australia, Australia
[d] Department of Molecular Imaging, School of Medicine and Pharmacology, University of Western Australia, Sir Charles Gairdner Hospital, Hospital Avenue, Nedlands 6009, Western Australia, Australia
* Corresponding author.
E-mail address: vgerbaudo@partners.org

PET Clin 6 (2011) 275–297
doi:10.1016/j.cpet.2011.04.001

epithelioid MPM at histologic examination. Furthermore, the differential diagnoses for the sarcomatoid subtype include metastatic sarcoma to the pleura, sarcomas originating in the chest wall or lung parenchyma, and sarcomatoid carcinoma. Mixed subtypes need to be differentiated from carcinosarcomas, biphasic synovial sarcomas of the lung or chest wall, and pulmonary blastomas. Lastly, yet importantly, it is also a challenge to differentiate desmoplastic MPMs from chronic fibrous pleuritis.[10,11] Therefore, immunohistochemical procedures serve as valuable adjuncts to distinguish MPM from their neoplastic look-alikes.[9] The most sensitive immunohistochemical markers for MPM are mesothelin, calretinin, and cytokeratin 5/6. However, the specificity of these markers is far from perfect, as certain squamous cell carcinomas can be mesothelin, calretinin, and cytokeratin positive, whereas adenocarcinomas might also test positive for calretinin and cytokeratin.[12] To increase the diagnostic accuracy to differentiate epithelioid MPM from adenocarcinoma, 2 markers with positive diagnostic value for MPM (eg, anti-calretinin, anti-mesothelin) and 2 with negative diagnostic value (eg, anti-CEA, anti-B71-3) should be used.[13]

CLINICAL PRESENTATION OF MALIGNANT PLEURAL MESOTHELIOMA

Symptoms of MPM are nonspecific and include dyspnea, chest pain, systemic symptoms of malignancy, or combinations of these. The type of chest pain may be pleuritic and/or neuropathic, due to involvement of autonomic, brachial, or intercostal nerves by tumor. Although dyspnea is commonly related to a pleural effusion at diagnosis, as the disease progresses it is often due to the restrictive respiratory effects of pleural thickening. As the disease advances, symptoms of cardiac tamponade may signify the presence of pericardial involvement.[14]

STAGING SYSTEMS FOR MALIGNANT PLEURAL MESOTHELIOMA

The pattern of MPM invasion is first locoregional with the disease manifesting as small plaques on the parietal pleura, resulting in diffuse thickening and subsequent fusion of the pleurae, which eventually leads to encasement and possible compression and/or invasion of the ipsilateral lung. Nodal involvement is not infrequent, and as the tumor grows, the chest wall, mediastinal organs, contralateral lung, diaphragm, and peritoneum may become involved.

Defining the extent of disease at the time of diagnosis has important implications for treatment and prognosis. Accurate tumor staging is of utmost importance to enable assessment of response to treatment and to be used as a common denominator during the information exchange among treatment and research centers across the globe. Several staging systems have been proposed over the years. Of these, the one introduced by the International Mesothelioma Interest Group in 1995[15] and adopted by the American Joint Committee on Cancer (AJCC) was recently revised and published in the seventh edition of the AJCC manual in 2010.[16] **Table 1** summarizes the revised AJCC staging system for MPM and its corresponding anatomic groupings. In brief, when compared with the previous edition the only change in the seventh edition is the addition of peridiaphragmatic nodes to the N2 category. A revised version of the Brigham and Women's Hospital (BWH) staging system was proposed in 1999. The BWH surgical staging system has been shown to stratify survival; it considers tumor histology, resectability, and nodal status with definition of 4 stages as follows. Stage I: disease confined within the capsule of the ipsilateral parietal pleura without adenopathy, lung, pericardium, diaphragm, or chest wall disease limited to previous biopsy sites; Stage II: same as stage I with positive resection margins, and/or positive intrapleural lymph nodes; Stage III: local extension of disease into chest wall, mediastinum, heart, or through the diaphragm to the peritoneum, with or without extrapleural lymph node involvement; Stage IV: presence of distant metastatic disease. The BWH staging system defers from that of the AJCC by grouping intrapleural nodes (N1) as Stage II and extrapleural nodes (N2) as Stage III disease.[17] Both staging systems consider the disease to be unresectable when there is evidence of mediastinal, contralateral pleural, transdiaphragmatic, spinal, and/or diffuse chest wall invasion with or without rib destruction, and with or without associated systemic metastases (corresponding to AJCC Stage IV and BWH Stages III and IV).

IMPLICATIONS OF STAGE AND TREATMENT SELECTION IN MALIGNANT PLEURAL MESOTHELIOMA

The implications of stage on treatment selection depend entirely on whether surgical intervention will be a treatment possibility for the individual. In patients who have performance status or comorbidities precluding surgery, who specifically decline surgery, or for whom surgery is geographically unavailable, stage is arguably unimportant in treatment selection, with the choice of symptom palliation or systemic chemotherapy being unaffected

Table 1
Malignant pleural mesothelioma: 2010 anatomic stage groupings and TNM descriptors

Stage	TNM Description
I	T1: Tumor in ipsilateral parietal pleura, with or without mediastinal and/or diaphragmatic pleural involvement N0: No regional lymph node metastases M0: No distant metastasis
IA	T1A: No visceral pleural involvement N0: No regional lymph node metastases M0: No distant metastasis
IB	T1B: Visceral pleural involvement N0: No regional lymph node metastases M0: No distant metastasis
II	T2: Tumor involving all ipsilateral pleural surfaces plus involvement of the diaphragm or pulmonary parenchyma N0: No regional lymph node metastases M0: No distant metastasis
III	T1, T2, with N1: Involves ipsilateral hilar or bronchopulmonary nodes T1, T2, with N2: Involves subcarinal or ipsilateral mediastinal nodes including internal mammary and peridiaphragmatic nodes T3: Locally advanced but potentially resectable tumor Involves all ipsilateral pleural surfaces plus the endothoracic fascia, mediastinal fat, chest wall in a solitary resectable focus, or nontransmural pericardium T3, N1 or N2 M0: No distant metastasis
IV	T4: Locally advanced technically unresectable tumor Involves all ipsilateral pleural surfaces plus chest wall diffusely or multifocally, with or without rib destruction, or peritoneum, contralateral pleura, mediastinal organs, or spine via direct extension N3: Involves contralateral mediastinal, contralateral internal mammary, or ipsilateral or contralateral supraclavicular nodes M1: Distant metastasis present

Data from Edge SB, Byrd DR, Compton CC, et al. American Joint Committee on Cancer (AJCC) Cancer Staging Manual. 7th edition. New York: Springer; 2010. p. 271–7.

by anatomic location of tumor or presence of metastases. The role of surgery in MPM remains controversial, with as yet no published randomized evidence that any surgical procedure for MPM provides benefits for survival or quality of life.[17] Nevertheless, a recent Surveillance Epidemiology and End Results analysis found that 22% of patients with MPM received cancer-directed surgery.[18] In patients for whom surgery is considered, careful staging is important in reducing the risk of finding unresectable tumor at operation or of performing futile surgery on a patient with extrapleural disease.[19]

Pleurectomy/Decortication and Extrapleural Pneumonectomy

The controversy surrounding surgery in MPM now goes beyond *whether* surgery is indicated to *which* surgical procedure, whether pleurectomy/decortication (P/D) or extrapleural pneumonectomy (EPP), is indicated in particular patients. EPP

consists of en bloc resection of both visceral and parietal pleura, as well as the lung, pericardium, and diaphragm. P/D removes gross tumor via visceral and parietal pleurectomy, and is considered "extended" if the diaphragm and/or pericardium are also resected. Partial pleurectomy removes a variable portion of pleura but leaves evident tumor in situ (Rice and colleagues, personal communication, 2010). There is also lack of consensus between expert groups on which patients, in terms of disease stage, would be suitable for a particular surgical procedure. Nevertheless, surgeons performing these procedures need accurate staging to be able to match the appropriate procedure, in their opinion, with the anatomic extent of disease in that patient.[20–22]

Most controversy surrounds the selection of EPP versus P/D in patients with epithelioid tumors who are fit for either procedure. In general, patients with T4 disease will not be considered for either procedure.[20] When pleural disease is staged as T2 or T3, EPP may be the only procedure to achieve macroscopic disease resection.

Patients with extrapleural lymph node (N2) disease appear to have worse survival following EPP in at least two large series,[23,24] and many surgeons will exclude patients from this procedure on the basis of positive N2 nodes, should these be identified preoperatively. It is certainly critical to avoid morbid surgery in patients with metastatic disease, and preoperative staging should be adequate to identify macroscopic metastases. One rigorous approach to patient selection is to perform bilateral thoracoscopy, mediastinoscopy, and laparoscopy in addition to imaging to exclude patients with occult contralateral or subdiaphragmatic disease.[25]

Chemotherapy and Radiotherapy

There is no randomized evidence to suggest that either preoperative or surgical stage should determine the use of adjuvant or neoadjuvant chemotherapy in resected MPM. Similarly, there is no evidence that surgical staging should alter the use of postoperative radiotherapy. Although use of conventional doublet chemotherapy is not altered by staging information, staging does provide important prognostic information that should be documented for all patients, particularly those enrolled in clinical trials.

INDICATIONS FOR MEDIASTINOSCOPY AND ENDOBRONCHIAL ULTRASONOGRAPHY FOR STAGING OF MALIGNANT PLEURAL MESOTHELIOMA

PET/computed tomography (CT) has substantial limitations in staging nodal disease,[26–28] and CT imaging does not perform any better.[29] Because of this, there are advocates for routine surgical staging by mediastinoscopy in all patients prior to surgical resection.[29,30] However, further small surgical series suggest that negative mediastinoscopy has poor predictive value for N2 involvement and patient outcomes.[31]

Newer techniques such as endobronchial ultrasonography (EBUS) and esophageal endoscopic ultrasonography (EUS) have performed well in non–small cell lung cancer. In MPM, EBUS improved the detection of N2 metastatic disease, demonstrating malignancy in 13 of 38 patients who had previously had a negative mediastinoscopy. Nevertheless, in this small series nodal metastatic disease was found at surgery in 10 of 22 patients with negative EBUS and mediastinoscopy who proceeded to surgery.[32]

ROLE OF MULTIMODALITY IMAGING IN THE DIAGNOSIS AND STAGING OF MALIGNANT PLEURAL MESOTHELIOMA

Early diagnosis and an accurate disease staging in patients with MPM are essential in classifying them into prognostic subgroups to allow delivery of stage-specific therapies, or to carry out the necessary steps to improve their quality of life.

Local control of the disease improves following prompt diagnosis, accurate staging, and trimodality therapy.[23] Unfortunately, the noninvasive selection of patients who could benefit from therapy still remains a diagnostic challenge. Cytologic examination of pleural fluid is relatively insensitive and, in most cases, a pleural biopsy is often performed to arrive at the diagnosis. Closed pleural biopsy is useful when positive, but often yields negative or inaccurate results. Therefore, open lung biopsy or thoracoscopy are performed.[23,33–35] Thoracoscopy is highly sensitive for the diagnosis of MPM, but carries the risk of known complications such as air leaks, empyema, subcutaneous emphysema, hemorrhage, and the probability of disease relapse at the incision site.[35] Furthermore, open pleural biopsy is less sensitive in characterizing histologic types, particularly the mixed and sarcomatoid subtypes.[36]

In patients with a suspicion of MPM, there is a need for accurate noninvasive distinction between benign and malignant pleural disease as well as for the differentiation between resectable and nonresectable disease. Because of its complex biology and asymmetric growth pattern, MPM is a challenging disease to image by all modalities, each of which has specific advantages and limitations. The following sections expand on the roles that CT, magnetic resonance imaging (MRI), and PET/CT play in the diagnosis, staging, and restaging of MPM.

Computed Tomography

As with most other malignancies, CT plays a central role in the diagnosis and staging of MPM. In general, the advantages of CT in oncologic imaging include its high-resolution cross-sectional images, its noninvasive nature, relatively low cost, abundant access, and short duration of examination. CT resolution has rapidly improved over the last decade, with unprecedented submillimeter spatial resolution and temporal resolution conferring the ability to freeze cardiac and respiratory motion.

Despite these impressive major advances in CT image quality, a major limitation remains: CT imaging relies on differential tissue attenuation between lesions and background tissues to provide contrast, which is problematic because diagnosis and staging relies on differentiating normal gross tissue composition and morphology from abnormal findings. This differentiation is not as difficult when lesions are located in structures with inherently different attenuation values from soft tissue such as the lung, bone, or fat. Rather, the limitation manifests within solid organs and juxtaposed soft tissues where the attenuation of tumor and normal background parenchymal tissues are similar, with little differential contrast to assist in defining the presence, size, and boundaries of disease. Intravenous contrast material is often administered to mitigate this limitation by homogeneously increasing the attenuation of the blood pool, which then flows into vascular organs such as the liver, brain, kidneys, and porous tumor neovasculature at differential rates, thus raising tumor conspicuity. Specifically, CT detection and quantitation of MPM is challenging because the attenuation values of adjacent pleura, postinflammatory fibrotic pleural tissue, chest wall musculature, airless adjacent atelectatic lung, and proteinaceous pleural effusions can be quite similar. Furthermore, despite intrinsically elevated levels of vascular endothelial growth factor (VEGF) receptor in MPM and histologic evidence of neovascularity, MPM generally does not demonstrate robust tumoral enhancement with routine contrast-enhanced CT techniques, although there is anecdotal evidence that acquisition of delayed postcontrast images may improve tumoral enhancement. Finally, MPM usually coexists with inflammatory benign partially calcified pleural plaques and has a discontinuous multiplanar geometry of growth, which further complicates CT evaluation. As a result, early detection of MPM requires a multifaceted approach that includes clinical assessment, CT imaging, and tissue confirmation (either via biopsy or pleural fluid sampling). Staging further employs [^{18}F]fluorodeoxyglucose (FDG)-PET or FDG-PET/CT, which contributes a keen sensitivity for the detection of subtle metastatic disease, and is especially useful in interrogating equivocal mediastinal and hilar lymph nodes detected on CT and for the detection of occult distant metastases.

CT findings that are suggestive of MPM include rind-like pleural thickening (specificity 54%, sensitivity 95%), mediastinal pleural involvement (specificity 70%, sensitivity 83%), pleural nodularity (specificity 38%, sensitivity 96%), and pleural thickness greater than 1 cm (specificity 47%, sensitivity 64%).[37] Other suspicious findings include a unilateral pleural effusion in the setting of pleural plaques, significant pleural plaque soft tissue growth, nodules in the pleural fissures, and gross evidence of local invasion or mediastinal/hilar adenopathy. In the case of equivocal CT findings of subtle chest wall invasion or diaphragmatic transgression, adjunctive MRI can often be helpful for more definitive evaluation and is considered superior to CT for accurate characterization of these findings.[38] To improve the sensitivity of detection of malignant mediastinal, supraclavicular, and hilar lymphadenopathy, particularly in lymph nodes of normal size (<1 cm in short axis), and of distant metastases, FDG-PET/CT or FDG-PET are routinely employed.

Magnetic Resonance Imaging

MRI is typically used as adjunctive imaging in the staging of MPM, most often to resolve equivocal findings on staging CT. Specifically, MRI is typically employed to further evaluate for potential transgression of tumor through the diaphragm or into the chest wall. Although MRI does not yet reach the exquisite spatial and temporal resolution of CT, it does not rely on differential tissue attenuation to provide tissue contrast. Rather, MRI is a functional imaging modality that produces images based on the inherent magnetic properties of the tissue of interest.

MRI sequences are tailored to differentiate certain tissue types. For example, T2-weighted sequences are highly sensitive for the detection of water and for characterizing pleural fluid as simple or complex, thus differentiating between pleura, pleural effusion, and lung. T2-weighted imaging is also very sensitive in characterizing soft tissue edema. T1-weighted sequences typically accentuate fatty tissue allowing for definition of musculature, body wall, mediastinum, retroperitoneum, and pelvis, and to confirm macroscopic fat within tissue using fat-suppression techniques. T1-weighted images are very helpful in discriminating diaphragmatic muscle (typically low in T1-weighted signal intensity), invasive tumor (typically intermediate in signal intensity on T1-weighted imaging), and subdiaphragmatic fat (high in signal intensity on T1-weighted images) (**Fig. 1**). These differing tissue types can be easily discriminated, even without the use of intravenous contrast material.

Other specialized MRI techniques can be helpful in addressing clinical questions in the staging of MPM. Heavily T2-weighted image sequences, parallel imaging techniques, and respiratory gating using mechanical bellows or navigator sequences can assist in minimizing imaging artifacts from respiratory motion. A recent article by Gill and colleagues[39] demonstrated that diffusion-weighted

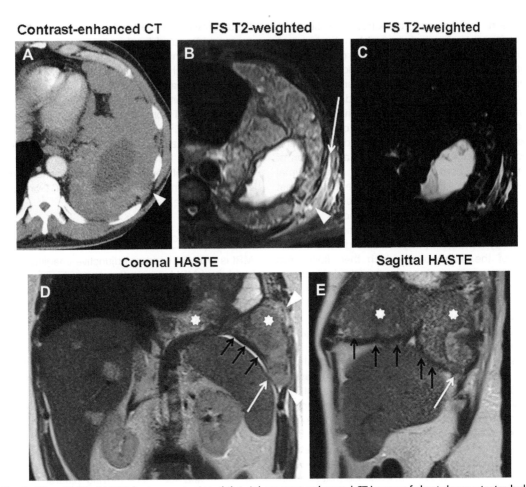

Fig. 1. CT and MRI of MPM for tumor staging. (*A*) Axial contrast-enhanced CT image of chest demonstrates bulky rind of tumor in pleural space with central proteinaceous fluid. Focal protrusion of tumor along posterolateral wall (*white arrowhead*) suggests possibility of chest wall invasion. (*B*) Axial fat-suppressed (FS) T2-weighted image reveals intermediate signal intensity tissue exiting chest wall at suspected location in posterolateral wall, spreading out within chest wall musculature admixed with reactive fluid visible as high T2-weighted signal intensity (*thin arrow*). By adjusting the window and level settings to optimize evaluation of high T2-weighted signal intensity fluid (*C*), internal septations are visible that are not seen on CT. (*D, E*) Coronal (*D*) and sagittal (*E*) slices of upper abdomen with unenhanced MRI using heavily T2-weighted sequences (half-Fourier acquisition single-shot turbo spin echo [HASTE]). Images show bulky heterogeneous MPM (*white stars*) in left pleural space, central septated fluid (high signal intensity rounded area within tumor), and focal diaphragmatic invasion (*white arrow*) involving near-complete full thickness of posterolateral diaphragm (*black arrows*), which is visible as low signal intensity band highlighted by thin curvilinear high signal intensity ascites below it on coronal image. On coronal image, left lateral chest wall invasion is also present, with tumor crossing parietal pleura to invade chest wall musculature (*white arrowheads*).

imaging, a means to measure intratumoral restriction of water molecule diffusivity, can differentiate between the more favorable epithelial and less favorable nonepithelial subtypes of MPM. Hierholtzer and colleagues[40] reported an MRI sensitivity and specificity of 100% and 93%, respectively, for the diagnosis of MPM using traditional sequences. While these studies do not suggest that MRI can replace tissue diagnosis, they do demonstrate the specificity of tissue signal intensity that can be obtained with the technique.

For the usual intended purpose of detecting transdiaphragmatic spread of tumor or chest wall invasion, MRI demonstrates remarkable specificity and sensitivity. A study by Heelan and colleagues[38] revealed the superiority of MRI over CT to detect chest wall and transdiaphragmatic invasion. Another study by Stewart and colleagues[41] showed that MRI is a valuable adjunct to differentiate T3 from T4 disease (sensitivity 85%, specificity 100%), to evaluate for resectability including evidence of transdiaphragmatic spread, full-thickness pericardial/mediastinal invasion, multifocal chest wall invasion, or direct extension into the spinal canal. Transdiaphragmatic and chest wall invasion manifests as focal irregularity of normal fat planes, focally intermediate T1-weighted and T2-weighted signal intensity foci of tumor extending through the low T1-weighted signal intensity musculature (see **Fig.** 1), and abnormal tissue enhancement. Entwisle[42] proposed that contrast-enhanced MRI is more accurate at diagnosing MPM than unenhanced MRI. In Heelan's study,[38] the accuracy of MRI versus CT for the detection of diaphragmatic

involvement was 82% versus 55%, respectively, and 69% versus 46%, respectively, in diagnosing chest wall invasion.

Mediastinal structures are generally well visualized by MRI, and MRI appears to have an advantage over CT primarily in the region of the pericardium. In this location, particularly in the left hemithorax, the pericardium comes in close approximation to the pleura, resulting in several layers of thin soft-tissue interfaces that may or may not be well defined by adjacent fat (**Fig.** 2). Such anatomic features are generally advantages

Double Inversion Recovery   **Pre-contrast FS GRE**   **Post-contrast FS GRE**

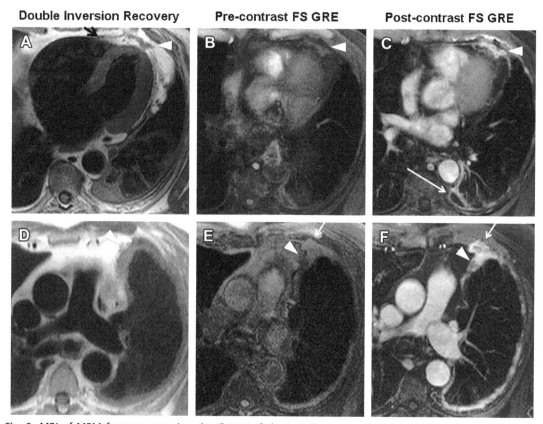

Fig. 2. MRI of MPM for tumor staging. (A–C) MRI of chest at the same level of thorax including axial double inversion recovery (A), axial fat-suppressed (FS) gradient echo (GRE) T1-weighted (B), and axial postcontrast fat-suppressed gradient echo T1-weighted images (C), revealing pericardial invasion near cardiac apex (white arrowhead) by MPM in left hemithorax. Note that pericardium is silhouetted by pericardial fluid and mediastinal fat, both of which are high in signal intensity on double inversion recovery sequence compared with pericardium, which has low signal intensity (black arrow) and tumor, which has intermediate signal intensity relative to skeletal muscle. Precontrast-enhanced and postcontrast-enhanced images reveal robust enhancement of tumor invading pericardium (white arrowhead), and demonstrate excellent tissue contrast between visceral and parietal pleural enhancing tumor and low signal intensity small posteromedial pleural fluid (thin white arrow). (D–F) MRI of chest, all obtained at same level of thorax, including axial double-inversion recovery (D), axial fat-suppressed gradient echo T1-weighted (E), and axial postcontrast fat-suppressed gradient echo T1-weighted (F) images. These images reveal tumor invasion of anterior mediastinal fat from MPM in left hemithorax (white arrowheads). Also seen is invasion of anterior chest wall musculature (thin white arrow). Fat-suppressed gradient echo image reveals robust tumor enhancement. Note excellent tissue contrast between enhancing nodular tumor-laden pleural surface, lung, and chest wall.

for MRI, as demonstrated by Kaminaga and colleagues,[43] who reported on the usefulness of MRI to characterize the presence or absence of pericardial invasion in the setting of MPM. However, in the rest of the mediastinum, the excellent inherent tissue contrast on CT resulting from the disparate tissue attenuations of fat and soft tissue renders CT superior, most likely due to better spatial resolution. For example, in a small study by Plathow and colleagues,[44] MRI was observed to miss mediastinal invasion in several cases, probably due to the lower spatial resolution of MRI relative to CT.

MRI is highly limited in the evaluation of the lung parenchyma, due to image distortion arising from artifact produced by the numerous air/soft tissue interfaces, termed "susceptibility artifact." Therefore, CT is needed to evaluate the lung parenchyma so as to identify pulmonary metastasis, lymphangitic spread of tumor, and pleural tumor in the pleural fissures.

Although MRI is excellent in discriminating between pleural fluid and solid tissue, in the presence of a large pleural effusion internal motion of the swirling pleural fluid generated during respiration can produce image distortion from motion artifact. This artifact can be minimized with measures to reduce respiratory motion as already mentioned, including the use of breath-hold heavily T2-weighted sequences, parallel imaging, and respiratory gating. Similarly, cardiac motion artifact can be mitigated with heavily T2-weighted sequences and electrocardiogram gating.

Therefore, in cases where there is a questioned chest wall or diaphragmatic extension of MPM with equivocal staging CT, MRI should be considered as adjunctive imaging. In cases where intravenous contrast cannot be administered, such as in severe allergy or renal insufficiency, MRI in addition to staging CT may be considered to optimize anatomic definition, taking advantage of the relative strengths of these two modalities. Finally, 3-dimensional imaging using segmentation techniques can allow for anatomic representations that may be helpful for surgical planning.[45]

PET and PET/CT

The most common PET radiotracer used in today's clinical oncology practice is FDG, due to the favorable half-life of ^{18}F (109 minutes) and the increased glucose metabolism of cancer cells as compared with normal tissues.[46]

Reports on the role and value of FDG-PET imaging of pleural malignancies are limited in number but encouraging. FDG-PET and PET/CT have been explored: (1) to characterize benign versus malignant pleural disease; (2) for the assessment of intrathoracic disease extent, tumor resectability, and prognosis in patients with MPM; (3) to characterize nodal status; (4) for the noninvasive assessment of extrathoracic invasion and recurrence of MPM; and (5) to monitor metabolic response to MPM therapy (discussed by Nowak and colleagues in an article elsewhere in this issue).

BENIGN VERSUS MALIGNANT PLEURAL DISEASE

Functional imaging with FDG-PET has come of age with today's practice of oncology because of the technique's inherent capacity to interrogate tumoral biological behavior and metabolism noninvasively, without reliance solely on lesion size and shape to characterize a lesion as being benign or malignant. In addition, the information gathered by whole-body PET images enhances findings observed on conventional imaging modalities during the diagnosis, preoperative staging, and postoperative restaging of MPM.

FDG tumoral uptake is a function of blood flow, facilitated transport by GLUT receptors across the plasma membrane, and the differential ratio of intracellular phosphorylation and dephosphorylation of the radiotracer.[47-51] The expression of GLUT-1 receptors in MPM and their diagnostic utility to differentiate MPM from benign reactive mesothelium have in fact been recently documented by Kato and colleagues.[52] These investigators performed immunohistochemical staining for GLUT-1 in 40 cases of reactive mesothelium, in 58 lung carcinomas, and in 48 MPMs. Immunohistochemical plasma membrane–based GLUT-1 expression was observed in all MPMs, and in 56 of 58 (96.5%) lung cancers. On the other hand, reactive mesothelium did not express the transporter. The investigators concluded that GLUT-1 is a sensitive and specific immunohistochemical marker for MPM, although it could not discriminate MPM from lung carcinoma.[52] This finding explains in part why the majority of mesotheliomas are FDG avid, with the intensity of uptake ranging from moderate to high, depending on the cell type.[53,54] Epithelial subtypes tend to be less metabolically active than their mixed and sarcomatoid counterparts, and in a small number of cases epithelial avidity can be very mild or absent.[53,55]

FDG-PET imaging accurately differentiates benign from malignant pleural disease. Bury and colleagues[56] were the first to report on the accuracy of FDG-PET to differentiate benign from malignant pleural disease in 25 patients. Of these, 16 (64%) had histologically confirmed pleural malignancies (13 metastatic lesions and 3 MPMs), and the remainder 9 (36%) had benign disease. All malignant lesions were FDG avid (intense in 14 and moderate in 2), with 7 of 9 benign lesions being FDG negative. There were 2 false-positive cases, with focal and moderate FDG uptake in a parapneumonic effusion and a tuberculous pleuritis. The investigators concluded that FDG-PET could reduce the number of futile invasive procedures in patients with benign pleural disease.

Bénard and colleagues[53] studied 28 patients using dedicated PET imaging to characterize pleural lesions and suspected MPM. Visual FDG image analysis yielded a sensitivity of 92%, a specificity of 75%, and an accuracy of 89% for the detection of MPM. When using a standardized uptake value (SUV) cutoff of greater than 2.0 to diagnose malignant disease, the sensitivity, specificity, and overall accuracy increased to 91%, 100%, and 92%, respectively. Schneider and colleagues[57] reported their results on 18 consecutive patients with biopsy-proven MPM, indicating that all MPMs were FDG avid. Gerbaudo and colleagues[54] reported similar results, with an overall sensitivity, specificity, and accuracy of FDG imaging to diagnose MPM of 97%, 80% and 94%, respectively, compared with 83%, 80%, and 82% for diagnostic CT. FDG imaging correctly identified 28 of 29 malignant tumors confirmed histologically, and yielded negative results in 4 of 5 benign lesions. The only false-positive finding was an area of diffusely low uptake in the right costophrenic sulcus of a patient treated with talc pleurodesis.

Furthermore, FDG-PET imaging has been of great value in guiding needle or thoracoscopic biopsy to the highest area of uptake within the thickened pleura.[54] PET/CT-guided biopsies of a variety of tumor types have increased the yield of positive findings by minimizing sampling errors from specimens containing only reactive fibrous changes and not viable tumor.[58,59]

Sources of known false-positive uptake in FDG-PET images of patients with pleural lesions include asbestos-related plaques, benign inflammatory pleuritis, tuberculous pleuritis, parapneumonic effusion, and bronchopleural fistulas.[53,56,57] On the other hand, mild pleural inflammatory reactions, benign asbestos pleural disease, benign angiolipoma, chronic fibrosing pleuritis, and pleural fibroma have been reported as true-negative findings.[53,54,56] As mentioned earlier, some epithelioid tumors might not be FDG avid and therefore may be a source of false-negative results.[53,55]

Recent results from studies employing hybrid technology (PET/CT) have confirmed those of earlier investigations previously conducted using dedicated PET. Yildirim and colleagues[60] examined the accuracy of FDG-PET/CT to differentiate MPM from asbestos-related benign pleural disease. The gold standards used were histopathology and/or a 3-year clinical follow-up. The investigators reported a sensitivity, specificity, and overall accuracy of FDG-PET/CT of 88.2%, 92.9%, and 90.3%, respectively. The mean SUV of MPM lesions was 6.5 ± 3.4, compared with 0.8 ± 0.6 for benign pleural disease. Using an SUV cutoff value of 2.2 the sensitivity, specificity, and positive and negative predictive values rose to 94.1%, 100%, 100%, and 93.3%, respectively.

Orki and colleagues[61] reported on the diagnostic accuracy of FDG-PET/CT compared with histopathology in a large cohort with undiagnosed pleural findings. These investigators studied 83 patients with CT evidence of pleural effusion (n = 63) and pleural thickening (n = 20) over a period of 2 years. Malignancy was considered when lesional SUV_{max} was greater than 3. Histopathological diagnosis was obtained with video-assisted thoracoscopic surgery in 76 patients and with mini-thoracotomy in the remaining 7. Forty-four malignant cases were confirmed by histopathology, of which 25 were due to MPM. FDG-PET/CT was 100% sensitive, 94.8% specific, and 97.5% accurate in diagnosing pleural malignancy, with 2 false-positive results due to pleural tuberculosis.

The potential of using dual time-point FDG-PET imaging to differentiate benign from malignant pleural disease was recently proposed by Mavi and colleagues.[62] These investigators concluded that as FDG uptake increased over time in pleural malignancies and stayed stable or decreased in benign pleural disease, the technique appeared to be an effective approach to noninvasively characterize pleural disease. By contrast, Yamamoto and colleagues[63] showed that although the mean values of early and late SUV in MPM were significantly higher than in benign pleural disease, the diagnostic performance of delayed PET was the same as that for early PET. Gerbaudo and colleagues[64,65] had a similar experience, and added that factoring in the increase of FDG uptake in the primary tumor as a function of time in MPM during image interpretation increases the PET and PET/CT accuracy in assessing disease extent and aggressiveness, and has prognostic value.

There is no doubt that FDG-PET and PET/CT are effective techniques for the noninvasive differentiation of benign from malignant pleural disease, and that they help reduce the number of futile surgical procedures in patients with a negative test. One of the major drawbacks of FDG imaging, however, is that neither the intensity of lesion avidity nor the pattern of uptake can be used to reliably differentiate between the different subtypes of MPM, or to differentiate adenocarcinoma and sarcoma from the epithelioid and sarcomatoid MPM subtypes, respectively. Lastly, a negative FDG-PET does not absolutely exclude the presence of MPM.

PREOPERATIVE STAGING

The imprecise anatomic detail of FDG images and their low spatial resolution, coupled to the irregular, nonspherical growth and invasion patterns of MPM, make T staging challenging with PET. Although earlier studies using dedicated PET scanners and coincidence gamma cameras showed good agreement between FDG and surgical findings, and that in many cases the metabolic images correctly predicted unresectable disease, they also brought to the surface some of the limitations of the technique.[53–55] It is not a simple task to differentiate uptake in the parietal pleura from that in the visceral pleura in the absence of a pleural effusion. Similarly, in many instances uptake in the basal pleura cannot be distinguished from diaphragmatic uptake. Diaphragmatic involvement can be unequivocally diagnosed only when transdiaphragmatic spread is grossly evident. In some cases, focal chest wall uptake may not be differentiated from pleural uptake. On many occasions, diffuse chest wall involvement can be unequivocally diagnosed only when FDG uptake is intense and its pattern causes distortion of the thoracic contour in the images. Furthermore, when the tumor's invasive front reaches mediastinal organs, it can be very difficult to resolve FDG uptake in individual structures.

Hybrid PET/CT systems have been introduced recently and have rapidly been incorporated into cancer imaging.[66] The technique provides metabolic and anatomic information in a single imaging session, and has improved the diagnostic and staging accuracy as compared with PET or CT alone in different thoracic malignancies, by enhancing the sensitivity of CT and the specificity of PET.[67,68] Furthermore, the technique has been shown to be helpful in differentiating atelectasis from tumor.[69,70]

The advantages and limitations of integrated PET/CT imaging for staging and assessing resectability of MPM have been reported recently by different groups.

Ambrosini and colleagues[71] indicated that despite the fact that FDG-PET/CT did not provide additional information about the primary tumor compared with CT, it was able to identify metastatic lymph nodes in 6 patients (40%) who were negative by CT criteria, as well as unexpected systemic metastases in 3 patients (20%). In addition, treatment planning was altered in 5 cases (33.3%) based on PET/CT findings alone.

Erasmus and colleagues[26] reported that FDG-PET/CT increased the accuracy of overall MPM staging by improving the selection of patients for extrapleural pneumonectomy, and providing additional information in 11 of 29 cases. The technique detected more extensive disease involvement, and identified occult distant metastases not seen in conventional images, assigning the correct overall TNM stage in 21 of 29 (72.4%) patients. The T stage was correctly assigned in 15 of 24 (63%) patients, 6 of whom had nonresectable disease, and was understaged in 7 (29%), 3 of whom had undetected transdiaphragmatic (T4) disease, with the remaining 4 patients having focal chest, lung, and/or diaphragmatic compromise. The main limitation of the technique was its inaccuracy for the detection of nodal disease, which was staged accurately only in 6 of 17 (35%) patients. N disease was overstaged in 5 (29%) patients and understaged in 6 (35%) (the majority with pathologically confirmed N2 disease), yielding a sensitivity of 38% and a specificity of 78%. However, the accuracy of PET/CT was significantly higher than the 19% and 11% sensitivities for T and N status, respectively, previously reported by Flores and colleagues[27] using a dedicated PET imaging without CT correlate, in 63 patients with MPM.

Pilling and colleagues[28] studied 20 consecutive patients who underwent 24 PET/CT scans over a median of 119 days (range 2–229) before EPP. The intrathoracic stage of MPM assigned by PET/CT was compared with histopathology results. The investigators indicated that PET/CT staged 3 patients correctly, overstaged 4, and understaged 17 patients, not detecting tumor in 6 patients, who were subsequently confirmed to have T4 disease. The technique did poorly in N2 staging, with a sensitivity of 11.1%, a specificity of 93%, and an accuracy of 66%. It was concluded that FDG-PET/CT is not accurate enough to identify advanced T4 or N2 disease, and that its preoperative staging role is to detect extrathoracic disease.

Plathow and colleagues[44] compared CT, PET, PET/CT, and MRI to stage 54 patients with epithelial MPM. The reference standard was surgery in 52 of the patients, and clinical follow-up for the remaining 2, with the N stage defined by mediastinoscopy. The results revealed that FDG-PET/CT was more accurate in early-stage disease when compared with all other modalities, and detected systemic metastases missed by CT and MRI in 2 patients.

Sørensen and colleagues[72] studied 42 patients with MPM undergoing FDG-PET/CT for preoperative staging following 3 to 6 courses of neoadjuvant platinum-based chemotherapy. The investigators found that futile surgery was avoided in 29% of the patients based on PET/CT findings, and in an additional 14% based on mediastinoscopy. PET/CT improved staging when compared with CT alone, with a slightly higher accuracy than in previous studies. The sensitivity and specificity of FDG-PET/CT for T4 disease were 78% and 100%, and for N2 disease 50% and 75%, respectively.

In summary, the currently available evidence suggests that FDG-PET/CT is superior to FDG-PET alone for staging MPM, with limitations to stage T4 and N2 disease, and remains superior to conventional imaging modalities for the detection of extrathoracic metastasis. The main advantage of fused PET/CT images is largely attributed to the coupling between the biological characterization of disease by PET, with the ability of CT to determine tumor extension into adjacent tissue. For example, assessment of diaphragmatic invasion with CT alone is sometimes difficult, because the images are limited to the transverse plane. MRI allows for image evaluation in multiple planes, although cardiac and respiratory motion affects image resolution. Transdiaphragmatic spread tends to be highly FDG avid and thus easily detectable in PET images, provided the size of the lesion falls within the system's resolution. It is usually better visualized in the sagittal and coronal planes as an area of intense and diffuse uptake extending from the lower thorax into the abdomen (**Fig. 3**). In this setting, FDG-PET accurately confirms tumor viability in areas of questionable diaphragmatic compromise in CT and MRI images. However, the irregular, nonspherical growth and invasion patterns of mesothelioma can make T staging challenging with PET/CT as well. The technique's limitations are evident when attempting to assess subtle, yet unresectable invasive disease.

Intrathoracic lymph nodes metastases are not infrequent and occur in 22% to 50% of patients.[23,73] The MPM pattern of lymphatic spread is different from that in lung cancer. MPM arises primarily from the parietal and diaphragmatic pleurae, and drains to the extrapleural (N2) nodal stations first, whereas this tumor has to affect the lung parenchyma before draining to the N1 nodes.[74] Flores and colleagues[24] recently confirmed this in a study of 348 patients with MPM who underwent EPP (n = 223) and P/D (n = 125). MPM was found to drain preferentially to N2 rather than to N1 lymph nodes.

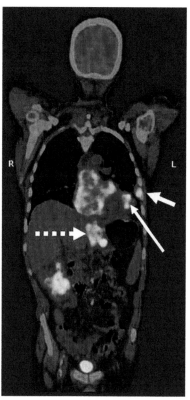

Fig. 3. FDG-PET/CT of epithelioid MPM for staging. Coronal PET/CT image demonstrates highly FDG-avid left parietal pleural nodularity (*short arrow*). Discrete FDG activity is also seen adjacent to left ventricle, with probable pericardial involvement (*long arrow*), subsequently confirmed by MRI (not shown). In addition, there is evidence of FDG-avid transdiaphragmatic disease, with diffuse and focal intense patterns of uptake extending into upper abdomen (*dotted arrow*).

FDG-PET and PET/CT have been found to be superior to CT or MRI in assessing N status, due to the ability of PET to demonstrate metabolic tumor viability in enlarged as well as in normal-size diseased lymph nodes (**Figs. 4** and **5**). However, the overall advantage of PET/CT for N staging in MPM appears to be marginal. Not infrequently, N1 nodes are a source of false-negative results. N1 uptake has to be very intense to be differentiated as a distinct entity from pleural uptake, especially in cases with bulky invasive tumor affecting the hilum. N2 nodes harboring micrometastatic disease have also been reported as another source of false-negative findings. Furthermore, the authors have encountered cases in which enlarged metastatic nodes were not FDG avid. Moreover, little is known about the accuracy of FDG-PET and PET/CT for the detection of metastases to extrapleural peridiaphragmatic

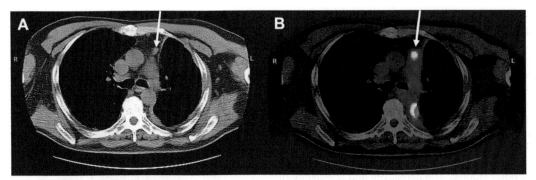

Fig. 4. FDG-PET/CT of MPM for tumor staging. Transverse CT (*A*) and PET/CT (*B*) images demonstrate encasing pattern of FDG uptake in left pleura due to MPM, with higher FDG uptake observed in thickened mediastinal pleura. Note small anterior mediastinal prevascular (N2) lymph node that is highly FDG avid (*arrows*).

nodes, whose involvement is not infrequent. On the other hand, false-positive results are not uncommon in granulomatous lymphadenitis.

These are important limitations, and caution should be exercised when using PET or PET/CT for N staging in MPM. Sugarbaker and colleagues[23,74] demonstrated that N2-positive nodes are always associated with poor survival, particularly the superior mediastinal nodes.[75] Therefore, both false-negative and false-positive extrapleural nodes could contribute misleading information with regard to optimal treatment strategy and prognosis. Histologic confirmation of nodal disease is still warranted with a negative or positive mediastinum in FDG-PET.

Systemic metastases from MPM have been reported in the adrenal glands, liver, bone, kidneys,

contralateral lung, abdominal wall, lymph nodes, peritoneum, brain, and leptomeninges.[76–78]

The available data from earlier and recent studies show that an important advantage of FDG-PET and PET/CT over conventional imaging modalities is their greater accuracy for the detection of occult distant metastases caused by MPM.[26,27,53,54,57,64] FDG images correctly define the presence or absence of extrathoracic disease, improving the selection of patients with resectable tumors (**Figs. 6** and **7**). In addition, the fused images allow for better characterization of extrathoracic findings as physiologic or pathologic by anatomically localizing areas of FDG uptake to specific structures.

Gerbaudo and colleagues[54,64] have observed that MPM sites of extrathoracic spread and

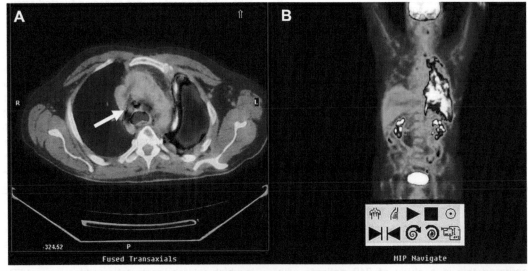

Fig. 5. FDG-PET/CT of biphasic MPM for tumor staging. Transverse PET/CT image (*A*) and coronal maximal intensity projection (MIP) PET/CT image (*B*) demonstrate highly FDG-avid circumferential left pleural thickening, with abnormal FDG uptake in contralateral right paratracheal lymph node, consistent with histologically confirmed N3 metastatic disease (*arrow*).

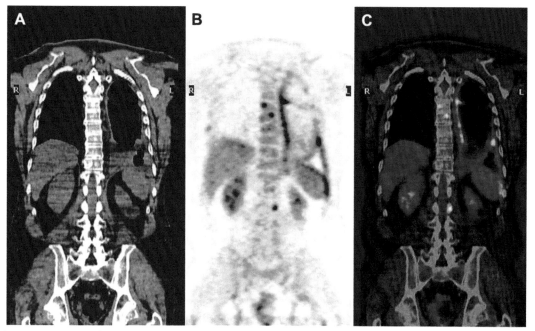

Fig. 6. FDG-PET/CT of epithelioid MPM for tumor staging. Coronal CT (*A*), PET (*B*), and PET/CT (*C*) images reveal FDG uptake in left pleural soft tissue due to MPM. PET also shows multiple foci of increased FDG uptake in thoracic and lumbar vertebrae, consistent with bone marrow metastases, indicating M1 disease.

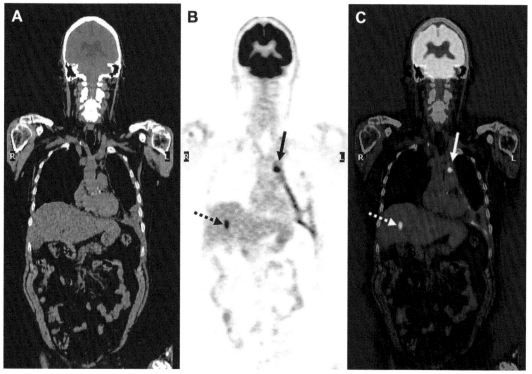

Fig. 7. FDG-PET/CT of sarcomatoid MPM for tumor staging. Coronal CT (*A*), PET (*B*), and PET/CT (*C*) images show increased FDG uptake in left pleural tumor. Note FDG-avid liver metastasis (*dotted arrows*) not evident on CT image as well as highly FDG-avid aortopulmonary window (N2) malignant lymph node (*arrows*).

metastases tend to be more FDG avid than primary lesions, and that FDG uptake in primary lesions of patients with extensive disease tends to be higher than in patients at lower stages. In addition, these investigators interrogated the value of the increment of lesion FDG uptake over time as a predictor of disease aggressiveness and prognosis in a pilot PET/CT study of 40 patients (22 untreated, 18 during restaging) with histologically confirmed MPM.[65] Semiquantitative image analysis was performed by calculating lesional SUV_{max} and the increment of FDG uptake over time in the primary tumor (malignant metabolic potential index [T-MMPi]) as: late SUV_{max} minus early SUV_{max}/ early $SUV_{max} \times 100\%$. The investigators found that the FDG lesion uptake increased over time at a higher rate in patients with more advanced disease. While the degree of histologic differentiation of the primary tumor did not always give a reliable estimation of tumor aggressiveness, high FDG uptake was a more reliable indicator of disease extent. In fact, the T-MMPi correlated better with the surgical stage, and was a better predictor of disease extent and aggressiveness than the SUV_{max} or histologic grade. The T-MMPi was greater in Brigham Stage IV (52.7% $\pm$ 12.5%) and Stage III-N2 disease (61.6% $\pm$ 59%), compared with Stages III-N1 (42.7% $\pm$ 14.7%), II (31.9% $\pm$ 6.4%), and I (21.4% $\pm$ 0.42%). Of interest, primary tumor SUV_{max} was significantly higher in patients with N2 disease ($P = .038$). Receiver operating characteristic curve analysis showed that a T-SUV_{max} greater than 12.37% identified pathologically confirmed N2 disease with a sensitivity of 88.9% and a specificity of 84.6% ($P = .001$). On the other hand, a T-MMPi greater than 47.8% identified patients harboring systemic metastases with a sensitivity of 100% and a specificity of 83.3%. Kaplan-Meier analysis showed that a high T-MMPi had a statistically significant relationship with worse survival ($P = .03$). These findings suggest that MPM tumors with high metastatic potential have higher energy requirements and poor prognosis. The results provide an interesting insight into the metabolic behavior of MPM, and further research is under way in Gerbaudo's laboratory in an attempt to elucidate the meaning of these observations.

POSTOPERATIVE RESTAGING AND PET/CT PATTERNS OF RECURRENT MPM

MPM recurrence can present as locoregional and/ or distant disease. Depending on the type of treatment algorithm used, local recurrence rates have been reported to range from 12% to 88%, and distant failure rates from 9% to 100% of cases.[76,78,79] Local recurrence tends to be more

common following P/D, whereas a combination of local and distant failure is found following EPP.[76,79]

Baldini and colleagues[76] reported a median time to first recurrence of 20 months in patients treated with trimodality therapy (EPP, chemotherapy, and radiation therapy) versus 11 months for those who did not receive all 3 treatment modalities. Sixty-seven percent of all recurrences occurred in the ipsilateral hemithorax, 33% in the contralateral hemithorax, 50% in the abdomen, and 8% as distant disease. Intrathoracic sites of recurrence included the surgical incision site, chest wall, neo-pleura, malignant effusion, pericardium, mediastinum, and diaphragm. Abdominal sites of recurrence included retroperitoneal masses and lymphadenopathy, ascites, transdiaphragmatic spread of chest disease, and peritoneal nodules. Distant recurrence was also present in the central nervous system.

At present, CT and MRI are considered the imaging modalities of choice for the assessment of MPM recurrence. The typical findings include enlarging soft tissue masses along the resection margins, new pulmonary nodules with or without mediastinal lymphadenopathy, peritoneal thickening, and ascites.[80] However, these imaging findings often cannot reliably distinguish recurrent tumor from benign post-therapeutic changes. Granulation tissue along the resection margins can present with a nodular pattern, and may therefore be concerning for relapse as seen on CT or MR images. FDG-PET/CT has been proposed as a valuable technique worth exploring in this setting.[80,81]

Tan and colleagues[82] published their results from an FDG-PET/CT study of 25 patients following multimodality treatment of MPM. These investigators reported a sensitivity of 94% and a specificity of 100% in diagnosing MPM recurrence. In their study there was one false-negative case, confirmed histopathologically as small nodules of recurrent MPM in the parietal and visceral pleura.

Gerbaudo and colleagues[78] recently confirmed that FDG-PET/CT is an accurate modality for the diagnosis and estimation of the extent of locoregional and distant MPM relapse, and that it affects management after treatment failure of MPM. In their 50-patient study, FDG-PET/CT was true positive for recurrence in 41 cases and true negative in 6, with only 1 false-negative and 2 false-positive findings, yielding a sensitivity of 97.6%, a specificity of 75%, and an accuracy of 94%. The only false-negative finding was a non–FDG-avid lesion of epithelial histology confirmed as relapse 3.5 months later by the presence of ascites and small peritoneal nodules on follow-up CT images. The first false-positive finding was an FDG-avid focus secondary to radiation pneumonitis confirmed at autopsy 3 months later. The other false-positive case was a linear area of intense uptake extending to the right chest wall, confirmed by biopsy as a bronchopleural fistula with empyema. The investigators found a significant difference in the intensity of radiotracer uptake between malignant lesions and benign changes in relapse-free patients. The intensity of uptake and the observed metabolic patterns of relapse in FDG-PET images (focal, linear, mixed [focal + linear], and encasing) proved to be highly reliable, unlike CT, in distinguishing recurrent tumor from benign post-therapeutic changes. Twenty patients (74%) recurred after EPP and 22 (96%) recurred after P/D. FDG-PET/CT evidence of a single site of recurrence was observed in 44% of the patients, with bilateral thoracic relapse in 7%, simultaneous recurrence in one hemithorax and in the abdomen in 24%, and disease detection in all 3 cavities in 17%. FDG-PET/CT demonstrated 20 unsuspected distant metastases in 11 patients (27%), with distant relapse being more frequent following EPP (35%) than following P/D (18.2%) (P = .04). Gerbaudo and colleagues indicated that FDG-PET/CT changed management in 12 patients (29%) who benefited from additional treatment at the time of failure.

PROGNOSTIC VALUE OF TUMOR METABOLISM AND TUMOR BULK
Standard Uptake Value

The fact that FDG uptake in primary pleural lesions is a function of the number of cancer cells, cellular proliferation, and the expression of GLUT receptors, all of which have been correlated with poor outcome in other thoracic tumors (eg, lung cancer, esophageal cancer), has led investigators to study the prognostic value of FDG uptake in MPM.

Bénard and colleagues[83] published the first study addressing the prognostic value of FDG-PET in MPM patients. In 17 patients with histologically confirmed MPM, it was demonstrated that high levels of FDG uptake in tumor were associated with an unfavorable prognosis. The investigators used a primary tumor SUV of 4.03 as a cutoff to define two patient groups with low and high lesion SUVs. The mean SUV of survivors was 3.2 ± 1.6, compared with 6.6 ± 2.9 for nonsurvivors. The high SUV group had a 1-year cumulative survival estimate of 17%, which was significantly shorter than the 86% observed in the low SUV group (P<.01). However, multivariate analysis was not performed.

Years later, Flores and colleagues[84] reported on the prognostic value of FDG-PET imaging from a study conducted in 137 patients with MPM. Multivariate analysis demonstrated that a primary lesion SUV greater than 10 (hazard ratio for death of 1.9), nonepithelial histology (hazard ratio of 2.9), and stages III and IV (hazard ratio of 1.8) were independent predictors of poorer survival. Of note, those patients with epithelioid tumors and a low SUV were alive beyond 5 years.

Krüger and colleagues[85] confirmed the previous findings using PET/CT in 17 patients with histologically confirmed MPM (9 epithelial, 2 sarcomatoid, and 6 biphasic subtypes). The mean epithelial SUV was 5.9 ± 1.9 compared with 15.1 ± 10.2 in sarcomatoid MPM. The investigators confirmed that the mean survival time tended to be higher in the subgroup of patients with lower mean SUV.

In a recent FDG-PET/CT study of 50 patients with MPM, Gerbaudo and colleagues[78] reported that epithelial histology, lack of nodal disease at presentation (pN0), a preoperative lesion SUV_{max} less than 10.7, and focal or linear patterns of FDG uptake were significantly associated with prolonged recurrence-free survival in univariate analysis. Cox proportional hazards analysis revealed that a lesion SUV_{max} of 10.7 was the only independent predictor of overall survival in their patient cohort (SUV of 10.7 or greater was associated with median overall survival of 7 months whereas an SUV <10.7 was associated with median overall survival of 41 months; P = .017; relative risk of 7.78). Their study population had a median survival time after relapse of 6 months (range 1–48 months), with univariate analysis revealing that a negative restaging FDG-PET/CT, a focal pattern of lesion uptake, lack of nodal uptake, and a recurrent lesion SUV_{max} of less than 3 were significantly associated with prolonged survival following restaging FDG-PET/CT. Multivariate analysis showed that the only independent predictors of survival following recurrence were the intrathoracic PET pattern of uptake in recurrent disease (relative risk 2.34; P = .01) and the PET N status (relative risk 2.26; P = .05).

Morphologic and Metabolic Tumor Bulk

Mesothelioma lesion volume is a critical factor that is always considered when making management decisions. Preoperative tumor bulk in part defines the type of surgical procedure to be used (EPP vs P/D), and has been shown to be a predictor of overall and progression-free survival.

Pass and colleagues[86] were the first group to report on the relationship between tumor morphologic volumes, recurrence, and prognosis in the setting of MPM. A total of 48 patients enrolled in a phase 3 randomized trial met the inclusion criteria (5 mm thickness of residual tumor after surgery). Preoperative morphologic tumor bulk was quantified using CT images and was expressed in cubic centimeters (cc). The investigators indicated that a preoperative volume of 100 cc or more was significantly associated with a worse prognosis, and that tumor bulk could serve as a potential alternative to clinical estimation of T stage. A very interesting finding was that those patients without nodal metastasis had significantly smaller primary tumor volumes than those with confirmed N1 and N2 disease. The results of multivariate analysis revealed that gender, platelet count, and preoperative as well as post-cytoreduction tumor bulk were independent predictors of outcome in their patient population.

Nowak and colleagues[87] reported on 89 eligible prospectively recruited patients with MPM who had FDG-PET and CT imaging at presentation. A semiautomated region growing algorithm was used to define 3-dimensional volumes of interest from which the tumor's total glycolytic volume (TGV) was derived (TGV = SUV × volume). TGV is a composite measure of both metabolic activity and tumor volume, and reflects the metabolically active tumor mass. A range of potential prognostic variables were evaluated in the patient group, of which sarcomatoid histology was found to be the strongest independent prognostic factor. Imaging variables that showed prognostic significance for survival included CT stage (P = .013), TGV (P = .003), and metabolic volume (P = .008).[87] SUV_{max} did not reach statistical significance for survival, but showed a trend toward a worse prognosis (P = .055). A prognostic nomogram was developed for patients with nonsarcomatoid disease, and the prognostic variables of weight loss and TGV were found to contribute significantly to the model and were incorporated into the nomogram. A correction factor for the increased metabolic activity related to previous talc pleurodesis was also incorporated into the model. This study illustrates the importance of metabolically active tumor burden on patient prognosis in MPM.

Lee and colleagues[88] evaluated the significance of metabolic tumor volume derived from FDG-PET/CT images of 13 patients with MPM, as a predictor of progression-free survival. Metabolic tumor volume (MTV), SUV_{max}, SUV_{mean}, and total lesion glycolysis (TLG = MTV × SUV_{mean}) were estimated from the FDG images. The study showed that there were significant differences in MTV and only marginal differences in TLG between patients with and without tumor progression following therapy. However, neither the SUV_{max} nor the SUV_{mean} were classified as predictors of disease progression. Multivariate analysis adjusted for treatment type demonstrated that the only significant predictors of time to progression were the MTV and the TLG.

These data suggest that MPM metabolic bulk-based parameters may be better indicators of primary tumor aggressiveness, and therefore more sensitive than the single-pixel–derived SUV_{max}. These small studies bring to the surface findings that have important treatment and prognostic implications for patients with MPM. Further research calls for their prospective validation as well as technique standardization in a larger patient cohort.

PLEURODESIS

Talc pleurodesis is commonly performed in patients with MPM for palliation of recurrent pleural effusions.[89,90] Talc induces an intense inflammatory reaction in pleura, resulting in chronic fibrosis.[91] The inflammatory effects of pleurodesis are evident on FDG-PET imaging and may persist for years.[92] The effect of talc pleurodesis on staging with CT or FDG-PET has not been well described. A recent study, however, suggests that talc pleurodesis may influence both CT and FDG-PET imaging. In a cohort of 89 patients, 28 (31%) had undergone previous talc pleurodesis at a median of 2 months before imaging.[93] The patient groups did not differ significantly in age, gender, pathology, performance status, or forced vital capacity, although the prior pleurodesis group reported more chest pain. Survival was the same in both groups. CT-based TNM classifications demonstrated that patients with prior pleurodesis were found to have more advanced nodal (N) stage, with more patients having N2 or N3 disease than in the nonpleurodesis group (P = .05).[93] There was no significant difference in stage when assessed by FDG-PET imaging in the prior pleurodesis or nonpleurodesis groups. The FDG-PET indices of TGV and SUV_{max} were higher in the prior pleurodesis group, although TGV remained strongly predictive of survival in both groups. CT-based TNM stage was only predictive of survival in the nonpleurodesis group. In summary, these data suggest that prior talc pleurodesis may confound the staging and the semiquantitative analysis of both CT and FDG-PET imaging, and that documentation of previous talc pleurodesis should be undertaken when assessing patients with MPM.

NOVEL PET PROBES

Novel PET radiotracers have been developed that may potentially allow the imaging of a variety of biological processes in mesothelioma. 3'-Deoxy-3'-[^{18}F]fluorothymidine (FLT) is a thymidine analogue, and as such a marker of cellular proliferation. FLT is transported into the cell and phosphorylated by thymidine kinase 1 (TK1), but not incorporated into DNA. Preclinical studies suggest that mesothelioma is a proliferative tumor and is likely to demonstrate FLT activity on PET imaging.[94] This suggestion has recently been confirmed in a small prospective clinical study in which 32 of 33 patients demonstrated FLT uptake in areas of MPM (Fig. 8).[95] FLT-PET T ($P<.001$), N ($P = .012$),

M ($P<.001$), and overall stage ($P = .001$) correlated well with FDG-PET stage, demonstrating the potential clinical utility of proliferation imaging in MPM.[95] Studies in other solid tumors, however, suggest that the predominant role of FLT-PET imaging is in response assessment rather than tumor detection or staging. Further studies are required to better define the role of proliferation imaging of mesothelioma.

Hypoxia imaging has predominantly been performed in head and neck cancers and in non–small cell lung carcinoma. Hypoxia is a marker of poor prognosis and is involved in tumor resistance to chemotherapy and radiotherapy. The most common PET radiotracer that has been used for hypoxia PET imaging is [^{18}F]fluoromisonidazole

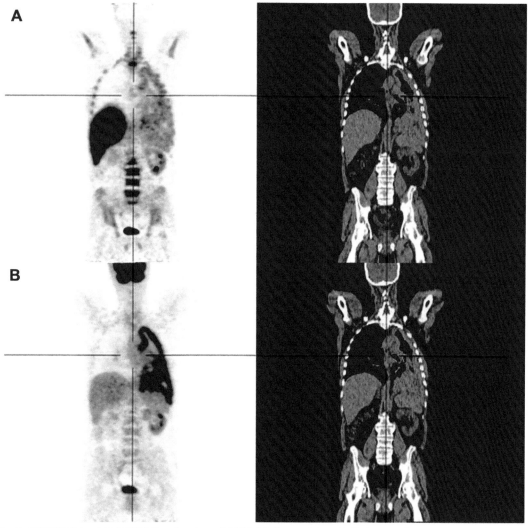

Fig. 8. FLT-PET/CT and FDG-PET/CT evaluation of MPM. (A) Coronal FLT-PET/CT images demonstrate moderate and diffuse FLT uptake in left thickened pleura due to tumor, with intense physiologic radiotracer uptake in liver (glucuronidation of FLT) and bone marrow (cell proliferation). (B) Coronal FDG-PET/CT images of same patient performed within 1 week of FLT-PET/CT scan. Note intense circumferential FDG uptake in left pleura due to tumor.

(FMISO). FMISO enters cells by passive diffusion, where it is reduced by nitroreductase enzymes to become trapped in cells with reduced tissue oxygen partial pressure. When oxygen is abundant in normally oxygenated cells the parent compound is quickly regenerated by reoxidation, and metabolites do not accumulate. However, in hypoxic cells the low partial pressure of oxygen prevents reoxidation of FMISO metabolites, resulting in radiotracer accumulation. Of importance, because FMISO only accumulates in hypoxic cells with functional nitroreductase enzymes, it targets viable cells and cannot accumulate in necrotic cells.[96] Preliminary unpublished work by Francis and colleagues demonstrated that mesothelioma appears to show FMISO activity, suggesting that it is a tumor with significant hypoxia (**Fig. 9**). This finding may have prognostic value, or may potentially lead to development and monitoring of therapies targeting hypoxia and/or neovascularization.

Ceresoli and colleagues[97] have demonstrated in a case report that mesothelioma may take up the amino acid PET radiotracer [^{11}C]methionine (MET). MET activity in tumors appears to be related to upregulation of amino acid transporters. This case report demonstrates MET uptake in a patient with MPM that did not appear to be FDG avid. ^{11}C PET radiotracers have a very short half-life (20 minutes), necessitating an onsite cyclotron. ^{18}F-based amino acid PET imaging agents have been developed, although there are no published cases of their use in MPM to date.

The role of non-FDG PET radiotracers in mesothelioma is likely to continue to evolve as a greater understanding of the tumor biology develops. PET allows for the noninvasive imaging of biologic processes, although establishing the potential clinical utility of novel agents in a relatively uncommon tumor is challenging, resource intensive, and expensive. PET-based biomarkers may, however, play an important role in the near future in patient prognosis and individualization of patient therapy.

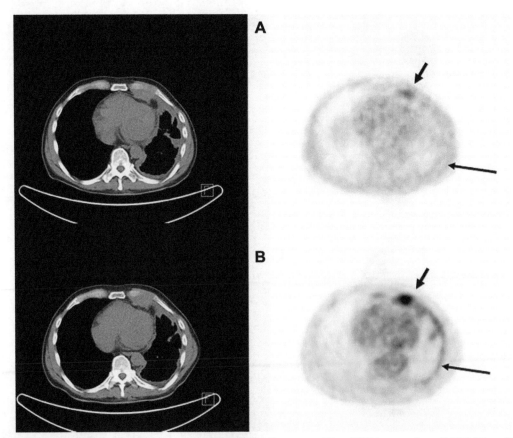

Fig. 9. FMISO-PET/CT and FDG-PET/CT evaluation of MPM. Transverse CT and PET images show FMISO (*A*) and FDG uptake (*B*) in left pleural tumor. Moderate FMISO activity (a marker of hypoxia) is demonstrated anteriorly in area of thickened pleura (*short arrow in A*), which also demonstrates intense FDG (metabolic) activity (*short arrow in B*). A thin rim of tumor along costal and mediastinal pleural surfaces is FDG avid (*long arrows*) but without significant FMISO activity, indicating metabolic/hypoxic incongruence.

Pearls and pitfalls and take home messages

- Early diagnosis and accurate staging in patients with MPM are essential in order to classify them into prognostic subgroups and to allow delivery of stage-specific therapies.
- CT and MRI are successful at predicting tumor resectability but have limitations for characterization of pleural lesions as benign or malignant.
- CT findings suggestive of MPM include rind-like pleural thickening, mediastinal pleural involvement, pleural nodularity, pleural thickness greater than 1 cm, unilateral pleural effusion in the setting of pleural plaques, significant pleural plaque soft tissue growth, nodules in the pleural fissures, gross evidence of local invasion of adjacent structures, and mediastinal or hilar lymphadenopathy.
- MPM generally does not demonstrate robust tumoral enhancement with routine CT techniques. Acquisition of delayed enhanced images may improve tumoral enhancement.
- MRI is typically employed as adjunctive imaging in the staging of MPM, most often to resolve equivocal findings on staging CT.
- MRI is typically used to further evaluate for potential transgression of tumor through the diaphragm or into the chest wall or pericardium.
- MRI is highly limited in the evaluation of the lung parenchyma, due to image distortion from artifact produced by the numerous air/soft tissue interfaces termed "susceptibility artifact."
- In cases where intravenous contrast cannot be administered, MRI in addition to staging CT should be considered to optimize anatomic definition, taking advantage of the relative strengths of these two modalities.
- FDG-PET imaging is an accurate tool for the noninvasive metabolic characterization of pleural lesions as benign or malignant. However, neither the pattern nor the intensity of FDG uptake is useful in differentiating MPM from other pleural malignancies.
- FDG-PET imaging is useful for guiding needle or thoracoscopic biopsy to the highest area of uptake within the thickened pleura.
- FDG-PET and PET/CT reduce the number of futile surgical procedures in patients with a negative test. However, it should be kept in mind that a negative FDG-PET does not absolutely exclude the presence of MPM. In particular, some epithelioid tumors may not be FDG avid.
- FDG-PET and PET/CT imaging are complementary to CT and MRI in the assessment intrathoracic disease extent and tumor resectability. The limitations of FDG-PET/CT become evident when attempting to assess subtle, yet unresectable, invasive disease.
- FDG-PET/CT increases the accuracy of overall MPM staging, by detecting more extensive disease involvement and identifying occult distant metastases not seen on CT and MRI.
- FDG-PET and PET/CT are superior to CT and MRI for the characterization of intrathoracic nodal status, but are less than perfect. The overall advantage of PET/CT for N staging in MPM appears to be marginal, due to the high number of false-negative and false-positive results. Histologic confirmation of nodal disease is still warranted with a negative or positive mediastinum in FDG-PET.
- FDG-PET/CT imaging accurately predicts or confirms the presence or absence of systemic metastases.
- FDG-PET/CT is an accurate modality in diagnosing and estimating the extent of locoregional and distant MPM recurrence.
- High levels of FDG uptake and tumor morphologic and metabolic bulk are associated with an unfavorable prognosis in patients with MPM.
- Prior talc pleurodesis may confound the staging and semiquantitative analysis of both CT and FDG-PET imaging, and documentation of previous talc pleurodesis should be undertaken when assessing patients with MPM.
- MPM appears to be FLT, FMISO, and MET avid. The role of these novel PET probes remains to be defined in patients with MPM.

REFERENCES

1. Connelly RR, Spirtas R, Myers MH, et al. Demographic patterns for mesothelioma in the United States. J Natl Cancer Inst 1987;78(6):1053–60.
2. Price B, Ware A. Time trend of mesothelioma incidence in the United States and projection of future cases: an update based on SEER data for 1973 through 2005. Crit Rev Toxicol 2009;39(7):576–88.
3. Wagner JC, Sleggs CA, Marchand P. Diffuse pleural mesothelioma and asbestos exposure in the North Western Cape Province. Br J Ind Med 1960;17: 260–7.
4. Bianchi C, Giarelli L, Grandi G, et al. Latency periods in asbestos-related mesothelioma of the pleura. Eur J Cancer Prev 1997;6(2):162–6.
5. Travis WD. Sarcomatoid neoplasms of the lung and pleura. Arch Pathol Lab Med 2010;134(11): 1645–58.
6. Lopez-Rios F, Illei PB, Rusch V, et al. Evidence against a role for SV40 infection in human mesotheliomas and high risk of false-positive PCR results

owing to presence of SV40 sequences in common laboratory plasmids. Lancet 2004;364:1157–66.

7. Manfredi JJ, Dong J, Liu WJ, et al. Evidence against a role for SV40 in human mesothelioma. Cancer Res 2005;65:2602–9.

8. Klebe S, Brownlee NA, Mahar A, et al. Sarcomatoid mesothelioma: a clinical-pathologic correlation of 326 cases. Mod Pathol 2010;23(3):470–9.

9. Corson JM. Pathology of diffuse malignant pleural mesothelioma. Semin Thorac Cardiovasc Surg 1997;9(4):347–55.

10. Inai K. Pathology of mesothelioma. Environ Health Prev Med 2008;13(2):60–4.

11. Mangano WE, Cagle PT, Churg A, et al. The diagnosis of desmoplastic malignant mesothelioma and its distinction from fibrous pleurisy: a histologic and immunohistochemical analysis of 31 cases including p53 immunostaining. Am J Clin Pathol 1998;110(2):191–9.

12. Marchevsky AM. Application of immunohistochemistry to the diagnosis of malignant mesothelioma. Arch Pathol Lab Med 2008;132(3):397–401.

13. Scherpereel A, Astoul P, Baas P, et al. European Respiratory Society/European Society of Thoracic Surgeons Task Force. Guidelines of the European Respiratory Society and the European Society of Thoracic Surgeons for the management of malignant pleural mesothelioma. Eur Respir J 2010;35(3): 479–95.

14. British Thoracic Society Standards of Care Committee. Statement on malignant mesothelioma in the United Kingdom. Thorax 2001;56:250–65.

15. Rusch VW. A proposed new international TNM staging system for malignant pleural mesothelioma. From the International Mesothelioma Interest Group. Chest 1995;108(4):1122–8.

16. Pleural mesothelioma. In: Edge SB, Byrd DR, Compton CC, et al, editors. AJCC cancer staging manual. 7th edition. New York: Springer; 2010. p. 271–7.

17. Treasure T. Surgery for mesothelioma: MARS landing and future missions. Eur J Cardiothorac Surg 2010;37(3):509–10.

18. Flores RM, Riedel E, Donington JS, et al. Frequency of use and predictors of cancer-directed surgery in the management of malignant pleural mesothelioma in a community-based (Surveillance, Epidemiology, and End Results [SEER]) population. J Thorac Oncol 2010;5(10):1649–54.

19. Zielinski M, Hauer J, Hauer L, et al. Staging algorithm for diffuse malignant pleural mesothelioma. Interact Cardiovasc Thorac Surg 2010;10(2):185–9.

20. Kent M, Rice D, Flores R. Diagnosis, staging, and surgical treatment of malignant pleural mesothelioma. Curr Treat Options Oncol 2008;9(2–3):158–70.

21. Rice D. Surgery for malignant pleural mesothelioma. Ann Diagn Pathol 2009;13(1):65–72.

22. Sugarbaker DJ, Wolf AS. Surgery for malignant pleural mesothelioma. Expert Rev Respir Med 2010;4(3):363–72.

23. Sugarbaker DJ, Flores RM, Jaklitsch MT, et al. Resection margins, extrapleural nodal status, and cell type determine postoperative long-term survival in trimodality therapy of malignant pleural mesothelioma: results in 183 patients. J Thorac Cardiovasc Surg 1999;117:54–65.

24. Flores RM, Routledge T, Seshan VE, et al. The impact of lymph node station on survival in 348 patients with surgically resected malignant pleural mesothelioma: implications for revision of the American Joint Committee on Cancer staging system. J Thorac Cardiovasc Surg 2008;136(3):605–10.

25. Alvarez JM, Hasani A, Segal A, et al. Bilateral thoracoscopy, mediastinoscopy and laparoscopy, in addition to CT, MRI and PET imaging, are essential to correctly stage and treat patients with mesothelioma prior to trimodality therapy. ANZ J Surg 2009;79(10):734–8.

26. Erasmus JJ, Truong MT, Smythe WR, et al. Integrated computed tomography-positron emission tomography in patients with potentially resectable malignant pleural mesothelioma: staging implications. J Thorac Cardiovasc Surg 2005;129(6): 1364–70.

27. Flores RM, Akhurst T, Gonen M, et al. Positron emission tomography defines metastatic disease but not locoregional disease in patients with malignant pleural mesothelioma. J Thorac Cardiovasc Surg 2003;126(1):11–6.

28. Pilling J, Dartnell JA, Lang-Lazdunski L. Integrated positron emission tomography-computed tomography does not accurately stage intrathoracic disease of patients undergoing trimodality therapy for malignant pleural mesothelioma. Thorac Cardiovasc Surg 2010;58(4):215–9.

29. Schouwink JH, Kool LS, Rutgers EJ, et al. The value of chest computer tomography and cervical mediastinoscopy in the preoperative assessment of patients with malignant pleural mesothelioma. Ann Thorac Surg 2003;75(6):1715–8 [discussion: 1718–9].

30. Pilling JE, Stewart DJ, Martin-Ucar AE, et al. The case for routine cervical mediastinoscopy prior to radical surgery for malignant pleural mesothelioma. Eur J Cardiothorac Surg 2004;25(4):497–501.

31. de Perrot M, Uy K, Anraku M, et al. Impact of lymph node metastasis on outcome after extrapleural pneumonectomy for malignant pleural mesothelioma. J Thorac Cardiovasc Surg 2007;133(1): 111–6.

32. Rice DC, Steliga MA, Stewart J, et al. Endoscopic ultrasound-guided fine needle aspiration for staging of malignant pleural mesothelioma. Ann Thorac Surg 2009;88(3):862–8 [discussion: 868–9].

33. Sugarbaker DJ, Garcia JP, Richards WG, et al. Extrapleural pneumonectomy in the multimodality therapy of malignant pleural mesothelioma. Results in 120 consecutive patients. Ann Surg 1996;224:288–96.

34. Sugarbaker DJ, Norberto JJ, Swanson SJ. Extrapleural pneumonectomy in the setting of multimodality therapy for diffuse malignant pleural mesothelioma. Semin Thorac Cardiovasc Surg 1997;9:373–82.

35. Kaiser LR, Bavaria JE. Complications of thoracoscopy. Ann Thorac Surg 1993;56:796–8.

36. Bueno R, Reblando J, Glickman J, et al. Pleural biopsy: a reliable method for determining the diagnosis but not subtype in mesothelioma. Ann Thorac Surg 2004;78(5):1774–6.

37. Metintas M, Ucgun I, Elbek O, et al. Computed tomography features in malignant pleural mesothelioma and other commonly seen pleural diseases. Eur J Radiol 2002;41(1):1–9.

38. Heelan RT, Rusch VW, Begg CB, et al. Staging of malignant pleural mesothelioma: comparison of CT and MR imaging. AJR Am J Roentgenol 1999; 172(4):1039–47.

39. Gill RR, Umeoka S, Mamata H, et al. Diffusion-weighted MRI of malignant pleural mesothelioma: preliminary assessment of apparent diffusion coefficient in histologic subtypes. AJR Am J Roentgenol 2010;195(2):W125–30.

40. Hierholzer J, Luo L, Bittner RC, et al. MRI and CT in the differential diagnosis of pleural disease. Chest 2000;118(3):604–9.

41. Stewart D, Waller D, Edwards J, et al. Is there a role for pre-operative contrast-enhanced magnetic resonance imaging for radical surgery in malignant pleural mesothelioma? Eur J Cardiothorac Surg 2003;24(6):1019–24.

42. Entwisle J. The use of magnetic resonance imaging in malignant mesothelioma. Lung Cancer 2004; 45(Suppl 1):S69–71.

43. Kaminaga T, Takeshita T, Kimura I. Role of magnetic resonance imaging for evaluation of tumors in the cardiac region. Eur Radiol 2003;13(Suppl 6):L1–10.

44. Plathow C, Staab A, Schmaehl A, et al. Computed tomography, positron emission tomography, positron emission tomography/computed tomography, and magnetic resonance imaging for staging of limited pleural mesothelioma: initial results. Invest Radiol 2008;43(10):737–44.

45. Plathow C, Schoebinger M, Fink C, et al. Quantification of lung tumor volume and rotation at 3D dynamic parallel MR imaging with view sharing: preliminary results. Radiology 2006;240(2):537–45.

46. Warburg O, Posener K, Negelein E. The metabolism of the carcinoma cell. In: Warburg O, editor. The metabolism of tumors. New York: Richard R. Smith, Inc; 1931. p. 129–69.

47. Gallagher BM, Fowler JS, Gutterson NI, et al. Metabolic trapping as a principle of radiopharmaceutical design: some factors responsible for the biodistribution of [^{18}F] 2-deoxy-2-fluoro-D-glucose. J Nucl Med 1978;19:1154–61.

48. Nelson CA, Wang JQ, Leav I, et al. The interaction among glucose transport, hexokinase, and glucose-6-phosphatase with respect to ^{3}H-2-deoxy-glucose retention in murine tumor models. Nucl Med Biol 1996;23:533–41.

49. Waki A, Fujibayashi Y, Yokoyama A. Recent advances in the analyses of the characteristics of tumors on FDG uptake. Nucl Med Biol 1998;25: 589–92.

50. Wiebe LI. FDG metabolism: quaecumque sunt vera. J Nucl Med 2001;42:1679–81.

51. Zhao S, Kuge Y, Mochizuki T, et al. Biologic correlates of intratumoral heterogeneity in ^{18}F-FDG distribution with regional expression of glucose transporters and hexokinase-II in experimental tumor. J Nucl Med 2005;46(4):675–82.

52. Kato Y, Tsuta K, Seki K, et al. Immunohistochemical detection of GLUT-1 can discriminate between reactive mesothelium and malignant mesothelioma. Mod Pathol 2007;20(2):215–20.

53. Bénard F, Sterman D, Smith RJ, et al. Metabolic imaging of malignant pleural mesothelioma with fluorodeoxyglucose positron emission tomography. Chest 1998;114:713–22.

54. Gerbaudo VH, Sugarbaker DJ, Britz-Cunningham S, et al. Assessment of malignant pleural mesothelioma with ^{18}F-FDG dual-head gamma-camera coincidence imaging: comparison with histopathology. J Nucl Med 2002;43:1144–9.

55. Carretta A, Landoni C, Melloni G, et al. ^{18}F-FDG positron emission tomography in the evaluation of malignant pleural diseases—a pilot study. Eur J Cardiothorac Surg 2000;17:377–83.

56. Bury T, Paulus P, Dowlati A, et al. Evaluation of pleural diseases with FDG-PET imaging: preliminary report. Thorax 1997;52:187–9.

57. Schneider DB, Clary-Macy C, Challa S, et al. Positron emission tomography with F18-fluorodeoxyglucose in the staging and preoperative evaluation of malignant pleural mesothelioma. J Thorac Cardiovasc Surg 2000;120:128–33.

58. Tatli S, Gerbaudo VH, Mamede M, et al. Abdominal masses sampled at PET/CT-guided percutaneous biopsy: initial experience with registration of prior PET/CT images. Radiology 2010;256(1): 305–11.

59. Tatli S, Gerbaudo VH, Tuncali K, et al. PET/CT-guided percutaneous biopsy of abdominal masses: initial experience. J Vasc Interv Radiol 2011;22(4): 507–14.

60. Yildirim H, Metintas M, Entok E, et al. Clinical value of fluorodeoxyglucose-positron emission tomography/computed tomography in differentiation of malignant mesothelioma from asbestos-related

benign pleural disease: an observational pilot study. J Thorac Oncol 2009;4(12):1480–4.

61. Orki A, Akin O, Tasci AE, et al. The role of positron emission tomography/computed tomography in the diagnosis of pleural diseases. Thorac Cardiovasc Surg 2009;57(4):217–21.

62. Mavi A, Basu S, Cermik TF, et al. Potential of dual time point FDG-PET imaging in differentiating malignant from benign pleural disease. Mol Imaging Biol 2009;11(5):369–78.

63. Yamamoto Y, Kameyama R, Togami T, et al. Dual time point FDG PET for evaluation of malignant pleural mesothelioma. Nucl Med Commun 2009; 30(1):25–9.

64. Gerbaudo VH, Britz-Cunningham S, Sugarbaker DJ, et al. Metabolic significance of the pattern, intensity and kinetics of ^{18}F-FDG uptake in malignant pleural mesothelioma. Thorax 2003;58(12):1077–82.

65. Gerbaudo VH, Mamede M, Bueno R, et al. Increment of FDG uptake as a function of time in malignant pleural mesothelioma: relationship to tumor invasion, metastasis, and prognosis. J Nucl Med 2006;47(Suppl 1):474P.

66. Beyer T, Townsend DW, Brun T, et al. A combined PET/CT scanner for clinical oncology. J Nucl Med 2000;41(8):1369–79.

67. Lardinois D, Weder W, Hany TF, et al. Staging of non-small-cell lung cancer with integrated positron-emission tomography and computed tomography. N Engl J Med 2003;348:2500–7.

68. Mamede M, Abreu-E-Lima P, Oliva MR, et al. FDG-PET/CT tumor segmentation-derived indices of metabolic activity to assess response to neoadjuvant therapy and progression-free survival in esophageal cancer: correlation with histopathology results. Am J Clin Oncol 2007;30(4):377–88.

69. Gerbaudo VH, Julius B. Anatomo-metabolic characteristics of atelectasis in F-18 FDG-PET/CT imaging. Eur J Radiol 2007;64(3):401–5.

70. Britz-Cunningham S, Millstein J. Improved discrimination of benign and malignant lesions on FDG PET/CT, using comparative activity ratios to brain, basal ganglia or cerebellum. Clin Nucl Med 2008; 33(10):681–7.

71. Ambrosini V, Rubello D, Nanni C, et al. Additional value of hybrid PET/CT fusion imaging vs. conventional CT scan alone in the staging and management of patients with malignant pleural mesothelioma. Nucl Med Rev Cent East Eur 2005;8(2):111–5.

72. Sørensen JB, Ravn J, Loft A, et al, Nordic Mesothelioma Group. Preoperative staging of mesothelioma by ^{18}F-fluoro-2-deoxy-D-glucose positron emission tomography/computed tomography fused imaging and mediastinoscopy compared to pathological findings after extrapleural pneumonectomy. Eur J Cardiothorac Surg 2008;34(5):1090–6.

73. Rusch VW. A proposed new international TNM staging system for malignant pleural mesothelioma from the International Mesothelioma Interest Group. Lung Cancer 1996;14:1–12.

74. Sugarbaker DJ, Strauss GM, Lynch TJ, et al. Node status has prognostic significance in the multimodality therapy of diffuse, malignant mesothelioma. J Clin Oncol 1993;11:1172–8.

75. Richards WG, Godleski JJ, Yeap BY, et al. Proposed adjustments to pathologic staging of epithelial malignant pleural mesothelioma based on analysis of 354 cases. Cancer 2010;116(6):1510–7.

76. Baldini EH, Recht A, Strauss GM, et al. Patterns of failure after trimodality therapy for malignant pleural mesothelioma. Ann Thorac Surg 1997;63(2):334–8.

77. Oksuzoglu B, Yalcin S, Erman M, et al. Leptomeningeal infiltration of malignant mesothelioma. Med Oncol 2002;19:167–9.

78. Gerbaudo VH, Mamede M, Trotman-Dickenson B, et al. FDG PET/CT patterns of treatment failure of malignant pleural mesothelioma: relationship to histologic type, treatment algorithm, and survival. Eur J Nucl Med Mol Imaging 2011;38(5):810–21.

79. Jänne PA, Baldini EH. Patterns of failure following surgical resection for malignant pleural mesothelioma. Thorac Surg Clin 2004;14(4):567–73.

80. Gill RR, Gerbaudo VH, Sugarbaker DJ, et al. Current trends in radiologic management of malignant pleural mesothelioma. Semin Thorac Cardiovasc Surg 2009;21(2):111–20.

81. Yamamuro M, Gerbaudo VH, Gill RR, et al. Morphologic and functional imaging of malignant pleural mesothelioma. Eur J Radiol 2007;64(3):356–66.

82. Tan C, Barrington S, Rankin S, et al. Role of integrated 18-fluorodeoxyglucose position emission tomography-computed tomography in patients surveillance after multimodality therapy of malignant pleural mesothelioma. J Thorac Oncol 2010;5(3):385–8.

83. Bénard F, Sterman D, Smith RJ, et al. Prognostic value of FDG PET imaging in malignant pleural mesothelioma. J Nucl Med 1999;40(8):1241–5.

84. Flores RM, Akhurst T, Gonen M, et al. Positron emission tomography predicts survival in malignant pleural mesothelioma. J Thorac Cardiovasc Surg 2006;132(4):763–8.

85. Krüger S, Pauls S, Mottaghy FM, et al. Integrated FDG PET-CT imaging improves staging in malignant pleural mesothelioma. Nuklearmedizin 2007;46(6):239–43.

86. Pass HI, Temeck BK, Kranda K, et al. Preoperative tumor volume is associated with outcome in malignant pleural mesothelioma. J Thorac Cardiovasc Surg 1998;115:310–8.

87. Nowak AK, Francis RJ, Phillips MJ, et al. A novel prognostic model for malignant mesothelioma incorporating quantitative FDG-PET imaging with clinical parameters. Clin Cancer Res 2010;16(8):2409–17.

88. Lee HY, Hyun SH, Lee KS, et al. Volume-based parameter of (18)F-FDG PET/CT in malignant pleural mesothelioma: prediction of therapeutic response and prognostic implications. Ann Surg Oncol 2010; 17(10):2787–94.

89. Lombardi G, Zustovich F, Nicoletto MO, et al. Diagnosis and treatment of malignant pleural effusion: a systematic literature review and new approaches. Am J Clin Oncol 2010;33(4):420–3.

90. Jones GR. Treatment of recurrent malignant pleural effusion by iodized talc pleurodesis. Thorax 1969; 24(1):69–73.

91. Bethune N. Pleural poudrage: a new technique for the deliberate production of pleural adhesions as a preliminary to lobectomy. J Thorac Surg 1935; 4:251.

92. Kwek BH, Aquino SL, Fischman AJ. Fluorodeoxyglucose positron emission tomography and CT after talc pleurodesis. Chest 2004;125(6):2356–60.

93. Nowak AK, Armato SG 3rd, Ceresoli GL, et al. Imaging in pleural mesothelioma: a review of imaging research presented at the 9th International Meeting of the International Mesothelioma Interest Group. Lung Cancer 2010;70(1):1–6.

94. Tsuji AB, Sogawa C, Sugyo A, et al. Comparison of conventional and novel PET tracers for imaging mesothelioma in nude mice with subcutaneous and intrapleural xenografts. Nucl Med Biol 2009;36(4):379–88.

95. Francis RJ, Nowak AN, Segard T, et al. FLT PET imaging in malignant pleural mesothelioma (MPM). International Mesothelioma Interest Group Meeting proceedings. 2010. p. 132, S08-3.

96. Lee ST, Scott AM. Hypoxia positron emission tomography imaging with ^{18}F-fluoromisonidazole. Semin Nucl Med 2007;37(6):451–6.

97. Ceresoli GL, Chiti A, Santoro A. ^{11}C-labeled methionine and evaluation of malignant pleural mesothelioma. N Engl J Med 2007;357:1982–4.

A Multimodality Imaging Review of Malignant Pleural Mesothelioma Response Assessment

Anna K. Nowak, MBBS, FRACP, PhD[a,b,*],
Roslyn J. Francis, MBBS, FRACP, PhD[a,b], Sharyn I. Katz, MD[c],
Victor H. Gerbaudo, PhD[d]

KEYWORDS

- Mesothelioma • Tumor response assessment • PET/CT
- Total glycolytic volume • Computed tomography
- Magnetic resonance imaging

Assessment of tumor response is a surrogate for patient benefit, allowing clinical trialists to share one language when discussing the activity of new agents and combinations. Implicit in this language is an understanding that tumor response may correspond to other benefits, such as improved survival, decreased symptoms, or better quality of life. Although tumor response is a corroborative end point in phase III clinical trials, in phase II studies it often assumes primary importance and, even if end points such as time to progression or progression-free survival are used, there is a reliance on tumor measurement to assign progression dates.

The first standardized response assessment criteria were developed 30 years ago following recognition by the World Health Organization (WHO) that standardizing tumor responses was important for interpretation of clinical trials results.[1] An updated alternative set of response criteria was subsequently developed by the Southwest

Oncology Group (SWOG) in response to perceived shortcomings in the WHO criteria.[2] However, these response criteria called for the measurement of "bidimensionally measurable lesions with clearly defined margins." With the publication of the Response Evaluation Criteria in Solid Tumors (RECIST) in 2000, although only unidimensional measurements were now required, these criteria still best applied to lesions that were spherical.[3] The updated RECIST 1.1 recently refined RECIST 1.0 and addressed some shortcomings and ambiguities, but did not improve on the usefulness of these criteria for mesothelioma.[4]

Unlike the spherical growth pattern of most primary tumor lesions, malignant pleural mesothelioma (MPM) does not grow concentrically from a central nidus, but instead grows as a sheet within the pleural cavity, eventually encasing the entire lung, contracting the chest wall, growing within the interlobar fissures, and often infiltrating the chest wall and mediastinum. Where disease takes

[a] School of Medicine and Pharmacology, University of Western Australia, 35 Stirling Highway, Nedlands, Perth 6009, Western Australia, Australia
[b] Department of Medical Oncology, Sir Charles Gairdner Hospital, Verdun Street, Nedlands, Perth 6009, Western Australia, Australia
[c] Department of Radiology, Hospital of the University of Pennsylvania, University of Pennsylvania School of Medicine, 1 Silverstein Building, 3400 Spruce Street, Philadelphia, PA 19104, USA
[d] Division of Nuclear Medicine and Molecular Imaging, Brigham and Women's Hospital, Harvard Medical School, 75 Francis Street, Boston, MA 02115, USA
* Corresponding author. School of Medicine and Pharmacology, University of Western Australia, 35 Stirling Highway, Nedlands, Perth 6009, Western Australia, Australia.
E-mail address: anowak@meddent.uwa.edu.au

PET Clin 6 (2011) 299–311
doi:10.1016/j.cpet.2011.04.002
1556-8598/11/$ – see front matter © 2011 Elsevier Inc. All rights reserved.

pet.theclinics.com

on a spherical morphology, it may not be representative of the tumor, or may be found in special locations such as the interlobar fissures. The location and growth pattern of this disease creates unique challenges for radiologists and clinicians assessing response to treatment when relying on the usual standard metrics. Nevertheless, the rarity of the disease and the paucity of phase III clinical trials make valid and reliable response assessment particularly important. This article reviews the current standards and emerging technologies for response assessment in MPM, and highlights controversies and areas for further research.

PRINCIPLES OF RESPONSE ASSESSMENT

The general principles of response assessment in mesothelioma are similar to the guidelines laid down by the RECIST 1.0 and 1.1 in that imaging is performed at baseline and repeated at relevant intervals using identical imaging techniques. Lesions at baseline are classified as measurable or nonmeasurable, with pleural and pericardial effusions considered as nonmeasurable disease. The size of measurable target lesions is documented at baseline, with nontarget lesions recorded as present. Superficial clinical lesions, such as skin nodules at sites of intervention, may be measured with calipers and should ideally be photographed. Response is then categorized at successive time points as complete response (CR), partial response (PR), stable disease (SD), or progressive disease (PD). Although these general principles apply readily to MPM, the details of how to measure tumor rind were open to a wide range of interpretation after the RECIST 1.0 were published.[5–7]

RADIOLOGICAL RESPONSE ASSESSMENT USING COMPUTED TOMOGRAPHY

Computed tomography (CT) is the most widely available technique that is routinely used for response assessment in MPM. Although chest radiography (CXR) is allowed for response assessment in the RECIST 1.0 and 1.1, RECIST 1.1 specifies that measurable lesions on CXR should be surrounded by aerated lung, thus making it unsuitable to assess pleural thickness in MPM. The CT measurement of MPM in clinical trials became better standardized following publication of the Modified RECIST in 2004.[8] Rather than truly modifying the RECIST, Modified RECIST sets out guidelines for applying the RECIST 1.0 to the unique growth pattern of MPM. Chief among these is the directive to measure pleural rind unidimensionally as a tumor thickness perpendicular to the chest wall or mediastinum, rather than in the longest

diameter, which may be difficult to assess in this disease (**Fig. 1**). Although the original RECIST 1.0 calls for 5 target lesions per organ and up to 10 in total to be summated, Modified RECIST calls for measurement of 2 pleural lesions, at each of 3 levels on transverse slices at least 1 cm apart, for a sum of pleural measurements. The locally invasive nature of MPM means that these 6 lesions are commonly the only tumor measurements taken. Furthermore, nodal disease can be measured separately, especially in those cases in which there is no measurable pleural lesion. The definitions of response are applied exactly as per RECIST 1.0.[3]

In validating these criteria, response to therapy measured this way was shown to predict survival and to have functional implications, in that responding patients showed an improvement in forced vital capacity (FVC) in the course of 6 treatment cycles. Hence, although these criteria can be criticized on many levels, they have shown value as a surrogate of clinical benefit, which is one of the desired roles of any useful surrogate marker in clinical trials.

However, there are several issues that are not clarified by the Modified RECIST. The definition of measurable disease has not been stated, although the RECIST 1.0 and 1.1 definition of 10 mm for disease to be considered as measurable should be used. Similarly, there is no guidance on selection of measurement sites, or demonstration of interobserver and intraobserver reliability.

RECIST 1.0, RECIST 1.1, AND THE MODIFIED RECIST

With the publication of RECIST 1.1, there are now some aspects of the Modified RECIST that are not congruent with the new, accepted metric in other

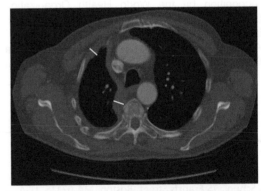

Fig. 1. The Modified RECIST specifies unidimensional measurement of tumor rind perpendicular to mediastinal structures or chest wall, rather than in the longest dimension. The white lines are examples of the placement of such measurement sites.

diseases. In particular, enlarged lymph nodes are now required to have a minimum short axis diameter of 15 mm, as opposed to 10 mm in RECIST 1.0,[9] and should be considered normal when they have decreased to a short axis diameter less than 10 mm. Individual clinical trials may consider adding this recommendation to response assessment guidelines to accord with RECIST 1.1. RECIST 1.1 also stipulates measurement of 5, rather than 10, target lesions, with no more than 2 per organ, and presents evidence that this does not change response assessment.[10] Similar evidence has been presented in other solid tumors.[11] At the moment, given that the Modified RECIST has been validated on 6 pleural unidimensional lesion measurements, and that measurement of only 2 lesions would not be representative of pleural bulk, there is no call to alter this in line with RECIST 1.1. RECIST 1.1 suggests that lesions that decrease to less than 5 mm but remain visible should be arbitrarily assigned a value of 5 mm. The main effect of this is to reduce the likelihood of premature determination of progression caused by observer variation while taking measurements at the lower limit of resolution. Again, individual trials could consider adding this recommendation in response assessment guidelines.

SPECIAL SITUATIONS IN RADIOLOGICAL RESPONSE ASSESSMENT FOR MESOTHELIOMA
Small Tumor Rind

An important problem facing clinical investigators is finding measurable disease in symptomatic patients with thin tumor rinds. The surface contact area of each visceral-parietal pleural pair is approximately 1000 cm^2. A 1-mm-thick rind of tumor throughout a unilateral pleural space would equate to a tumor volume of around 100 cm^3, similar to that of a spherical tumor between 6 and 7 cm in diameter. In most other organs, this would be considered a substantial local tumor mass. In MPM, this volume of tumor, if spread evenly throughout the pleural space, would not even approach measurability standards for a clinical trial, and would also be impossible to assess for the management of individual patients. This scenario is common in MPM, in which the pleura may be uniformly involved because of the field effect of asbestos exposure (Fig. 2). If there is no measurable pleural lesion, it can be helpful to find measurable nodal disease to allow patients to participate in a clinical trial.

Pleural Effusion

Pleural effusions are common in MPM, and can mask pleural tumor, or masquerade as tumor

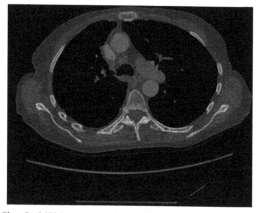

Fig. 2. MPM presentation with thin circumferential tumor rind represents substantial tumor bulk, but often does not provide any areas of tumor thickness suitable for assessment of response.

masses in the case of complex proteinaceous loculated effusions. Pleural effusion is never considered as a target or nontarget lesion, and an increase or decrease in the quantity of pleural fluid should not be used to assess disease response or progression. The use of intravenous (IV) contrast with CT, optimized for evaluation of the pleura, may assist in distinguishing pleural effusion from neoplastic pleural rind.[12] Investigators should always inspect all scan levels before selecting sites for measurement to avoid inadvertently selecting a site of loculated pleural effusion. In considering causes for new pleural effusion in patients with MPM, clinicians must be aware of other potential causes for pleural effusion including posttherapeutic hemorrhage, pneumonia, empyema, cardiogenic edema, and ascites.

Pleurodesis

Pleural effusions are a frequent cause of dyspnea in patients with MPM. Early treatment of recurrent pleural effusions is important for palliation and to prevent trapped lung syndrome. Bethune[13] introduced the technique of talc pleurodesis in 1935, although obliteration of the pleural space by inducing a chronic inflammatory response can be achieved through the instillation of talc, antibiotics, antiparasitics, or chemotherapeutic agents.[14] Talc pleurodesis is still considered the technique of choice to treat symptomatic malignant effusions and recurring spontaneous pneumothoraces.[15]

At postmortem examination, macroscopic patterns of pleural chemical sclerosis start with an early phase of purulent hemorrhagic exudate, followed by a collagenous phase coupled with a necrotic component and a talc granulomatous reaction. Six months later, the process evolves into a chronic inflammatory response leading to pleural fibrosis.[16] This process leads to imaging findings independent of the underlying malignant disease process. The CT features of talc pleurodesis consist of pleural areas of very high attenuation (mean CT attenuation values ranging from 140 to 380 HU), with single or multiple focal, nodular, or linear plaquelike areas of thickening, representing talc deposits and associated granulomatous reaction with hyaline fibrosis. In general, the pleural thickening associated with talc pleurodesis in the chronic setting is planar and minimal in thickness, although more exuberant and nodular configurations are common and typically occur in the posterobasilar pleural surfaces, often in the paramediastinal or paravertebral areas. One small study of 20 patients who received talc pleurodesis showed an uneven distribution of talc in 75% of patients, with 50% or more of the talc located in the posterior and posterobasilar hemithorax.[17]

In a study of 133 patients receiving talc pleurodesis to prevent pneumothorax in the setting of lymphangioleiomyomatosis (LAM), a nonmalignant cystic pulmonary disease condition, 14% of patients developed pleural nodules following talc pleurodesis, 65% developed pleural thickening, and 11% developed loculated pleural effusions.[18] The nodules that developed in this study enhanced with IV contrast administration and were stable or decreased in size in a 6-year period. Other investigators have reported that these talc-induced fibrotic lesions remain stable on subsequent CT scans, and usually do not enhance following contrast administration.[19,20] The disparity between reports regarding enhancement may be explained by differences in timing of IV contrast delivery. Rarely, these talc-containing nodules can grow slowly for a long period and mimic neoplasms, termed talcomas.[21]

Familiarization with the CT appearance of the pleura following pleurodesis is important when following therapeutic response in pleural malignancy. In MPM, this is further complicated by calcified pleural plaques related to asbestos exposure that also typically distribute along the lower third of the hemithorax. However, these are almost always bilateral and tend to be distributed circumferentially.[19] To prevent confusion in follow-up imaging, comparisons with prior imaging, including pretherapy imaging, and an accurate clinical history regarding pleurodesis are vital for accurate assessment of therapeutic response.

Atelectatic Lung

Atelectatic lung can cause difficulties in response assessment, particularly if atelectasis is mistakenly assessed as tumor at baseline. There are 2 types of atelectasis that are common in patients with MPM: compressive atelectasis and rounded atelectasis. Compressive atelectasis is the resultant loss of alveolar air caused by adjacent mass effect. It usually appears as a bandlike region of airless lung opposed to the cause of the mass effect, which in MPM is usually a combination of pleural fluid and pleural tumor. Because airless lung adjacent to high-attenuation pleural fluid or tumor can lead to inaccurate tumor measurement, tumor measurement should be performed away from areas of pleural fluid whenever possible.

Rounded atelectasis occurs in pleural thickening and is commonly observed in association with asbestos-related pleural plaques and MPM. Rounded atelectasis likely begins with a focal area of visceral pleuritis that matures into fibrosis, thickening, and retraction of the pleura. This process results in an inward curling of the pleural surface and subsequent collapse of the underlying lung parenchyma into a masslike focus seen on CT.[22] Rounded atelectasis can be easily recognized by the swirling bronchovascular structures that are rolled into this area of folded lung and pleural thickening with linear proximal tails radiating from the hilum in a configuration termed the comet-tail sign. In most cases, pleural effusion is either minimal or not present.[23,24] Considering that rounded atelectasis commonly coexists with asbestos-related disease, including MPM, it is important to be aware of avoiding areas of rounded atelectasis in measurements for response assessment.[25]

DIFFICULTIES AND CONTROVERSIES IN CT RESPONSE ASSESSMENT

The Modified RECIST have been criticized for high interobserver variability, and by studies modeling different mesothelioma growth patterns.[26,27] Armato and colleagues[26] assessed variability while measuring unidimensional tumor thickness between 5 observers and intraobserver variability within 3 observers. Measurements of the 5 observers were highly correlated, and most measurements were within 15% of each other. There was a higher degree of intraobserver correlation. However, there was a higher degree of variability in the angle of measurement, and this was even more problematic for computer-generated linear tumor measurements. Measured tumor thickness in MPM depends on the vector or angle at which it is taken (**Fig. 3**). Unless initial measurements are recorded and available for visual comparison of measurement vectors, such errors are to be anticipated. This group also showed that interobserver measurement agreement was better when observers were able to visualize previous measurements, rather

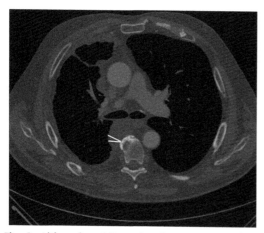

Fig. 3. Although unidimensional measurement lines originate from 1 point, differences in vectors of measurement have led to 15% increase in tumor measurement, from 18.7 to 21.4 mm.

than imputing the location of the measurement from a descriptive report, although response classification was little changed.[26] Unlike RECIST, which stipulates measurement of the longest diameter of the lesion irrespective of axis changes between examinations, Modified RECIST measurements should be taken at the same location on the pleura and in the same direction each time, and should be visually recorded to allow the investigator to reapply the same vector or angle at the same site on each assessment during and after therapy.

Armato and colleagues[26] also noted that selection of CT slices for unidimensional measurements was highly variable between 2 observers, with agreement on slice selection in only 24% of 66 slices. There can be no clear guideline on site selection that covers all possibilities. It is most important that slices selected contain reproducible anatomic landmarks (eg, the aortic arch, the carina, or the pulmonary artery) in order that the same anatomic site can be located for subsequent measurements. However, this may not always ensure that the same site is being measured on each examination, because the relationship of the chest wall and ribs to the mediastinum may alter as tumor bulk increases or decreases and as the chest wall contracts over time.

An important shortcoming of the unidimensional response criteria for MPM is that, in this disease, the relationship between unidimensional changes, -30% for response and $+20\%$ for progression, and change in the volume of the lesion, is undoubtedly different from that in spherical tumors. This difference was elegantly shown by Oxnard and colleagues,[27] who used geometric models to propose that use of the RECIST for PD and PR

corresponded to a 20% increase and 30% decrease in volume respectively when pleural thickness was measured, rather than the 73% increase and 66% decrease that corresponding changes in linear measurements elicit for a spherical lesion. In a study presented in abstract form, the same group showed that fewer than 50% of patients classified as having PD on unidimensional criteria had an increase in the two-dimensional (2D) area of tumor on the CT slices from which measurements were taken.[28] Contrary to the mathematical modeling data, this suggests that progression is being overestimated rather than underestimated. A more recent publication comparing volumetric response with Modified RECIST response suggested that volumetric response assessment, directly extrapolating response criteria from spherical tumors, resulted in more patients being assessed as having SD rather than PR, or PD rather than SD.[29] Nevertheless, the Modified RECIST have been validated as a surrogate for patient benefit in survival and lung function, suggesting that the aims of standardizing tumor measurement are being met, regardless of whether the volumetric changes accord with those in cancers with a spherical morphology. They remain the current, albeit imperfect, standard for radiological response assessment.

EMERGING TECHNOLOGIES IN CT RESPONSE ASSESSMENT

Although unidimensional measurements are used as the current standard, they are labor intensive, suffer from interobserver and intraobserver variability, and arguably do not truly represent the bulk of disease. Manual delineation of tumor bulk is even more time consuming. There are several groups working on automated or semiautomated measurement of tumor volume using CT imaging algorithms, which may have the advantage of standardizing and automating measurement techniques, although it is moving away from the prevailing paradigm of simple unidimensional measurements used in other tumors. Nevertheless, this approach is technically challenging and is still being optimized.[30] If these approaches are to be applied to clinical trial response measurements, they will require a new set of response criteria and careful validation with meaningful clinical outcomes such as survival, lung function, and quality of life.

METABOLIC RESPONSE ASSESSMENT USING [^{18}F]FLUORODEOXYGLUCOSE POSITRON EMISSION TOMOGRAPHY

[^{18}F]Fluorodeoxyglucose (FDG)-positron emission tomography (PET) is a functional imaging modality that is emerging as a potentially powerful imaging biomarker of cancer therapy in a broad range of solid tumors. For diseases in which CR can be achieved, FDG-PET seems more accurate than CT in differentiating residual viable tumor from fibrosis or necrosis in posttherapy residual CT masses.[31] This difference has been particularly apparent in the posttherapy assessment of lymphoma, and FDG-PET assessments are now incorporated into lymphoma response protocols.[32] FDG-PET has also been shown in multiple different solid tumor types to predict response to chemotherapy and patient outcomes early, often after only 1 or 2 cycles of chemotherapy. This finding may potentially lead to individualization of therapy, and may ultimately have a significant impact on subsequent patient management. However, despite the increasing clinical use of FDG-PET for response assessment, until recently there has been no clear standardization of imaging protocols, machine calibration, or reporting criteria, which has limited the use of FDG-PET in assessment of response in clinical trials, particularly those involving multiple sites.

The PET Response Criteria in Solid Tumors (PERCIST), published in 2009, provide guidelines for semiquantitative analysis of FDG-PET scans, in particular for application to multicenter clinical trials that incorporate FDG-PET for response assessment.[33] The PERCIST incorporate the principles of the RECIST for response categorization, and help define region placement for standardized uptake value (SUV) measurements. Additional guidelines for PET and PET/CT, as well as quality control procedures, have been published to ensure that optimal images are obtained, to facilitate semiquantitative assessments, and to allow for incorporation of FDG-PET response evaluations into multicenter clinical trials.[34,35]

FDG-PET RESPONSE ASSESSMENT IN MESOTHELIOMA

Once established, MPM is often intensely metabolically active on FDG-PET imaging, and is characteristically seen as a contiguous or semicontiguous rind of tumor around the pleural surface involving costal, diaphragmatic, and mediastinal pleura (Fig. 4). Infiltration of the fissures is commonly seen, and the differentiation between pleural fluid and active tumor is usually apparent.

In 2006, Ceresoli and colleagues[36] published the first study showing the potential value of FDG-PET in response assessment in MPM. This study used the maximum standardized uptake value (SUVmax) to assess response in 20 evaluable patients after 2 cycles of pemetrexed-based chemotherapy. A PR, as defined by a 25% reduction in SUVmax, was seen in 8 patients (40%), and this translated to an

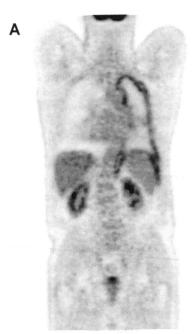
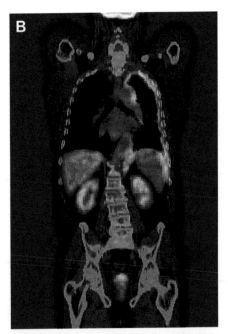

Fig. 4. Representative coronal FDG-PET (*A*) and fused PET/CT (*B*) images of left pleural mesothelioma. Abnormal FDG activity is visualized circumferentially around the pleural surface, involving costal, diaphragmatic, and mediastinal pleura, also with involvement of the major fissure.

improved time to progression (TTP) of 14 months versus 7 months for nonresponders ($P = .02$), and a trend to improved survival ($P = .07$). No correlation was found between radiological response after 2 cycles and TTP.

In a concurrent study, Francis and colleagues[37] used volumetric analysis of metabolic response in 23 evaluable patients with MPM. FDG-PET imaging was performed at baseline and after 1 cycle of chemotherapy with cisplatin and gemcitabine. A semiautomated region-growing algorithm was used to define three-dimensional (3D) volumes of interest (VOI), from which the total glycolytic volume (TGV) was obtained. TGV is a composite of metabolic activity and volume. The study showed a strong relationship between change in TGV after only 1 cycle of chemotherapy and survival ($P = .015$). Neither SUVmax on FDG-PET imaging or CT response using Modified RECIST after the first cycle of chemotherapy were predictive for survival ($P = .097$ and $P = .131$, respectively).

A recent publication reported experience with FDG-PET/CT performed at baseline and after 3 cycles of first-line or second-line pemetrexed and platinum chemotherapy in 41 patients.[38] PET/CT response parameters included SUVmax, mean standardized uptake value (SUVmean), PET-based volumetric measurement (PETvol), and tumor lesion glycolysis (TLG). The PETvol was derived using a rectangular VOI placed over the involved hemithorax, and voxels with SUV of greater than 2.5 included in the VOI. TLG was defined as SUVmean multiplied by PETvol. Neither SUVmax ($P = .61$) nor SUVmean ($P = .68$) were prognostic for overall survival. However, the volume-based measures of PETvol ($P = .0002$) and TLG ($P = .01$) were predictive of survival. CT response using Modified RECIST were also predictive of survival ($P = .001$) after 3 cycles of chemotherapy.

These 3 studies represent the largest published series of response assessment in MPM using FDG-PET. Several other studies have been published in abstract form only. The sample size in all studies to date is small (maximum 41 patients), the studies vary in timing of the PET scans in relation to chemotherapy (1–3 cycles), chemotherapy regimens, method of analysis (SUVmax, TGV, TLG), response criteria (European Organization for Research and Treatment of Cancer [EORTC], continuous variable) and outcome measures (TTP or survival). No published studies to date have analyzed FDG-PET response in MPM using the recently proposed PERCIST. However, despite the variability in the clinical studies to date, the emerging evidence is that obtaining a metabolic response seems to have prognostic value, often at a time point before radiological response.

THE ROLE OF VOLUMETRIC RESPONSE IN PET ASSESSMENT

The most commonly used measure of response in FDG-PET imaging is SUVmax, which represents the most intense FDG activity in the tumor and is a single-voxel value. Determining the SUVmax in MPM can be challenging because of the rindlike tumor growth around the pleural cavity. SUVmax also can be influenced by technical factors, and therefore PERCIST propose using the SUVmean of a 1.1-cm diameter VOI placed at the most intense region of tumor, in order that the measure of intensity is not just dependent on 1 voxel.[33] Whether it is a single-voxel value or a 1.1-cm diameter VOI, it could be argued that SUV intensity measures alone are an underrepresentation of change in a tumor that often encompasses the entire pleural cavity.

Volume-based measures of response (TGV/TLG) may be more sensitive than single-voxel values, such as SUVmax, because they provide a better overall representation of tumor burden. Volume-based measures take into account both tumor volume and intensity. An important variable then becomes the method for region generation of the VOI, because this may substantially influence the TGV/TLG. Two proposed methods in MPM include a semiautomated, iterative, region growing algorithm[37] and a fixed threshold approach (SUV>2.5).[38] The semiautomated region-growing algorithm applies an adaptive threshold that is influenced by the SUV intensity measure of adjacent background (ie, liver). This method is more sophisticated than fixed threshold approaches and has less chance of including adjacent normal tissue, although it does require software and time, and may have problems with interuser reproducibility. Veit-Heichbach and colleagues apply a fixed threshold of SUV greater than 2.5 in the user-determined hemithorax.[38] The fixed threshold method is simple and does not require sophisticated software. However, it may include nontumor in the VOI, provided the SUV is greater than 2.5. This problem may potentially occur for the liver, which is immediately adjacent to the pleural surface. The myocardium can usually be separated using a dedicated VOI. Both methods seem more sensitive than SUVmax for prediction of response to chemotherapy in the published studies to date. Volume-based approaches (TGV/TLG) seem to be more sensitive to change within the tumor mass and, therefore, larger reductions in TGV/TLG may be required for a meaningful response, compared with SUV measures.

In summary, there are insufficient data currently in FDG-PET imaging in response assessment in MPM to recommend either a definite method for response assessment (SUV vs TLG/TGV) or to identify a percentage reduction cutoff that could be used in clinical trials to categorize patients as metabolic responders. However, the data that are emerging are extremely encouraging for the potential value of FDG-PET imaging in response assessment in MPM. Larger clinical trials, ideally multicenter, are required to ascertain the value of FDG-PET for response assessment in MPM.

ISSUES IN FDG-PET RESPONSE ASSESSMENT IN MESOTHELIOMA
Pleurodesis

Increased FDG uptake is common in inflammatory processes, and is related to the expression of the rate-limiting steps of FDG uptake, mainly GLUT receptors and hexokinase, by activated macrophages and other inflammatory cells.[39,40] Therefore, areas affected by talc pleurodesis are often FDG avid.[20,41,42] Kwek and colleagues[20] described focal and diffuse patterns of FDG uptake in pleurodesis. Focal (single or multiple) patterns were observed in both plaquelike and nodular areas of high-attenuation pleural thickening, and, although not as common, a diffuse pattern of uptake was also seen in some patients. Recognition of the known anatomometabolic patterns of pleurodesis on CT and PET images is essential to be able to characterize the nonmalignant nature of high FDG uptake in pleurodesis-induced granulomatous reactions. This ability in turn will help minimize false-positive interpretations of benign foci of pleural densities and/or uptake during the diagnostic, staging, and monitoring of response to therapy in patients with MPM.

The inflammatory effect of pleurodesis may confound the assessment of response on FDG-PET imaging in patients with MPM, which is likely to be particularly problematic with recent pleurodesis because the inflammatory effects of pleurodesis may be increasing (shortly after pleurodesis) or decreasing over time, and reduction in metabolic activity may not be able to be reliably discriminated from the effects of chemotherapy on tumor. The intensity of inflammatory activity from pleurodesis is usually similar to tumor activity. The distribution of activity also usually cannot be discriminated. Assessing the time course of inflammatory effects of pleurodesis in patients with MPM is difficult, because, even in the absence of treatment, there are 2 concurrent processes: tumor growth over time and changes caused by pleurodesis.

Consequently, the confounding effects of pleurodesis on metabolic activity in the pleura have resulted in several investigators either recommending exclusion of all patients with previous pleurodesis from clinical trials of FDG-PET imaging for response assessment, or exclusion of patients with recent pleurodesis.[36,37] The definition of recent pleurodesis has not been determined, although in some cases it has been arbitrarily assigned as 6 months. This topic therefore remains an area of controversy of which clinicians need to be aware, and it makes the use of FDG-PET response as an end point in clinical trials difficult. Accurate data collection on patients' history of talc pleurodesis is essential when considering response assessment with FDG-PET in this patient group.

Atelectasis

Recently, metabolic imaging with FDG-PET and PET/CT has proved helpful to differentiate atelectatic lung not involved by tumor from tumor-infiltrated atelectatic lung and from normal lung.[43–45] In addition to its diagnostic value, the accurate differentiation between tumor and atelectasis achieved by PET has proved beneficial for the creation of appropriate size portals during radiation therapy planning, to minimize radiation dose to normal tissue,[46] and could potentially be useful in ensuring that selection of sites for response assessment avoids atelectatic areas. McAdams and colleagues[44] reported their results on 9 patients with rounded atelectasis who underwent dedicated FDG-PET imaging. None of the 10 lesions were FDG avid, so the investigators concluded that FDG-PET imaging might play a role in differentiating rounded atelectasis from malignancy in those cases with atypical patterns encountered on chest radiographs and CT.

Gerbaudo and Julius[45] studied the anatomometabolic characteristics of atelectasis with FDG-PET/CT using qualitative and semiquantitative analysis. The pattern of uptake in atelectasis was described as diffuse and homogeneous, and, in some cases, heterogeneous uptake was observed in the larger areas of collapse.[45] The investigators indicated that, regardless of the size of collapse, the intensity of FDG uptake in atelectasis was low to moderate, always higher than in the normal lung, and generally lower than in malignant lesions. FDG avidity was higher in relaxation and resorptive atelectasis compared with the dependent and rounded subtypes of atelectasis, but the difference was not statistically significant. However, a positive relationship was found between the attenuation of collapse and FDG uptake in the atelectatic lung, which in turn had a negative effect on specificity. Although tumors had significantly higher SUVs, in 3 out of 21 (14%) patients, FDG uptake in the collapsed lung overlapped with SUVs at the low end of the range for malignancies in this patient cohort. Kikuchi and colleagues[47] reported a case in which rounded atelectasis had moderate FDG uptake with a baseline SUV of 2.56 that increased to 3.47 after dual-time-point PET imaging, which could have been interpreted as malignant. Careful inspection of the anatomometabolic patterns observed on the fused PET/CT images can prove helpful in these types of cases. The complementary information from both sets of images regarding lesion size, lesion shape, a diffuse pattern of uptake, and a low degree of FDG avidity facilitates the distinction of atelectasis from tumor in those cases with equivocal findings on CT and/or PET.

NOVEL PET RADIOTRACERS FOR RESPONSE ASSESSMENT

A wide range of novel PET radiotracers are currently being developed and may find application for the assessment of therapeutic response in MPM. PET probes of cell proliferation, amino acid transport, apoptosis, hypoxia, and angiogenesis have already been developed and are being tested in other tumor types.

Of particular interest is the radiotracer 3'-deoxy-3'-[^{18}F]fluorothymidine (FLT), which is an analogue of thymidine and an established probe of cellular proliferation. FLT is transported into the cell and phosphorylated by thymidine kinase 1 (TK1), but is not incorporated into DNA. Its tissue kinetics are analogous to those for FDG, with phosphorylation as the rate-limiting step of FLT, which in most conditions correlates with DNA synthesis rate. FLT-PET has shown promise in several malignancies as an early marker of response to therapy, as early as 24 to 48 hours following initiation of chemotherapy. However, because of its modest sensitivity in most malignancies, FLT might have limited usefulness in following response to therapy in tumors less than 2 cm. A preclinical study has recently showed that murine mesotheliomas are FLT avid. Tsuji and colleagues[48] compared the biodistribution and uptake of FDG, FLT, and 4'-methyl-[^{11}C]thiothymidine (S-[^{11}C]dThd) using nude mouse models of epithelioid and sarcomatoid mesothelioma. The investigators found that FLT and S-[^{11}C]dThd uptake was higher in the epithelioid subtype, whereas sarcomatoid tumors were more avid for FDG. Clinical studies have confirmed mesothelioma to be a proliferative tumor, with FLT tumor activity seen in 32 of 33 prospectively recruited patients (**Fig. 5**).[49] Early response data after 1 cycle of chemotherapy suggest that FLT-PET visual response correlates with CT response, although these results are preliminary and the final analysis is pending.[50]

Although primarily used for imaging cerebral gliomas, [^{11}C]methionine (MET) has shown great potential in imaging head and neck cancers, melanoma, non-Hodgkin lymphoma, and, recently, to assess breast cancer response to therapy.[51–56] Amino acid radiotracers such as MET have advantages compared with FDG because of higher tumor-to-background contrast and less uptake in benign inflammatory processes.[57] In a case report, Ceresoli and colleagues[58] showed the usefulness of MET imaging in a patient with epithelioid MPM that was FDG negative but positive with MET imaging. The investigators successfully used MET imaging to monitor response to therapy after 2 cycles of pemetrexed plus carboplatin. Based on this experience, Ceresoli and colleagues[58] proposed that MET-PET may be used as an alternative modality to image those MPMs that are not FDG avid. The main limitation of MET is its short (20 minutes) half-life, which limits its use to PET imaging facilities that have an on-site cyclotron.

Radiolabeled annexin V is currently being studied as a marker of tumor cell apoptotic death in response to therapy. Annexin V binds to phosphatidylserine (PS), which becomes exposed on the cell surface once cellular commitment to apoptosis has begun. As a programmed cell death marker, Annexin V promises tumor death–specific imaging that may give timely definitive evidence of therapeutic response. Annexin V has recently been labeled with fluorine 18 and used as a probe to image apoptosis in preclinical models, with encouraging results.[59,60] Furthermore, a malonic acid derivative, [^{18}F]ML-10 (ApoSense), has recently been shown to accumulate in a cerebral artery occlusion model that correlated with histologic evidence of cell death. Presently, this agent is undergoing testing in phase II trials to monitor response to radiotherapy in other tumor types,[61] and pilot testing of this agent in MPM is also underway.

Tumor growth and metastasis require adequate blood supply. The importance of the angiogenic process in MPM is well documented. MPM cells express and respond to many angiogenic factors, including vascular endothelial growth factor (VEGF).[62,63] VEGF expression in MPM is correlated with microvascular density, and is associated with poor survival.[64] Antiangiogenic therapy is mainly cytostatic, inhibiting the development of tumor vascularity and affecting the existing vessels. A reduction in tumor size does not entirely represent the expected outcome of this type of treatment. Thus, evaluation of tumor response relying solely on changes in tumor size can lead to erroneous evaluation of the effects of antiangiogenic therapy. The assessment of tumor perfusion, vascularity, permeability, and the intrinsic biologic processes of angiogenesis should prove superior in assessing

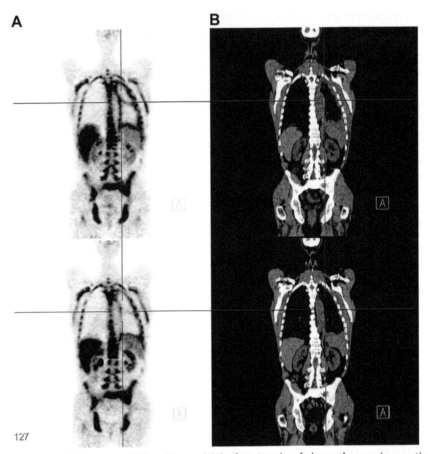

A

B

127

Fig. 5. FLT-PET/CT coronal images at (*A*) baseline and (*B*) after 1 cycle of chemotherapy in a patient with left pleural mesothelioma. Reduction in FLT activity (tumor proliferation) is seen in circumferential pleural tumor. Physiologic bone marrow activity is seen both at baseline and after treatment.

therapeutic response to antiangiogenic treatment. Tumor angiogenesis is facilitated by the upregulation of a family of cell surface receptors called integrins.[65] Antiangiogenesis probes, such as [^{18}F]galacto-arginine-glycine-aspartic acid (RGD), have been successfully developed by targeting the integrin $\alpha_v\beta_3$ via the tripeptide sequence RGD.[66] [^{18}F]Galacto-RGD has stable accumulation in $\alpha_v\beta_3$-expressing tumors, giving a high signal/noise ratio, and has been used with success to image tumor-associated angiogenesis and to estimate microvascular density.[67] There are several clinical trials currently assessing the addition of antiangiogenic agents to pemetrexed-based chemotherapy, but the clinical benefit of this approach is as yet unknown. To the best of our knowledge, there are no studies assessing the role of angiogenesis-targeted radiotracers to monitor response to MPM treatment. In addition to general markers of tumor metabolism, a specific imaging marker for MPM is also under development. The labeled antibody to mesothelin, K1,

may serve as a specific marker for mesothelioma when evaluating response to therapy.[68,69]

All these probes could represent the future of clinical molecular imaging in oncology beyond FDG. However, their availability is still limited, and much remains to be learned about the role of these novel radiotracers in the setting of monitoring response to MPM therapy.

CURRENT RESEARCH IN MESOTHELIOMA RESPONSE ASSESSMENT

In addition to implementing novel PET radiotracers, advances in response to therapy in MPM include further evaluation of existing technologies already in clinical use in this setting, including CT, FDG-PET, and magnetic resonance (MR) imaging. Volumetric FDG-PET measurement of MPM has been shown to provide robust prognostic predictive value[70] and a more accurate measure of therapeutic response than CT or conventional use of FDG-PET SUVmax.[37] CT techniques to improve the accuracy of tumor quantitation and tumor conspicuity are under development and are areas of active research in therapeutic response assessment. Also under investigation is clarification of the role of MR imaging in MPM, especially in light of novel techniques for mitigating the effects of respiratory and cardiac motion. Giesel and colleagues[71] evaluated the feasibility of perfusion delayed contrast enhancement MR imaging in 19 patients with MPM to monitor response to gemcitabine chemotherapy. Using a pharmacokinetic 2-compartment model, they estimated amplitude (Amp), redistribution rate constant (kep), and elimination rate constant (kel). Although Amp and kel successfully differentiated tumor from nontumor tissue ($P = .001$), nonresponders had a higher kep value (3.6 minutes) compared with responders (2.6 minutes), with significant correlation with survival after therapy (460 days vs 780 days, respectively). Plathow and colleagues[72] recently tested the value of 2D and 3D dynamic MR (dMR) imaging to evaluate lung motion and to monitor response after 3 and 6 cycles of chemotherapy in 22 patients with MPM, finding that dMR imaging using the 3D technique detected changes in lung motion and volume following therapy that were not evident by spirometry.

These results are promising and call for further testing in larger patient populations. The development of new probes and quantitative techniques should improve the ability of molecular imaging techniques and perfusion MR imaging to monitor the therapeutic effect of new therapies and to serve as useful and independent predictors of outcome.

SUMMARY

MPM continues to challenge clinical trialists, imaging specialists, and clinicians who wish to quantify and categorize response to treatment of clinical trials or for purposes of individualized patient care. The Modified RECIST remain the validated standard, but are acknowledged to be imperfect; improved techniques for assessing CT response are awaited, but must also be validated to ensure that imaging changes correspond with clinical outcomes. Given the difficulties in assessing radiological response in this disease, particularly for investigators who have little experience with MPM, independent central review of response or progression is recommended if response or progression-free survival is the primary end point of a clinical trial. FDG-PET is a promising technique for response assessment, but widespread implementation or use in clinical trials is hampered by uncertainty on the best metrics to use, lack of standardized validated response criteria, and difficulties interpreting FDG-PET after pleurodesis. International collaboration is required to gain adequate patient numbers for a large prospective validation study; this should be a priority for the MPM imaging research community.

ACKNOWLEDGMENTS

AKN acknowledges Professor Samuel Armato and Adam Starkey for use of the Abras software to produce **Figs. 1** to **3**.

REFERENCES

1. Miller A, Hoogstraten B, Staquet M, et al. Reporting results of cancer treatment. Cancer 1981;47:207.
2. Green S, Weiss GR. Southwest Oncology Group standard response criteria, endpoint definitions and toxicity criteria. Invest New Drugs 1992;10:239.
3. Therasse P, Arbuck SG, Eisenhauer EA, et al. New guidelines to evaluate the response to treatment in solid tumors. J Natl Cancer Inst 2000;92:205.
4. Eisenhauer EA, Therasse P, Bogaerts J, et al. New response evaluation criteria in solid tumours: revised RECIST guideline (version 1.1). Eur J Cancer 2009; 45:228.
5. Hillerdal G. Staging and evaluating responses in malignant pleural mesothelioma. Lung Cancer 2004;43:75.
6. van Klaveren RJ, Aerts JG, de Bruin H, et al. Inadequacy of the RECIST criteria for response evaluation in patients with malignant pleural mesothelioma. Lung Cancer 2004;43:63.
7. Monetti F, Casanova S, Grasso A, et al. Inadequacy of the new Response Evaluation Criteria in Solid Tumors (RECIST) in patients with malignant pleural mesothelioma: report of four cases. Lung Cancer 2004;43:71.
8. Byrne MJ, Nowak AK. Modified RECIST criteria for assessment of response in malignant pleural mesothelioma. Ann Oncol 2004;15:257.
9. Schwartz LH, Bogaerts J, Ford R, et al. Evaluation of lymph nodes with RECIST 1.1. Eur J Cancer 2009; 45:261.
10. Moskowitz CS, Jia X, Schwartz LH, et al. A simulation study to evaluate the impact of the number of lesions measured on response assessment. Eur J Cancer 2009;45:300.
11. Hillman SL, An MW, O'Connell MJ, et al. Evaluation of the optimal number of lesions needed for tumor evaluation using the response evaluation criteria in solid tumors: a north central cancer treatment group investigation. J Clin Oncol 2009;27:3205.
12. Helm EJ, Matin TN, Gleeson FV. Imaging of the pleura. J Magn Reson Imaging 2010;32:1275.

13. Bethune N. Pleural poudrage: a new technique for the deliberate production of pleural adhesions as a preliminary to lobectomy. J Thorac Surg 1935;4:251.

14. Adler RH, Sayek I. Treatment of malignant pleural effusion: a method using tube thoracostomy and talc. Ann Thorac Surg 1976;22:8.

15. Lombardi G, Zustovich F, Nicoletto MO, et al. Diagnosis and treatment of malignant pleural effusion: a systematic literature review and new approaches. Am J Clin Oncol 2010;33:420.

16. Jones GR. Treatment of recurrent malignant pleural effusion by iodized talc pleurodesis. Thorax 1969;24:69.

17. Mager HJ, Maesen B, Verzijlbergen F, et al. Distribution of talc suspension during treatment of malignant pleural effusion with talc pleurodesis. Lung Cancer 2002;36:77.

18. Avila NA, Dwyer AJ, Rabel A, et al. CT of pleural abnormalities in lymphangioleiomyomatosis and comparison of pleural findings after different types of pleurodesis. AJR Am J Roentgenol 2006;186:1007.

19. Murray JG, Erasmus JJ, Bahtiarian EA, et al. Talc pleurodesis simulating pleural metastases on 18F-fluorodeoxyglucose positron emission tomography. AJR Am J Roentgenol 1997;168:359.

20. Kwek BH, Aquino SL, Fischman AJ. Fluorodeoxyglucose positron emission tomography and CT after talc pleurodesis. Chest 2004;125:2356.

21. Hemdan Abdalla AM, White D. A 29-year-old woman with a remote history of osteosarcoma and positron emission tomography-positive pleurally based masses. Chest 2008;134:640.

22. Menzies R, Fraser R. Round atelectasis. Pathologic and pathogenetic features. Am J Surg Pathol 1987;11:674.

23. Blesovsky A. The folded lung. Br J Dis Chest 1966;60:19.

24. Schneider HJ, Felson B, Gonzalez LL. Rounded atelectasis. AJR Am J Roentgenol 1980;134:225.

25. Mintzer RA, Gore RM, Vogelzang RL, et al. Rounded atelectasis and its association with asbestos-induced pleural disease. Radiology 1981;139:567.

26. Armato SG 3rd, Ogarek JL, Starkey A, et al. Variability in mesothelioma tumor response classification. AJR Am J Roentgenol 2006;186:1000.

27. Oxnard GR, Armato SG 3rd, Kindler HL. Modeling of mesothelioma growth demonstrates weaknesses of current response criteria. Lung Cancer 2006;52:141.

28. Nowak AK, Armato SG 3rd, Ceresoli GL, et al. Imaging in pleural mesothelioma: a review of imaging research presented at the 9th International Meeting of the International Mesothelioma Interest Group. Lung Cancer 2010;70:1.

29. Frauenfelder T, Tutic M, Weder W, et al. Volumetry – an alternative to assess therapy response for malignant pleural mesothelioma? Eur Respir J 2011. [Epub ahead of print].

30. Armato SG 3rd, Entwisle J, Truong MT, et al. Current state and future directions of pleural mesothelioma imaging. Lung Cancer 2008;59:411.

31. Weber WA. Assessing tumor response to therapy. J Nucl Med 2009;50(Suppl 1):1S.

32. Cheson BD, Pfistner B, Juweid ME, et al. Revised response criteria for malignant lymphoma. J Clin Oncol 2007;25:579.

33. Wahl RL, Jacene H, Kasamon Y, et al. From RECIST to PERCIST: evolving considerations for PET Response Criteria in Solid Tumors. J Nucl Med 2009;50(Suppl 1):122S.

34. Boellaard R, O'Doherty MJ, Weber WA, et al. FDG PET and PET/CT: EANM procedure guidelines for tumour PET imaging: version 1.0. Eur J Nucl Med Mol Imaging 2010;37:181.

35. Delbeke D, Coleman RE, Guiberteau MJ, et al. Procedure guideline for tumor imaging with 18F-FDG PET/CT 1.0. J Nucl Med 2006;47:885.

36. Ceresoli GL, Chiti A, Zucali PA, et al. Early response evaluation in malignant pleural mesothelioma by positron emission tomography with [18F] fluorodeoxyglucose. J Clin Oncol 2006;24:4587.

37. Francis RJ, Byrne MJ, van der Schaaf AA, et al. Early prediction of response to chemotherapy and survival in malignant pleural mesothelioma using a novel semiautomated 3-dimensional volume-based analysis of serial 18F-FDG PET scans. J Nucl Med 2007;48:1449.

38. Veit-Haibach P, Schaefer NG, Steinert H, et al. Combined FDG-PET/CT in response evaluation of malignant pleural mesothelioma. Lung Cancer 2010;67(3):311–7.

39. Jones HA, Clark RJ, Rhodes CG, et al. In vivo measurement of neutrophil activity in experimental lung inflammation. Am J Respir Crit Care Med 1994;149:1635.

40. Jones HA, Cadwallader KA, White JF, et al. Dissociation between respiratory burst activity and deoxyglucose uptake in human neutrophil granulocytes: implications for interpretation of (18)F-FDG PET images. J Nucl Med 2002;43:652.

41. Strauss LG. Fluorine-18 deoxyglucose and false-positive results: a major problem in the diagnostics of oncological patients. Eur J Nucl Med 1996;23:1409.

42. Gerbaudo VH, Sugarbaker DJ, Britz-Cunningham S, et al. Assessment of malignant pleural mesothelioma with (18)F-FDG dual-head gamma-camera coincidence imaging: comparison with histopathology. J Nucl Med 2002;43:1144.

43. Kawabe J, Okamura T, Shakudo M, et al. Thallium and FDG uptake by atelectasis with bronchogenic carcinoma. Ann Nucl Med 1999;13:273.

44. McAdams HP, Erasums JJ, Patz EF, et al. Evaluation of patients with round atelectasis using 2-[18F]-fluoro-2-deoxy-D-glucose PET. J Comput Assist Tomogr 1998;22:601.

45. Gerbaudo VH, Julius B. Anatomo-metabolic characteristics of atelectasis in F-18 FDG-PET/CT imaging. Eur J Radiol 2007;64:401.

46. Nestle U, Walter K, Schmidt S, et al. 18F-deoxyglucose positron emission tomography (FDG-PET) for the planning of radiotherapy in lung cancer: high impact in patients with atelectasis. Int J Radiat Oncol Biol Phys 1999;44:593.

47. Kikuchi N, Kodama T, Satoh H. Positron emission tomography findings in rounded atelectasis. Tuberk Toraks 2009;57:483.

48. Tsuji AB, Sogawa C, Sugyo A, et al. Comparison of conventional and novel PET tracers for imaging mesothelioma in nude mice with subcutaneous and intrapleural xenografts. Nucl Med Biol 2009;36:379.

49. Nowak AK, Francis RJ, Segard T, et al. Early experience with [18F] fluorothymidine positron emission tomography (FLT PET) for response assessment in malignant pleural mesothelioma (MPM). J Thorac Oncol 2009;4:S389.

50. Francis RJ, Segard T, Philips MJ, et al. FLT PET imaging in malignant pleural mesothelioma (MPM). In: International Mesothelioma Interest Group Meeting. Kyoto, Japan, September 1, 2011. p. 132 [abstract S08-3].

51. Bustany P, Chatel M, Derlon JM, et al. Brain tumor protein synthesis and histological grades: a study by positron emission tomography (PET) with C11-L-Methionine. J Neurooncol 1986;3:397.

52. Leskinen-Kallio S, Lindholm P, Lapela M, et al. Imaging of head and neck tumors with positron emission tomography and [11C]methionine. Int J Radiat Oncol Biol Phys 1994;30:1195.

53. Lindholm P, Leskinen S, Nagren K, et al. Carbon-11-methionine PET imaging of malignant melanoma. J Nucl Med 1806;36:1995.

54. Lindholm P, Leskinen-Kallio S, Grenman R, et al. Evaluation of response to radiotherapy in head and neck cancer by positron emission tomography and [11C]methionine. Int J Radiat Oncol Biol Phys 1995;32:787.

55. Leskinen-Kallio S, Ruotsalainen U, Nagren K, et al. Uptake of carbon-11-methionine and fluorodeoxyglucose in non-Hodgkin's lymphoma: a PET study. J Nucl Med 1991;32:1211.

56. Lindholm P, Lapela M, Nagren K, et al. Preliminary study of carbon-11 methionine PET in the evaluation of early response to therapy in advanced breast cancer. Nucl Med Commun 2009;30:30.

57. Jager PL, Vaalburg W, Pruim J, et al. Radiolabeled amino acids: basic aspects and clinical applications in oncology. J Nucl Med 2001;42:432.

58. Ceresoli GL, Chiti A, Santoro A. 11C-labeled methionine and evaluation of malignant pleural mesothelioma. N Engl J Med 1982;357:2007.

59. Murakami Y, Takamatsu H, Taki J, et al. 18F-labelled annexin V: a PET tracer for apoptosis imaging. Eur J Nucl Med Mol Imaging 2004;31:469.

60. Yagle KJ, Eary JF, Tait JF, et al. Evaluation of 18F-annexin V as a PET imaging agent in an animal model of apoptosis. J Nucl Med 2005;46:658.

61. Reshef A, Shirvan A, Waterhouse RN, et al. Molecular imaging of neurovascular cell death in experimental cerebral stroke by PET. J Nucl Med 2008; 49:1520.

62. Ohta Y, Shridhar V, Bright RK, et al. VEGF and VEGF type C play an important role in angiogenesis and lymphangiogenesis in human malignant mesothelioma tumours. Br J Cancer 1999;81:54.

63. Kumar-Singh S, Weyler J, Martin MJ, et al. Angiogenic cytokines in mesothelioma: a study of VEGF, FGF-1 and -2, and TGF beta expression. J Pathol 1999;189:72.

64. Curran D, Sahmoud T, Therasse P, et al. Prognostic factors in patients with pleural mesothelioma: the European Organization for Research and Treatment of Cancer experience. J Clin Oncol 1998;16:145.

65. Clezardin P. Recent insights into the role of integrins in cancer metastasis. Cell Mol Life Sci 1998;54:541.

66. Haubner R, Wester HJ, Weber WA, et al. Noninvasive imaging of alpha(v)beta3 integrin expression using 18F-labeled RGD-containing glycopeptide and positron emission tomography. Cancer Res 2001;61:1781.

67. Drevs J, Schneider V. The use of vascular biomarkers and imaging studies in the early clinical development of anti-tumour agents targeting angiogenesis. J Intern Med 2006;260:517.

68. Hassan R, Wu C, Brechbiel MW, et al. 111Indium-labeled monoclonal antibody K1: biodistribution study in nude mice bearing a human carcinoma xenograft expressing mesothelin. Int J Cancer 1999;80:559.

69. Yoshida C, Sogawa C, Tsuji AB, et al. Development of positron emission tomography imaging by 64Cu-labeled Fab for detecting ERC/mesothelin in a mesothelioma mouse model. Nucl Med Commun 2010;31:380.

70. Nowak AK, Francis RJ, Phillips MJ, et al. A novel prognostic model for malignant mesothelioma incorporating quantitative FDG-PET imaging with clinical parameters. Clin Cancer Res 2010;16:2409.

71. Giesel FL, Bischoff H, von Tengg-Kobligk H, et al. Dynamic contrast-enhanced MRI of malignant pleural mesothelioma: a feasibility study of noninvasive assessment, therapeutic follow-up, and possible predictor of improved outcome. Chest 2006;129:1570.

72. Plathow C, Klopp M, Schoebinger M, et al. Monitoring of lung motion in patients with malignant pleural mesothelioma using two-dimensional and three-dimensional dynamic magnetic resonance imaging: comparison with spirometry. Invest Radiol 2006;41:443.

Cardiac Assessment with PET

Amol Takalkar, MD, MS[a,b,*], Anshul Agarwal, MD, PhD[c],
Scott Adams, MD[b], Abass Alavi, MD[d],
Drew A. Torigian, MD, MA[d]

KEYWORDS

- Myocardial perfusion imaging
- Coronary computed tomography angiography
- Cardiac imaging • Coronary artery calcium score
- Cardiac PET

PET, a nuclear medicine imaging technique that enables us to image functional processes occurring in the body, has now become an important imaging modality in the workup of several malignancies. Fluorine (F)-18–labeled fluorodeoxyglucose (FDG) is the main radiotracer used for oncologic imaging. Initially developed in the 1970s, it was applied for functional brain imaging and cardiac metabolism assessment. However, these applications did not progress to the routine clinical realm because the technology was limited mostly to research centers. In the last decade, the value of FDG-PET imaging in oncology was established, which has led to widespread use and availability of this modality across the United States and elsewhere in the world for this purpose. Along with the ease of accessibility, Food and Drug Administration (FDA) approval of PET cardiac perfusion radiotracers has led to a rebound in interest for cardiac PET applications. The recent shortage of technetium (Tc)-99m (the main radioisotope used for cardiac single-photon emission computed tomography [SPECT] imaging), the advantages of cardiac PET imaging over cardiac SPECT imaging, and the favorable reimbursement from Centers for Medicare and Medicaid for cardiac PET imaging have all resulted in a significant increase in routine clinical use of cardiac PET imaging for perfusion assessment.

PET has been very well validated for assessing myocardial viability, and a combination of myocardial perfusion imaging (MPI) using either PET or SPECT and metabolism imaging using FDG-PET has been considered the gold standard for noninvasive assessment of myocardial viability.[1] More recently, MPI with PET radiotracers (especially rubidium [Rb]-82) has increasingly been used in conjunction with or as an alternative to gated SPECT cardiac imaging with attenuation correction, the previous standard for MPI (which suffers from several disadvantages and can be particularly limited or equivocal in patients with a large body habitus). Advances in technology have led to development of integrated PET/computed tomography (CT) imaging systems, and there is potential for integrated PET/magnetic resonance (MR) imaging as well in the near future. These sophisticated hybrid imaging technologies offer tremendous promise for delivering an in-depth but noninvasive evaluation of cardiac perfusion and function in various pathologic conditions during a single imaging session. Moreover, there are several new PET radiotracers in the research and preclinical arena that are poised to enter the clinical setting

[a] PET Imaging Center, Biomedical Research Foundation of Northwest Louisiana, 1505 Kings Highway, Shreveport, LA 71103, USA
[b] Department of Radiology, Louisiana State University Health Sciences Center-Shreveport (LSUHSC-S), 1505 Kings Highway, Shreveport, LA 71103, USA
[c] Department of Nuclear Medicine, University of Texas Southwestern Medical Center, Dallas, TX, USA
[d] Department of Radiology, Hospital of the University of Pennsylvania, University of Pennsylvania School of Medicine, 3400 Spruce Street, Philadelphia, PA 19104, USA
* Corresponding author. PET Imaging Center, Biomedical Research Foundation of Northwest Louisiana, 1505 Kings Highway, Shreveport, LA 71103.
E-mail address: atakalka@biomed.org

PET Clin 6 (2011) 313–326
doi:10.1016/j.cpet.2011.05.002
1556-8598/11/$ – see front matter © 2011 Elsevier Inc. All rights reserved.

in the foreseeable future. With such exciting developments in noninvasive assessment of various cardiac pathologies on the horizon, cardiac PET and PET/CT imaging and potentially integrated cardiac PET/MR imaging have become the focus of the molecular imaging paradigm for comprehensive cardiovascular assessment.

PET MYOCARDIAL PERFUSION IMAGING

Myocardial perfusion has been traditionally assessed with cardiac SPECT imaging using either technetium- and/or thallium-based agents. Electrocardiogram gating and attenuation correction have led to significant improvement in myocardial perfusion evaluation with cardiac SPECT imaging. Despite this, SPECT cardiac perfusion imaging suffers from several limitations, and PET cardiac perfusion imaging offers several advantages over SPECT. By virtue of faster image acquisition and use of shorter-lived radionuclides, PET cardiac imaging protocols are more efficient, resulting in lower radiation exposure to patients. The superior attenuation correction algorithms in PET imaging makes it better suited for patients prone to attenuation artifacts. The better spatial and temporal resolution of PET imaging allows for detection of less apparent perfusion abnormalities, and facilitates absolute quantification of regional radiotracer uptake and detection of endothelial dysfunction. PET cardiac perfusion imaging permits more precise measurement of heart volumes and function with stress (unlike SPECT cardiac imaging with post-stress imaging), resulting in more accurate assessment.

At present, there are two FDA-approved PET radiotracers to assess myocardial perfusion: Nitrogen (N)-13 ammonia (NH_3) (cyclotron produced) and Rb-82 chloride (CI) (generator produced). A third agent commercially known as

flurpiridaz (BMS-747158-02 by Lantheus Medical Inc, North Billerica, MA, USA) recently completed a phase-2 multicenter clinical trial and is expected to enter phase-3 clinical trials in early to mid 2011.

Rb-82 was the first PET radiotracer to be FDA approved for MPI in 1989. It is obtained from a strontium (Sr)-82 generator and hence is readily available at imaging center sites. A single Sr-82 generator can be used for up to a month, as the physical half-life of Sr-82 is approximately 25 days. The expenses for a single generator are approximately \$35,000 a month, thus necessitating 4 to 5 studies a day (or at least 3 studies a day) to make this financially cost effective under current reimbursement rates. It has a very short physical half-life of 75 seconds that results in shorter duration of studies (generally <45 minutes for a rest-stress study), but also requires administration of higher doses of the radiotracer and excludes use of exercise stress. The physical characteristics of the positron emitted by Rb-82 (positron energy of 3.15 MeV and average positron range of 2.8 mm) are not quite optimal for imaging, resulting in slightly impaired spatial resolution (compared with other PET radioisotopes such as F-18 or N-13). Nevertheless, it produces high-resolution images (compared with SPECT). Rb-82 CI is transported into the cells by the active Na/K-ATPase pumps similar to potassium and thallium-201. **Fig. 1** shows a typical rest-stress myocardial perfusion study protocol using Rb-82 CI. **Fig. 2** illustrates the attenuation correction achieved by realigning the PET images with help of CT transmission images of the chest and subsequent processing. It is important to carefully confirm proper registration of the CT and PET images, as misregistration can lead to perfusion artifacts[2] and incorrect interpretation of the study. **Fig. 3** shows a normal PET MPI in rest and stress phases using Rb-82 with no perfusion defects. **Figs. 4–6** illustrate rest and stress myocardial perfusion PET images using

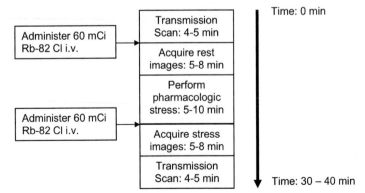

Fig. 1. Dose of rubidium is usually 30mCi for rest & stress each (total 60 mCi per study as per ASNC guidlines, the figure currently says 60 mCi for each part). (*Reproduced from* Takalkar A, Chen W, Desjardins B, et al. Cardiovascular imaging with PET, CT, and MR imaging. PET Clinics 2008;3(3):411–34; with permission.)

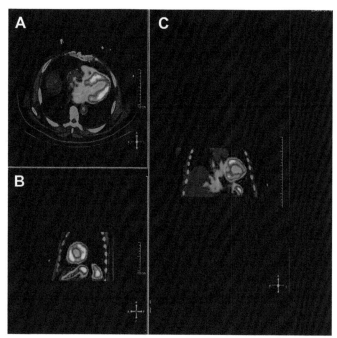

Fig. 2. Cardiac PET/CT attenuation correction. The selected images in transaxial (*A*), sagittal (*B*), and coronal (*C*) sections show attenuation correction achieved by realigning and processing the PET myocardial perfusion images with CT transmission images taken at stress phases. CT attenuation correction (CTAC) is done for both rest and stress phases, and final myocardial perfusion images are reconstructed in conventional short-axis, horizontal long-axis, and vertical long-axis projections for quantitative analysis.

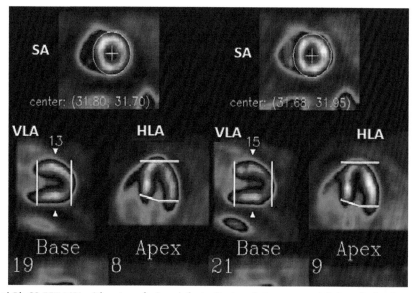

Fig. 3. Normal Rb-82 PET MPI without perfusion defects. Rest and stress myocardial perfusion imaging with PET using Rb-82 in a 56-year-old man with diabetes mellitus, hypertension, and morbid obesity complaining of exertional dyspnea and atypical chest pain. The patient was stressed pharmacologically with regadenoson. The images show myocardial perfusion in rest and stress phases without any perfusion defects in conventional short-axis (SA), horizontal long-axis (HLA), and vertical long-axis (VLA) projections.

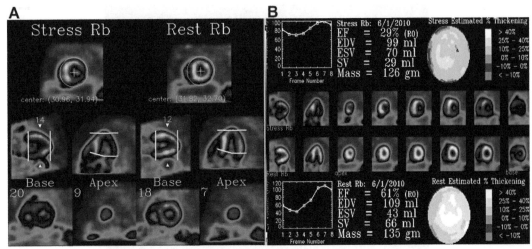

Fig. 4. Abnormal Rb-82 PET MPI with a reversible perfusion defect and reduced left ventricular ejection fraction (LVEF). The myocardial perfusion images are from an Rb-82 PET scan in a 59-year-old man with known coronary artery disease, and a history of percutaneous coronary intervention for the left anterior descending coronary artery (LAD). The patient was complaining of exertional arm and jaw pain, and the PET MPI was performed with 0.4 mg regadenoson as the pharmacologic stress agent. The perfusion images in conventional projections (A) show a large territory of moderately severe inferolateral reperfusion defect compatible with ischemia in an expected left circumflex distribution. Quantitative analysis (B) revealed a normal LVEF of 61% at rest, which fell to 29% at stress. There was evidence of transient ischemic dilation (TID) of the left ventricle between rest and stress imaging with a TID ratio abnormally elevated at 1.3 (normal <1.15). The summed stress score was calculated to be 15, and global hypokinesis was noted on stress-gated images. This patient also exhibited ST changes on electrocardiogram (ECG) and chest/jaw discomfort during the pharmacologic stress, which was reversed by aminophylline. EDV, end-diastolic volume; EF, ejection fraction; ESV, end-systolic volume; SV, stroke volume.

Rb-82 in diseased myocardium with reversible and nonreversible defects in different coronary territories. Such high-resolution and high-contrast images are commonly seen with PET Rb-82 MPI. It is noteworthy that these studies are typically completed in less than an hour. The ultra-short half-life requires imaging during pharmacologic stressor agent effect and permits acquisition of "pure" stress-related images uncontaminated by the prior rest radiotracer injection. Although the doses administered are slightly higher than those for SPECT imaging, the patient leaves the facility with only background radioactivity.

N-13 NH_3 is the other PET radiotracer that has been approved by the FDA for MPI. N-13 NH_3 is a cyclotron-produced radioisotope and has a physical half-life of 9.9 minutes, thus necessitating the presence of an on-site/in-house cyclotron for use of this radiotracer for PET MPI. The physical characteristics of its positron (positron energy of 1.19 MeV and average positron range of 0.4 mm) are similar to that of F-18 and hence it generates excellent PET images. It has a high extraction rate and exhibits prolonged myocardial retention by remaining metabolically trapped within the myocytes, due to the glutamine synthetase pathway. **Fig. 7** shows a typical rest-stress myocardial perfusion study protocol using N-13 NH_3. **Fig. 8** shows a PET MPI study with N-13 NH_3. Again, such images are not

atypical for PET with N-13 NH_3, demonstrating high-resolution and high-contrast images with this modality. Similar to Rb-82 cardiac PET, these stress images are also more "pure" with almost no residual contamination from the rest radiotracer injection. Although the protocol is longer than the PET MPI protocol with Rb-82, it is still shorter than the traditional SPECT study. However, a major advantage of N-13 NH_3 PET MPI as compared with Rb-82 PET MPI is the ability to perform exercise-induced stress MPI studies[3] in addition to pharmaceutical stress MPI studies (only the latter is possible with Rb-82 PET MPI).

There are other PET radiotracers that can be used for cardiac perfusion evaluation, such as O-15 water and Cu-64 pyruvaldehyde-bis(N4-methylthiosemicarbazone). These agents are mostly restricted to the research setting. However, there is another agent that has potential to be used in routine clinical practice, commercially known as flurpiridaz (BMS-747158-02 by Lantheus Medical Inc), which has just completed phase-2 clinical multicenter trial testing. Flurpiridaz binds to the mitochondrial complex 1 with high affinity. Preclinical studies and phase-1 trials have shown flurpiridaz to have a higher extraction, prolonged retention, and first-pass extraction fraction superior to Tc-99m-sestamibi.[4] Trials demonstrated that doses of flurpiridaz are

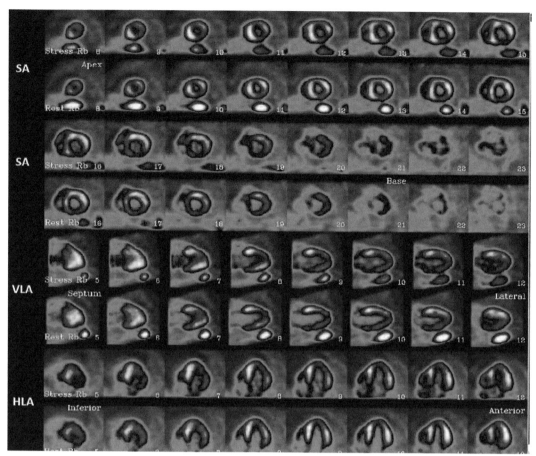

Fig. 5. Abnormal Rb-82 MPI with partially reversible defects in LAD and circumflex artery territories. The Rb-82 PET MPI in conventional projections shown are from a 57-year-old man with known coronary artery disease and a history of prior coronary artery bypass grafting with recent exertional chest pain. PET MPI was performed to assess for diminished vascular reserve and for risk stratification purposes. Images show a moderate-sized partially reversible perfusion defect involving the anteroseptal and inferolateral segments; this was compatible with a combination of viable ischemic myocardium and scar in the expected LAD and circumflex distribution.

within acceptable ranges and without any adverse events. Stress imaging is possible either with exercise or pharmacologic agents, and the myocardium perfusion defects are visualized more extensively as compared with Tc SPECT imaging.[5] If validated and approved by the FDA, this agent has the potential to become an alternative to Rb-82 and N-13 NH_3, as the half-life of the isotope (110 minutes) facilitates distribution of the radiotracer from a central cyclotron facility to the imaging centers just as is currently done with F-18 FDG. Moreover, ordering unit doses of F-18 flurpiridaz has the potential to be more cost effective for imaging centers with low volumes of PET MPI studies, as it will eliminate the financial pressures related to maintaining an Rb-82 generator or the precise scheduling restrictions encountered with N-13 NH_3 PET MPI studies. The imaging protocol may be more along the lines of traditional SPECT MPI studies.

PET MPI has similar indications to SPECT MPI: detection and evaluation of coronary artery disease (CAD) and risk assessment/stratification. In patients with a body habitus that is prone to lead to a suboptimal SPECT scan (eg, female patients with large breasts, significantly obese patients, and muscular patients with a thick chest wall), it is preferred over SPECT MPI. In patients who have had a prior inconclusive SPECT MPI study (ie, equivocal or technically uninterpretable study), PET MPI can be performed following the inconclusive SPECT MPI study when considered necessary to determine what medical or surgical intervention is required to treat the patient. PET MPI can also be performed following a SPECT MPI study in patients in whom the prior SPECT scan results were discordant and did not correlate with subsequent angiographic findings or with the clinical impression. PET MPI is also preferred over

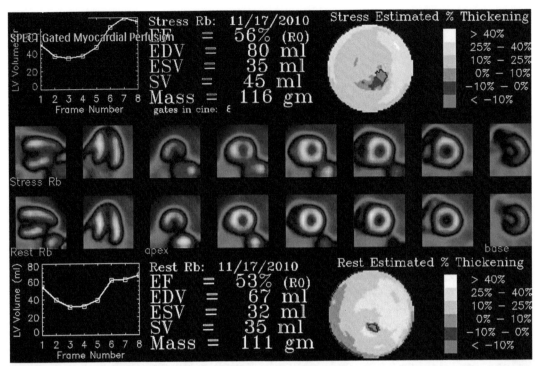

Fig. 6. Abnormal Rb-82 PET MPI showing nonreversible perfusion defects. The Rb-82 PET MPI is from a 50-year-old man with history of chronic chest pain, elevated risk factors for coronary artery disease, and an abnormal ECG. As shown in the conventional projections of myocardial perfusion, a severe nonreversible perfusion defect was noted in the distal inferior wall and apex, consistent with old myocardial infarction.

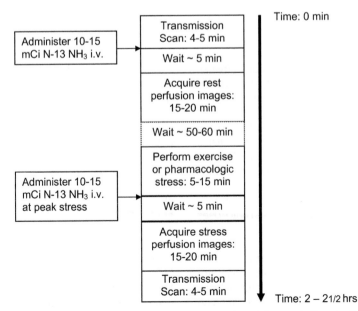

Fig. 7. N-13 NH_3 myocardial perfusion imaging protocol. (*Reproduced from* Takalkar A, Chen W, Desjardins B, et al. Cardiovascular imaging with PET, CT, and MR imaging. PET Clinics 2008;3(3):411–34; with permission.)

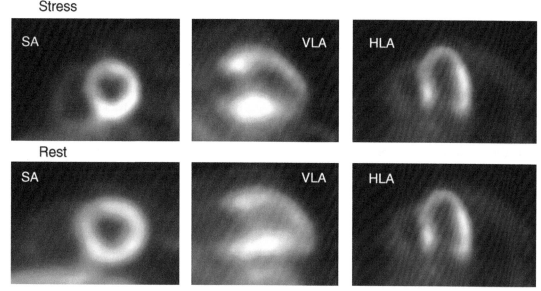

Fig. 8. Myocardial perfusion study with N-13 NH_3 PET. Rest and stress myocardial perfusion imaging with PET using N-13 NH_3 in a 47-year-old man with history of essential hypertension complaining of exertional chest pain. The selected images of stress and rest myocardial perfusion in SA, VLA, and HLA demonstrate a large area of moderate reduction in radiotracer uptake in the mid and distal anterior wall and apex at peak exercise stress with normal myocardial perfusion at rest. (*Reproduced from* Takalkar A, Mavi A, Alavi A, et al. PET in cardiology. Radiol Clin North Am 2005;43(1):107–19; with permission.)

SPECT MPI in patients in whom measurement of coronary flow reserve would be helpful in making management decisions and in those requiring serial studies for assessment of disease progression/regression.

Several investigators have validated the high sensitivity, specificity, and accuracy of PET MPI in CAD. Sampson and colleagues[6] reported a sensitivity of 93%, specificity of 91%, and overall diagnostic accuracy of 87% for diagnosis of CAD using coronary angiography as the gold standard. The high accuracy was maintained across various subgroups such as men and women as well as obese and nonobese individuals, affirming the overall robustness of this modality. PET MPI has been shown to be superior to SPECT with Thallium (Tl)-201[7,8] as well as with Tc-99m-sestamibi.[9] Nandalur and colleagues[10] performed a meta-analysis of studies from January 1977 through July 2008 that evaluated the diagnostic performance of PET in detection of CAD. Their data also confirmed a high sensitivity (92%) and specificity (85%) for detecting luminal stenoses 50% or greater, with excellent positive and negative likelihood ratios. The investigators concluded that PET MPI appeared not only superior to SPECT MPI with Tl-201 and Tc-99m-sestamibi, but also to anatomic imaging with coronary multidetector computed tomography (MDCT) angiography or magnetic resonance angiography (MRA). SPECT MPI has been an established modality for decades

with proven cost effectiveness, and concerns about cost effectiveness of PET MPI are considerations in the current health care fiscal environment. However, as early as 1995 PET was reported to be cost effective in the workup of CAD relative to exercise testing, SPECT, and immediate angiography.[11] The increased availability and use of PET in the oncologic setting have led to a gradual decrease in the costs associated with this imaging modality. A more recent study in 2006 by Merhige and colleagues[12] illustrated the cost effectiveness of PET MPI with Rb-82 in comparison with SPECT MPI. These investigators studied a group of 2159 patients with CAD who received PET MPI, and compared the frequency of diagnostic arteriography, revascularizations, outcomes, and the total cost, with two control groups of patients who received SPECT MPI, for a period of 1 year. Their results showed that diagnosis by PET MPI resulted in greater than 50% reduction of invasive coronary arteriography and coronary artery bypass grafting, and a total cost reduction of 30% as compared with the control groups.

INTEGRATED CARDIAC PET/CT-MPI/ CORONARY COMPUTED TOMOGRAPHIC ANGIOGRAPHY

Patients with suspected CAD and a positive stress MPI study generally are further evaluated by catheter-based coronary angiography to identify the diseased coronary vessel(s) and determine further management. When a critical culprit lesion amenable to percutaneous intervention is identified, this approach can then be used as a therapeutic procedure to address the stenosis. However, a majority of invasive catheter-based coronary angiograms remain diagnostic in nature (as opposed to therapeutic) for various reasons such as diffuse disease that requires medical management or normal coronaries without significant disease (and a false-positive MPI study). Coronary computed tomographic angiography (CCTA) using 64-slice CT scanners offers the ability to perform angiographic evaluation less invasively than traditional catheter-based angiography. Because integrated PET/CT scanners have the necessary hardware to perform functional and structural imaging in one session, recent integrated PET/CT scanners with a 64-slice CT scanner integrated with the PET scanner offer the ability to perform MPI studies with PET myocardial perfusion agents along with CCTA in one session. A dedicated CCTA study may not be feasible on integrated PET/CT scanners with a less than 16-slice CT scanner. An integrated PET/CT-MPI/CCTA study estimates the presence and severity of coronary artery luminal stenosis (by CCTA) along with its downstream hemodynamic consequences, such as stress-induced ischemia or microvascular dysfunction (by MPI), in a single imaging study. The volumetric assessment of the luminal stenosis provided by CCTA may not be a reliable indicator of its downstream hemodynamic effects, potentially leading to discordant coronary angiography and MPI findings. Specifically, a territory supplied by a coronary artery with significant stenosis may still have adequate perfusion from collateral blood supply and would not appear to be at risk for ischemia on MPI. Thus, the integrated cardiac PET/CT-MPI/CTA study providing functional and structural information offers several benefits in the management of CAD patients. It will accurately identify the culprit stenosis responsible for downstream ischemia and facilitate optimal management of offending lesions. In patients with endothelial/microvascular dysfunction without critical coronary artery stenosis, an integrated PET/CT-MPI/CCTA study will help avoid unnecessary invasive catheter-based coronary angiography and steer those patients to appropriate medical management. In addition, because the positive predictive value of CCTA for identifying hemodynamically significant coronary stenoses (those that produce stress-induced ischemia) is suboptimal, the integrated PET/CT-CCTA study provides the necessary complementary functional information to aid in determining further management of patients. This combined approach with an integrated PET/CT-MPI/CCTA study to determine optimal management of CAD patients has the potential to make a significant impact by reducing unnecessary therapeutic invasive coronary catheterizations and revascularization procedures done on the basis of angiographic findings alone.

At the same time, PET MPI may underestimate the extent of actual CAD, especially in the setting of multivessel disease CAD, because MPI relies strongly on relative perfusion abnormalities to detect ischemia in various coronary territories. Hence, it usually discerns ischemia only in the territory downstream to the most severe stenosis. Because the coronary vasodilator reserve is frequently diminished even in territories supplied by hemodynamically noncritical stenoses, the relative flow differences between normal, noncritical, and critical stenosis territories is frequently diminished, leading to underestimation of the extent of actual CAD.[13,14] Complementing the MPI findings with the high-resolution anatomic information supplied by the CCTA study in an integrated PET/CT-MPI/CCTA study can help avoid this pitfall. Thus, an integrated PET/CCTA cardiac evaluation overcomes limitations of each individual modality and provides a more comprehensive evaluation. **Fig. 9** shows a typical schema for an integrated cardiac PET/CT-MPI/CCTA protocol. Due to significant technical and professional resources demanded by these highly sophisticated studies and lack of uniform reimbursement for such studies, they are not yet in common use in clinical practice.

INTEGRATED CARDIAC PET/CT-MPI/ CORONARY ARTERY CALCIUM SCORING

Coronary artery calcium (CAC) scoring is increasingly being used after normal MPI to assess preclinical CAD.[15] A significant number of patients with normal MPI but other cardiac risk factors may have widespread underlying coronary artery atherosclerotic calcification.[16] These noncritical lesions may not cause detectable ischemia on MPI, and although a normal MPI study justifies no further invasive testing in most cases, this cohort of patients with a normal MPI study but high CAC score may benefit from aggressive risk factor modification to halt progression of the hemodynamically stable CAD. As it is possible to combine CAC scoring with PET MPI imaging, even with a 4-slice CT as a part of the PET/CT scanner, an integrated cardiac PET/CT-MPI/CAC scoring examination may provide a better approach toward risk stratification and management in this

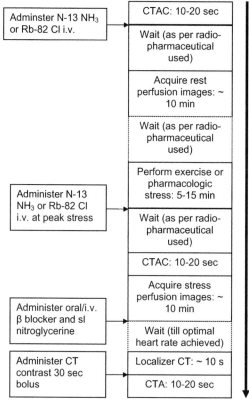

Fig. 9. Integrated cardiac PET/CT-MPI/CCTA protocol. (*Reproduced from* Takalkar A, Chen W, Desjardins B, et al. Cardiovascular imaging with PET, CT, and MR imaging. PET Clinics 2008;3(3):411–34; with permission.)

cohort of patients. The protocol would be almost similar to the protocol for a combined MPI/CCTA study on an integrated PET/CT scanner, except that a CAC scoring study would be performed instead of a CCTA study.

PET MYOCARDIAL VIABILITY EVALUATION

Precise determination of myocardial viability is of utmost importance in patients with severe left ventricular dysfunction and ischemic heart disease because therapeutic options are limited to medical management, revascularization (surgical or percutaneous), and cardiac transplantation.[17,18] Despite the considerable advances in medical management in this setting, when myocardial ischemia has been conclusively demonstrated, revascularization treatment definitely offers superior long-term survival rates as compared with medical management.[19–21] Because revascularization procedures are associated with significant periprocedural risks, it is critical to select appropriately only those patients who will benefit the most from revascularization treatment in order to optimize the risk-benefit ratio.

Scarred and infarcted myocardium is nonviable, and revascularization does not benefit in this situation. However, stunned or hibernating myocardium is dysfunctional but viable, and has the potential to revert to normal or show significant improvement in contractile function with revascularization. This reversibility of contractile dysfunction is the most crucial determinant of postrevascularization functional improvement and overall benefit to the patient. Hence, accurate identification of viable myocardium from nonviable myocardium is the single most decisive factor in determining the value and necessity of revascularization in this setting. Although there are several techniques for the assessment of myocardial viability, Tillisch and colleagues[22] were the first to successfully predict functional reversibility of myocardium on the basis on FDG-PET imaging in 1986. Several investigators have since extensively validated FDG-PET metabolism imaging to assess myocardial viability in an array of clinical scenarios.[23–30] When dysfunctional myocardium with an intermediate decline in blood flow is encountered, the presence of myocardial viability cannot be adequately assessed with regional myocardial blood flow alone. Hence, myocardial viability is typically determined by evaluating myocardial metabolism (using FDG-PET imaging) in combination with myocardial blood flow (using PET or SPECT MPI), and MPI combined with FDG-PET myocardial metabolic imaging has been considered as the gold standard for assessing myocardial viability.[1]

Although free fatty acids (FFA) are the primary myocardial substrate under normal circumstances, ischemic and hypoxic myocardium switches from FFA to glucose as the substrate of choice for its metabolic needs.[18,26,31–34] Hence, FDG is used for PET myocardial metabolic imaging. When ischemic myocardium has enough blood supply to keep it viable, it shows increased FDG uptake on FDG-PET myocardial metabolic imaging, and when there is no blood supply to the myocardium, there is no FDG uptake in that myocardial segment on FDG-PET myocardial imaging; this is the underlying principle for assessing myocardial viability with FDG-PET metabolic imaging combined with MPI. Because there is typically highly variable myocardial uptake of FDG, glucose loading is generally performed prior to FDG administration when performing myocardial metabolism studies with FDG, to overcome the variability in myocardial FDG uptake. Glucose loading increases plasma glucose and hence plasma insulin levels during the FDG uptake period, promoting increased intramyocardial FDG transport and thus ensuring good myocardial FDG uptake. Several methods are used to perform glucose loading. Specific details are beyond the scope of this text, but some of these protocols include oral glucose administration, intravenous glucose administration, drugs such as Acipimox, and other more complex techniques. **Fig. 10** depicts a myocardial viability assessment protocol using PET MPI with N-13 NH_3 at rest combined with PET myocardial metabolism imaging with FDG and use of oral glucose loading. Myocardial blood flow combined with myocardial glucose metabolism can have 3 distinct patterns, as depicted schematically in **Fig. 11**: (1) normal blood flow and normal glucose metabolism (normal viable myocardium), (2) decreased blood flow and decreased glucose metabolism (necrosed/scarred myocardium—nonviable), and (3) decreased blood flow but retained/normal glucose metabolism (the classic flow-metabolism mismatch—hallmark of dysfunctional but viable myocardium).[17,18]

In the setting of left ventricular failure with CAD, myocardial viability assessment provides several important prognostic implications regarding the clinical management of these patients. Specifically, pretreatment myocardial viability assessment can aid in predicting functional recovery and amount of expected improvement from congestive heart failure symptoms after revascularization.[22,35–38] The extent of ischemic but viable myocardium as determined by the size and number of viable

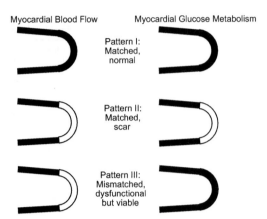

Fig. 11. Patterns of myocardial blood flow and myocardial metabolism for myocardial viability studies. (*Reproduced from* Takalkar A, Chen W, Desjardins B, et al. Cardiovascular imaging with PET, CT, and MR imaging. PET Clinics 2008;3(3):411–34; with permission.)

myocardial segments also positively affect functional outcome after revascularization.[39,40] Complementing the clinical and angiographic findings with myocardial viability information and using this in the decision-making process for revascularization results in less perioperative complications, less need for inotropic drugs, low early mortality, and better short-term survival.[41,42] In fact, identification of viable myocardium in a patient with left ventricular dysfunction due to CAD is an indication for prompt revascularization therapy, as delaying revascularization in the presence of documented viable myocardium usually leads to a suboptimal outcome, potentially with serious consequences including death.[43] Medical management of such patients without revascularization does not decrease the risk for future ischemic events.[44,45] Conversely, lack of significant viable myocardium on flow-metabolism imaging in this setting strengthens the decision to treat such patients medically or by cardiac transplantation, if warranted.

INTEGRATED CARDIAC PET/MR IMAGING

Advances in MR imaging have enabled this modality to provide excellent morphologic and functional evaluation of the heart, and it has the potential to be the "one-stop-shop" examination for cardiac imaging. Similar to the integration of PET and CT systems, it is theoretically possible to integrate PET and MR imaging systems as well. However, the hardware integration of PET and MR imaging is much more difficult than for PET and CT, due to the presence of an active magnetic field in which the PET imaging needs to occur. Nevertheless, a few prototype clinical PET/MR

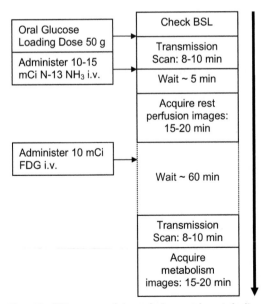

Fig. 10. PET myocardial perfusion and metabolism imaging protocol for myocardial viability. BSL, blood sugar level. (*Reproduced from* Takalkar A, Chen W, Desjardins B, et al. Cardiovascular imaging with PET, CT, and MR imaging. PET Clinics 2008;3(3):411–34; with permission.)

imaging systems are now in place at a few beta sites in the United States, but thus far no significant attention has been directed toward their use for integrated cardiac PET/MR imaging evaluation.

There are several potential areas of synergy between PET and MR imaging for cardiac evaluation. Both imaging modalities can assess myocardial viability and can potentially complement each other. PET imaging may be limited when there is variable FDG uptake in the heart, and MR imaging is an attractive alternative. Delayed enhancement on MR imaging is the basis for determining viable myocardium. However, Knuesel and colleagues[46] studied tissue classification with respect to functional recovery after revascularization, and showed the limitations of MR imaging in capturing the variability and biological complexity of involved segments. Assessment of cardiac innervation in patients with dilated cardiomyopathy or prior heart transplantation is another potential area where combined PET (using carbon [C]-11 hydroxyephedrine) and cardiac MR imaging (with high-resolution morphologic imaging and wall motion imaging) can be used to delineate cardiac regional innervation and control mechanisms.[47] Furthermore, cardiac PET and MR imaging can be complementary for the assessment of cardiac masses. In contrast to CT, MR imaging provides more precise anatomic delineation of a primary or metastatic cardiac tumor, and FDG-PET can characterize its metabolic activity. The more robust evaluation provided by a combined cardiac PET/MR imaging evaluation may provide a better initial assessment of the tumor for treatment planning purposes, and may also be useful for more accurate assessment of tumor response to therapy.

FDG-PET/CT OR FDG-PET/MR IMAGING IN CORONARY ARTERY ATHEROSCLEROSIS

Formation of atherosclerotic plaque is a dynamic inflammatory process involving interactions between atherogenic lipoproteins and macrophages. However, rupture of the atherosclerotic plaque and its downstream effects, such as thrombosis or embolism, are more important determinants of serious clinical complications such as sudden cardiac death or stroke (rather than the luminal narrowing of the atherosclerotic artery itself). Angiography, the current imaging gold standard for assessing the arterial lumen, is suboptimal for identifying inflamed plaque or nonstenotic plaque, which may be particularly prone to inflammation and rupture.[48] Angiography requires an imaging approach that can identify the inflammatory status and vulnerability of plaque along with the degree of luminal narrowing. Several molecular imaging

modalities are currently being evaluated to address the issue of identifying the vulnerable plaques. These techniques include intravascular ultrasonography, near-infrared fluorescence imaging, contrast-enhanced ultrasonography with targeted microbubbles, and FDG-PET or PET/CT imaging. Of the various strategies being employed to assess inflammatory and vulnerable atherosclerotic plaques, FDG-PET has been the most vigorously pursued and investigated.[49,50] FDG is known to accumulate in activated inflammatory cells including macrophages, and increased glucose uptake and metabolism in plaque macrophages is believed to account for the visualization of atherosclerotic lesions by FDG-PET imaging. Although a significant amount of studies have assessed vascular FDG uptake in atherosclerotic vessels, the evaluation has been mostly restricted to larger arteries such as the aorta and carotids. However, demonstration of atherosclerotic inflammation in the coronary vasculature with FDG-PET imaging, an area with potentially the greatest prognostic significance, has so far been limited by several technical and practical hurdles. The variable FDG uptake by cardiac myocytes may lead to high background uptake, making it difficult to separate uptake in coronary arteries from background activity. Atherosclerotic lesions are very small in size, and ongoing cardiac motion occurs during imaging, which makes imaging with current PET systems challenging. Moreover, the FDG uptake in these atherosclerotic lesions may not be significantly high enough, with an adequate target to background ratio, to facilitate easy detection of these lesions by routine visual evaluation of these images. However, investigators are addressing these issues, and have made progress in suppressing myocardial FDG uptake to facilitate visualization of coronary FDG uptake. A recent study by Rogers and colleagues[51] reported the feasibility of prospectively imaging coronary inflammation in humans, and found that patients with unstable coronary syndromes harbor greater inflammation than those with stable syndromes, demonstrating the potential utility of molecular imaging for evaluation of the coronary bed. Further advances in PET instrumentation and technology, along with potential development of more specific molecular imaging PET probes that target vulnerable plaque, hold promise for noninvasive and accurate imaging of vulnerable plaque prior to catastrophic clinical event occurrence.

FUTURE APPLICATIONS FOR PET IMAGING IN CARDIOVASCULAR CONDITIONS

Cardiac neuronal evaluation with PET to assess cardiac innervation and its impact on other cardiac parameters such as heart rate and contractility, as well as rhythm abnormalities, is another important area of research for cardiac PET imaging. There are several PET radiotracers in development for cardiac neuronal imaging that may be useful for assessment of the role of autonomic system dysfunction in patients with heart failure, dilated cardiomyopathy, or following cardiac transplantation. Catecholamine analogues labeled with PET radioisotopes such as F-18 fluorodopamine, C-11 epinephrine, C-11 metahydroxyephedrine, and C-11 phenylephrine are undergoing evaluation for their utility in assessing the cardiac sympathetic innervation, whereas vesamicol-based agents such as F-18 fluoroethoxybenzovesamicol can be used to assess the cardiac parasympathetic nervous system.[52] However, there is still a need to identify PET radiotracers with optimal tracer kinetics for cardiac neuronal imaging. Receptor imaging with PET is another avenue of interest for investigators engaged in drug development. Several PET radiotracers have been developed to image the adrenergic and muscarinic receptors in the heart. These agents act as PET radioligands for postsynaptic myocardial receptor proteins and offer true postganglionic receptor imaging. Examples include C-11 CGP 12177 for β1 and β2 adrenoceptors, C-11 GB67 for α1 adrenoceptors, and C-11 MQNB for M1 and M2 muscarinic receptors.[53–55] Noninvasive assessment of cardiac gene therapy with cardiac PET is another exciting investigational application. Imaging reporter gene expression is useful for noninvasive monitoring of gene therapy. Noninvasive imaging of cardiac PET reporter genes combined with PET reporter probes in small animals using dedicated micro-PET and micro-PET/CT systems affords determination of the location, magnitude, and time course of gene expression, thus offering the potential to monitor the expression of therapeutic genes in cardiac gene therapy expression.[56,57] However, progress in cardiac gene therapy clinical trials has suffered from lack of clear-cut demonstration of therapeutic effectiveness and improvement in clinical outcomes. Noninvasive gene-targeted imaging is expected to serve as a quantitative means of providing evidence of the usefulness of new gene therapy approaches as well as to provide an understanding of the underlying molecular mechanisms, thus enhancing the determination of therapeutic effects in cardiovascular molecular therapy in the future.[58–60]

The current applications of cardiac PET imaging for assessment of cardiac perfusion and metabolism along with the exciting future potential applications of cardiac PET, including detection and quantification of vulnerable atherosclerotic plaque,

evaluation of cardiac neuronal regulation, quantification of receptor expression, and monitoring of cardiac gene therapy, have brought cardiac PET imaging to the forefront of individualized molecular imaging assessment of patients with various cardiovascular pathologies.

REFERENCES

1. Bax JJ, Visser FC, van Lingen A, et al. Metabolic imaging using F18-fluorodeoxyglucose to assess myocardial viability. Int J Card Imaging 1997;13(2): 145–55 [discussion: 157–60].

2. Gould KL, Pan T, Loghin C, et al. Frequent diagnostic errors in cardiac PET/CT due to misregistration of CT attenuation and emission PET images: a definitive analysis of causes, consequences, and corrections. J Nucl Med 2007;48(7):1112–21.

3. Krivokapich J, Smith GT, Huang SC, et al. ^{13}N ammonia myocardial imaging at rest and with exercise in normal volunteers. Quantification of absolute myocardial perfusion with dynamic positron emission tomography. Circulation 1989;80(5):1328–37.

4. Nekolla SG, Saraste A. Novel F-18-labeled PET Myocardial perfusion tracers: bench to bedside. Curr Cardiol Rep 2011;13(2):145–50.

5. Thomas GS, Maddahi J. The technetium shortage. J Nucl Cardiol 2010;17(6):993–8.

6. Sampson UK, Dorbala S, Limaye A, et al. Diagnostic accuracy of rubidium-82 myocardial perfusion imaging with hybrid positron emission tomography/ computed tomography in the detection of coronary artery disease. J Am Coll Cardiol 2007;49(10):1052–8.

7. Go RT, Marwick TH, MacIntyre WJ, et al. A prospective comparison of rubidium-82 PET and thallium-201 SPECT myocardial perfusion imaging utilizing a single dipyridamole stress in the diagnosis of coronary artery disease. J Nucl Med 1990;31(12): 1899–905.

8. Stewart RE, Schwaiger M, Molina E, et al. Comparison of rubidium-82 positron emission tomography and thallium-201 SPECT imaging for detection of coronary artery disease. Am J Cardiol 1991;67(16):1303–10.

9. Bateman TM, Heller GV, McGhie AI, et al. Diagnostic accuracy of rest/stress ECG-gated Rb-82 myocardial perfusion PET: comparison with ECG-gated Tc-99m sestamibi SPECT. J Nucl Cardiol 2006; 13(1):24–33.

10. Nandalur KR, Dwamena BA, Choudhri AF, et al. Diagnostic performance of positron emission tomography in the detection of coronary artery disease: a meta-analysis. Acad Radiol 2008;15(4):444–51.

11. Patterson RE, Eisner RL, Horowitz SF. Comparison of cost-effectiveness and utility of exercise ECG, single photon emission computed tomography, positron emission tomography, and coronary angiography

for diagnosis of coronary artery disease. Circulation 1995;91(1):54–65.

12. Merhige ME, Breen WJ, Shelton V, et al. Impact of myocardial perfusion imaging with PET and (82)Rb on downstream invasive procedure utilization, costs, and outcomes in coronary disease management. J Nucl Med 2007;48(7):1069–76.

13. Uren NG, Crake T, Lefroy DC, et al. Reduced coronary vasodilator function in infarcted and normal myocardium after myocardial infarction. N Engl J Med 1994;331(4):222–7.

14. Yoshinaga K, Katoh C, Noriyasu K, et al. Reduction of coronary flow reserve in areas with and without ischemia on stress perfusion imaging in patients with coronary artery disease: a study using oxygen 15-labeled water PET. J Nucl Cardiol 2003;10(3):275–83.

15. Thompson RC, McGhie AI, Moser KW, et al. Clinical utility of coronary calcium scoring after nonischemic myocardial perfusion imaging. J Nucl Cardiol 2005;12(4):392–400.

16. Berman DS, Wong ND, Gransar H, et al. Relationship between stress-induced myocardial ischemia and atherosclerosis measured by coronary calcium tomography. J Am Coll Cardiol 2004;44(4):923–30.

17. Keng FY. Clinical applications of positron emission tomography in cardiology: a review. Ann Acad Med Singapore 2004;33(2):175–82.

18. Schelbert HR. ^{18}F-deoxyglucose and the assessment of myocardial viability. Semin Nucl Med 2002;32(1):60–9.

19. Ellis SG, Fisher L, Dushman-Ellis S, et al. Comparison of coronary angioplasty with medical treatment for single- and double-vessel coronary disease with left anterior descending coronary involvement: long-term outcome based on an Emory-CASS registry study. Am Heart J 1989;118(2):208–20.

20. Emond M, Mock MB, Davis KB, et al. Long-term survival of medically treated patients in the Coronary Artery Surgery Study (CASS) Registry. Circulation 1994;90(6):2645–57.

21. Mickleborough LL, Maruyama H, Takagi Y, et al. Results of revascularization in patients with severe left ventricular dysfunction. Circulation 1995;92(9 Suppl):II73–9.

22. Tillisch J, Brunken R, Marshall R, et al. Reversibility of cardiac wall-motion abnormalities predicted by positron tomography. N Engl J Med 1986;314(14):884–8.

23. Tamaki N, Ohtani H, Yamashita K, et al. Metabolic activity in the areas of new fill-in after thallium-201 reinjection: comparison with positron emission tomography using fluorine-18-deoxyglucose. J Nucl Med 1991;32(4):673–8.

24. Gropler RJ, Geltman EM, Sampathkumaran K, et al. Comparison of carbon-11-acetate with fluorine-18-fluorodeoxyglucose for delineating viable myocardium

by positron emission tomography. J Am Coll Cardiol 1993;22(6):1587–97.

25. Lucignani G, Paolini G, Landoni C, et al. Presurgical identification of hibernating myocardium by combined use of technetium-99m hexakis 2-methoxyiso-butylisonitrile single photon emission tomography and fluorine-18 fluoro-2-deoxy-D-glucose positron emission tomography in patients with coronary artery disease. Eur J Nucl Med 1992;19(10):874–81.

26. Marwick TH, MacIntyre WJ, Lafont A, et al. Metabolic responses of hibernating and infarcted myocardium to revascularization. A follow-up study of regional perfusion, function, and metabolism. Circulation 1992;85(4):1347–53.

27. Tamaki N, Yonekura Y, Yamashita K, et al. Prediction of reversible ischemia after coronary artery bypass grafting by positron emission tomography. J Cardiol 1991;21(2):193–201.

28. Tamaki N, Yonekura Y, Yamashita K, et al. Positron emission tomography using fluorine-18 deoxyglucose in evaluation of coronary artery bypass grafting. Am J Cardiol 1989;64(14):860–5.

29. vom Dahl J, Eitzman DT, al-Aouar ZR, et al. Relation of regional function, perfusion, and metabolism in patients with advanced coronary artery disease undergoing surgical revascularization. Circulation 1994;90(5):2356–66.

30. Tamaki N, Yonekura Y, Yamashita K, et al. Value of rest-stress myocardial positron tomography using nitrogen-13 ammonia for the preoperative prediction of reversible asynergy. J Nucl Med 1989;30(8):1302–10.

31. Liedtke AJ. Alterations of carbohydrate and lipid metabolism in the acutely ischemic heart. Prog Cardiovasc Dis 1981;23(5):321–36.

32. Liedtke AJ. The changing metabolic role of fatty acids in increasingly complex organisms: an evolutionary perspective. J Mol Cell Cardiol 1997;29(10):2611–9.

33. Liedtke AJ, Renstrom B, Hacker TA, et al. Effects of moderate repetitive ischemia on myocardial substrate utilization. Am J Physiol 1995;269(1 Pt 2):246–53.

34. Schelbert HR, Henze E, Phelps ME, et al. Assessment of regional myocardial ischemia by positron-emission computed tomography. Am Heart J 1982;103(4 Pt 2):588–97.

35. Baer FM, Voth E, Deutsch HJ, et al. Predictive value of low dose dobutamine transesophageal echocardiography and fluorine-18 fluorodeoxyglucose positron emission tomography for recovery of regional left ventricular function after successful revascularization. J Am Coll Cardiol 1996;28(1):60–9.

36. Bax JJ, Cornel JH, Visser FC, et al. F18-fluorodeoxyglucose single-photon emission computed tomography predicts functional outcome of dyssynergic myocardium after surgical revascularization. J Nucl Cardiol 1997;4(4):302–8.

37. Knuuti MJ, Saraste M, Nuutila P, et al. Myocardial viability: fluorine-18-deoxyglucose positron emission tomography in prediction of wall motion recovery after revascularization. Am Heart J 1994;127(4 Pt 1):785–96.

38. Schoder H, Campisi R, Ohtake T, et al. Blood flow-metabolism imaging with positron emission tomography in patients with diabetes mellitus for the assessment of reversible left ventricular contractile dysfunction. J Am Coll Cardiol 1999;33(5):1328–37.

39. Di Carli MF, Asgarzadie F, Schelbert HR, et al. Quantitative relation between myocardial viability and improvement in heart failure symptoms after revascularization in patients with ischemic cardiomyopathy. Circulation 1995;92(12):3436–44.

40. Marwick TH, Nemec JJ, Lafont A, et al. Prediction by postexercise fluoro-18 deoxyglucose positron emission tomography of improvement in exercise capacity after revascularization. Am J Cardiol 1992;69(9):854–9.

41. Haas F, Haehnel CJ, Picker W, et al. Preoperative positron emission tomographic viability assessment and perioperative and postoperative risk in patients with advanced ischemic heart disease. J Am Coll Cardiol 1997;30(7):1693–700.

42. Landoni C, Lucignani G, Paolini G, et al. Assessment of CABG-related risk in patients with CAD and LVD. Contribution of PET with [^{18}F]FDG to the assessment of myocardial viability. J Cardiovasc Surg (Torino) 1999;40(3):363–72.

43. Beanlands RS, Hendry PJ, Masters RG, et al. Delay in revascularization is associated with increased mortality rate in patients with severe left ventricular dysfunction and viable myocardium on fluorine 18-fluorodeoxyglucose positron emission tomography imaging. Circulation 1998;98(Suppl 19):51–6.

44. Allman KC, Shaw LJ, Hachamovitch R, et al. Myocardial viability testing and impact of revascularization on prognosis in patients with coronary artery disease and left ventricular dysfunction: a meta-analysis. J Am Coll Cardiol 2002;39(7):1151–8.

45. Di Carli MF, Maddahi J, Rokhsar S, et al. Long-term survival of patients with coronary artery disease and left ventricular dysfunction: implications for the role of myocardial viability assessment in management decisions. J Thorac Cardiovasc Surg 1998;116(6):997–1004.

46. Knuesel PR, Nanz D, Wyss C, et al. Characterization of dysfunctional myocardium by positron emission tomography and magnetic resonance: relation to functional outcome after revascularization. Circulation 2003;108(9):1095–100.

47. Bengel FM, Ueberfuhr P, Schiepel N, et al. Myocardial efficiency and sympathetic reinnervation after orthotopic heart transplantation: a noninvasive study with positron emission tomography. Circulation 2001;103(14):1881–6.

48. Pasterkamp G, Schoneveld AH, van der Wal AC, et al. Relation of arterial geometry to luminal narrowing and histologic markers for plaque vulnerability: the remodeling paradox. J Am Coll Cardiol 1998; 32(3):655–62.

49. Narula J, Chandrashekhar Y. Molecular imaging of coronary inflammation: overcoming hurdles one at a time. JACC Cardiovasc Imaging 2010;3(4):448–50.

50. Narula J, Garg P, Achenbach S, et al. Arithmetic of vulnerable plaques for noninvasive imaging. Nat Clin Pract Cardiovasc Med 2008;5(Suppl 2): S2–10.

51. Rogers IS, Nasir K, Figueroa AL, et al. Feasibility of FDG imaging of the coronary arteries: comparison between acute coronary syndrome and stable angina. JACC Cardiovasc Imaging 2010;3(4): 388–97.

52. Langer O, Halldin C. PET and SPET tracers for mapping the cardiac nervous system. Eur J Nucl Med Mol Imaging 2002;29(3):416–34.

53. Delforge J, Janier M, Syrota A, et al. Noninvasive quantification of muscarinic receptors in vivo with positron emission tomography in the dog heart. Circulation 1990;82(4):1494–504.

54. Delforge J, Le Guludec D, Syrota A, et al. Quantification of myocardial muscarinic receptors with PET in humans. J Nucl Med 1993;34(6):981–91.

55. Law MP, Osman S, Pike VW, et al. Evaluation of [^{11}C] GB67, a novel radioligand for imaging myocardial alpha 1-adrenoceptors with positron emission tomography. Eur J Nucl Med 2000;27(1):7–17.

56. Inubushi M, Wu JC, Gambhir SS, et al. Positron-emission tomography reporter gene expression imaging in rat myocardium. Circulation 2003; 107(2):326–32.

57. Wu JC, Inubushi M, Sundaresan G, et al. Positron emission tomography imaging of cardiac reporter gene expression in living rats. Circulation 2002; 106(2):180–3.

58. Bengel FM. Noninvasive imaging of cardiac gene expression and its future implications for molecular therapy. Mol Imaging Biol 2005;7(1):22–9.

59. Hiona A, Wu JC. Noninvasive radionuclide imaging of cardiac gene therapy: progress and potential. Nat Clin Pract Cardiovasc Med 2008;5(Suppl 2): S87–95.

60. Inubushi M, Tamaki N. Radionuclide reporter gene imaging for cardiac gene therapy. Eur J Nucl Med Mol Imaging 2007;34(Suppl 1):S27–33.

The Role of PET with [18-F] Fluorodeoxyglucose in the Diagnosis and Management of Thoracic Vascular Disease

YiDing Yu, BA^{a,}*, Drew A. Torigian, MD, MA^b,
Nehal N. Mehta, MD, MSCE^a

KEYWORDS

- FDG-PET • Vascular • Inflammation • Atherosclerosis
- Vasculitis

The role of positron emission tomography (PET) in thoracic vascular diseases has grown substantially since [18-F] Fluorodeoxyglucose uptake was first reported in large vessels. Although there were early reports of vascular FDG uptake in rabbit models,[1] the first case series reporting vascular FDG uptake in healthy human subjects by Yun and colleagues[2] helped launch FDG-PET in vascular imaging. Recent years have seen an expansion of FDG-PET technology for the investigation of a wide array of vascular pathologies, and this growing popularity necessitates an understanding of the proper role of FDG-PET compared to conventional imaging modalities in the diagnosis and management of vascular disease.

As FDG-PET technology has matured, several unique properties have helped FDG-PET play a unique role in vascular imaging owing to its exquisite sensitivity to inflammatory activity in the vasculature and to macrophage activity in particular. This unique ability to visualize and quantify vascular inflammation allows FDG-PET to differentiate labile active vascular lesions from chronic disease and to observe changes in vascular inflammation over time. When coregistered with computed tomography (CT) or magnetic resonance (MR) imaging, FDG-PET imaging may additionally offer detailed anatomic inflammation to aid surgical intervention and alert clinicians to the distribution of vascular involvement.

In this review, the authors discuss the development and role of FDG-PET imaging in the assessment of thoracic vascular disease, including atherosclerosis, acute aortic syndromes (AAS), large vessel vasculitis, vascular graft infections, and mycotic aneurysms, as well as novel and emerging applications for FDG-PET. For each of these applications, the authors discuss how FDG-PET has influenced the diagnostic and management approach to disease as well as future applications of FDG-PET technology.

This work is supported by a grant from the Doris Duke Charitable Foundation (Y.Y), a grant from the National Psoriasis Foundation (N.N.M.), and by grant K23HL097151-01 (N.N.M.).
^{a} Division of Cardiovascular Medicine, Department of Medicine, Cardiovascular Institute, University of Pennsylvania School of Medicine, 6 Penn Tower, 3400 Civic Center Boulevard, Philadelphia, PA 19104, USA
^{b} Department of Radiology, Hospital of the University of Pennsylvania, University of Pennsylvania School of Medicine, 3400 Spruce Street, Philadelphia, PA 19104, USA
* Corresponding author.
E-mail address: yiding.yu@uphs.upenn.edu

PET Clin 6 (2011) 327–338
doi:10.1016/j.cpet.2011.04.003
1556-8598/11/$ – see front matter © 2011 Elsevier Inc. All rights reserved.

pet.theclinics.com

ROLE OF FDG-PET FOR ASSESSMENT OF ATHEROSCLEROSIS AND PLAQUE VULNERABILITY

Since the earliest reports of vascular inflammation on FDG-PET, there has been intense interest in the role of FDG-PET for the assessment of atherosclerosis. Atherosclerotic diseases, including ischemic heart disease and cerebrovascular disease, affect millions of people each year and account for nearly a third of all deaths in the United States.[3] Up to 70% of sudden deaths occur secondary to rupture of macrophage-rich plaques[4,5] (compared with stable plaque erosion), and consequently, the technology able to identify at-risk plaques may have the most potential to significantly affect the diagnosis and management of cardiovascular disease. In the last decade, numerous groups have helped advance FDG-PET to achieve this goal.

Identifying Macrophage Infiltration and Plaque Vulnerability

There is substantial evidence that FDG uptake along the vessel wall represents macrophage infiltration in atherosclerotic plaques. Compared with neighboring cells, activated macrophages consume exogenous glucose avidly to maintain their inflammatory and phagocytic activities. Because FDG cannot be metabolized further by the cell after conversion to FDG-6-phosphate, FDG accumulates in the macrophage cytoplasm in its phosphorylated form. These features of macrophage metabolism favor the avid uptake of FDG and the accumulation of FDG radiotracer on FDG-PET imaging (**Fig. 1**).

Furthermore, numerous studies, in both animal models and humans, have shown that the uptake of exogenous glucose radiotracer is concentrated in macrophage-rich areas of lipid-laden plaques and correlates directly with macrophage density.[6–10] Rudd and colleagues[6] performed FDG-PET/CT scans on 8 patients with symptomatic carotid stenosis and found FDG uptake in symptomatic lesions 27% greater than asymptomatic lesions on the contralateral side. After autoradiography of endarterectomy samples from 3 patients, the investigators confirmed FDG uptake concentrated in CD68$^+$ macrophage–rich areas of the plaques. In another study by Tawakol and colleagues,[8] patients with severe carotid stenosis were scanned by FDG-PET and underwent subsequent carotid endarterectomy within 1 month. The investigators found that FDG uptake in the carotid artery was prospectively correlated with macrophage concentration but not plaque area, plaque thickness, vessel size, or smooth muscle density. Other studies comparing FDG-PET/CT imaging of carotid arteries with carotid ultrasonography[11] or carotid angiography[12] have found strong correlation between FDG uptake and degree of stenosis in symptomatic patients, but neither study included macrophage infiltration as an additional outcome. Taken together, these studies demonstrate that FDG uptake is greatest among symptomatic atherosclerotic lesions and in areas of

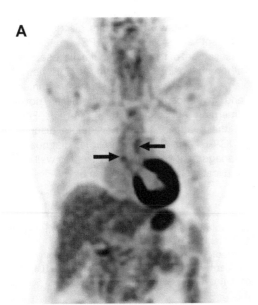

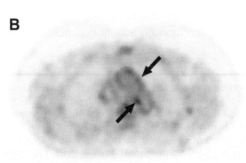

Fig. 1. A 49-year-old woman with a history of parotid malignancy undergoing staging evaluation. Coronal (A) and transverse (B) PET images from FDG-PET/CT examination show increased FDG uptake (arrows) in ascending aorta and aortic arch, in keeping with atherosclerosis.

macrophage infiltration in particular, demonstrating the promise FDG-PET imaging may hold for early detection of vulnerable atherosclerotic plaques.

Clinical Implications for FDG-PET in Atherosclerosis

Naturally, the potential of FDG-PET to detect plaque vulnerability and symptomatic stenosis has prompted several groups to explore the prognostic potential of FDG uptake on vascular events. The technique has been shown to have high interuser and intrauser reproducibility, promoting greater use in clinical research.[13,14] To explore the clinical utility of FDG-PET, several groups have investigated the relationship between FDG uptake and known cardiovascular risk factors, such as age, gender, hypertension, and hyperlipidemia. In a retrospective study of 149 patients by Bural and colleagues,[15] the percentage of vascular segments (aorta, iliac, and femoral) visualized on FDG-PET were directly correlated with age. In a follow-up pilot study by the same group, mean standardized uptake value (SUV), wall volume, wall calcification volume, and global metabolic activity in the aorta on FDG-PET and contrast-enhanced CT were all significantly associated with age.[16] Another study that analyzed the number and quality (FDG avid, inactive calcified, or mixed) of plaques in the aorta, iliac arteries, and carotid arteries also found a strong association of cardiovascular risk factor burden with both total plaque burden and number of FDG-avid plaques.[17]

Carotid inflammation on FDG-PET has also been linked to numerous known cardiovascular risk factors, including metabolic syndrome, by Tahara and colleagues.[18] In their study of 216 oncology patients, FDG uptake was significantly associated with waist circumference, antihypertensive medication, carotid intima-media thickness, high-density lipoprotein cholesterol, homeostasis model assessment of insulin resistance, and high-sensitivity C-reactive protein (CRP) after multiple stepwise regression. In addition to these risk factors, FDG uptake has also been linked to cardiovascular outcomes. In a retrospective study, Paulmier and colleagues[19] matched patients with enhanced arterial FDG uptake to patients with normal FDG uptake levels. The investigators found that FDG uptake was significantly associated with both historic (>6 months before scan) and recent (<6 months to scan) cardiovascular events, whereas arterial calcium index was only associated with historic cardiovascular events.

These studies naturally prompted efforts to investigate the ability of FDG-PET imaging to predict future cardiovascular events. In a study

using the rabbit model, Aziz and colleagues[10] induced atherosclerosis and subsequent thrombosis in 20 rabbits fed high-cholesterol diets. The rabbits were scanned using PET/CT angiography before feeding, at feeding midpoint, after feeding, and after thrombosis induction. The investigators found that maximal SUV in the aorta was strongly correlated with thrombosis and macrophage density at the same sites. In segments that developed thrombi, maximal SUV and macrophage density were more than 2 times greater than segments without thrombi.

Studies in humans have not been as conclusive. In a study of carotid artery stenosis, Arauz and colleagues[12] performed angiography and FDG-PET on 13 patients who had a recent carotid territory transient ischemic event or ischemic stroke. Patients received standard-of-care treatment (medical treatment, endarterectomy, or stent placement) and were followed prospectively for 6 months for stroke, death, or restenosis. There was significant correlation between FDG uptake and degree of stenosis by angiography (Spearman $r = 0.92$, $P = .0005$). However, although the 11 patients who had strong FDG uptake (defined as SUV ≥ 2.7) had a greater incidence of primary outcomes than the 2 patients who did not have strong uptake, the study could not determine the significance of this finding.

A more recent retrospective study of 932 oncology patients by Rominger and colleagues[20] examined FDG uptake and calcified plaque sum in the aorta, carotid arteries, and iliac arteries of patients undergoing FDG-PET/CT for cancer diagnoses. Rominger and colleagues used target-to-background ratio (TBR), defined as maximal SUV divided by blood pool SUV, as a marker of atherosclerosis. The investigators reviewed patient charts and found 15 vascular events after a mean follow-up of 29 months. An additional 319 patients had sufficient clinical data to be analyzed as controls. The investigators found a significant correlation between mean TBR and calcified plaque sum ($P<.001$) and reported both a TBR of 1.7 or greater (hazard ratio [HR], 14.1; $P<.001$) and a calcified plaque sum of 15 or greater (HR, 3.6; $P<.025$) as independent predictors of vascular events.

The large retrospective study by Rominger and colleagues generated considerable excitement for the prognostic value of FDG-PET imaging. However, the considerably large amount of missing clinical data (approximately one-third of all patients) in their retrospective study limited the investigators' ability to fully control for confounding. To fill the need for larger prospective studies to test the power of imaging to predict cardiovascular events, the High-Risk Plaque Initiative was recently developed as a prospective study of more than 6500 patients at risk of cardiovascular events.[21] Patients undergo baseline imaging using multiple modalities, including FDG-PET/CT, and are followed for 3 years for cardiovascular events. The investigators hope that their study and other prospective studies will help elucidate the prognostic potential of FDG-PET imaging on vascular outcomes, especially compared with traditional risk prediction tools.

Sensitivity of FDG-PET to Modulation of Inflammation

A feature of FDG-PET imaging that is garnering growing attention is its sensitivity to modulation of atherosclerotic inflammation, particularly for the study of medical intervention. In a study using the rabbit model by Worthley and colleagues,[9] the investigators performed serial FDG-PET imaging on rabbits (n = 8) after randomization to atherogenic or regular diet. Before the randomization, all rabbits were fed an atherogenic diet and exposed to balloon denudation of the aorta to induce atherosclerosis. Rabbits continued on the atherogenic diet demonstrated a steady and significant increase in FDG uptake ($P = .001$) in the thoracic aorta as feeding progressed, whereas rabbits moved from the atherogenic diet to a normal diet demonstrated a corresponding decline in FDG uptake ($P<.0001$) over time.

A similar study of a rabbit model by Ogawa and colleagues[22] also demonstrated FDG-PET sensitivity to inflammatory modulation. In this study, rabbits were fed either a regular diet or a regular diet with probucol, an antioxidant. After 3 months, there was significantly less FDG uptake among the rabbits that were administered probucol compared with controls, and after 6 months, no FDG uptake could be identified in the aorta of rabbits that were administered probucol. The investigators reported a concomitant decrease in macrophage infiltration after 6 months of probucol, correlating the decrease in FDG uptake with decrease in macrophage density.

Testing these same ideas in human subjects, Tahara and colleagues[23] randomized 43 patients undergoing FDG-PET for cancer screening to receive simvastatin (5 or 10 mg/day) or diet management. After 3 months of follow-up, patients were scanned using FDG-PET/CT. Low-dose simvastatin significantly attenuated FDG uptake ($P<.01$), whereas diet management resulted in no significant change. Previous studies using high-resolution MR imaging required 12 months to visualize atherosclerosis regression after simvastatin therapy,[24,25] suggesting that FDG-PET may be a more powerful and more sensitive tool for the assessment of atherosclerotic plaque modulation. In a later study by Lee and colleagues,[26] the investigators showed that 17 months of lifestyle modification was associated with a reduction in FDG uptake, further demonstrating modulation of FDG signal with atherogenic risk reduction. As a result of these studies, FDG-PET has emerged as a potential tool for studying numerous antiinflammatory or antiatherosclerotic interventions and may have a significant role in the evaluation of drug therapies on vascular inflammation.

ROLE OF FDG-PET IN AAS

AAS represent several conditions that may be rapidly fatal if untreated. AAS describe a range of conditions, including thoracic aortic aneurysm, thoracic aortic dissection, intramural hematoma, and penetrating aortic ulcer. AAS develop over a period driven by other underlying risk factors, such as atherosclerosis and hypertension. Despite appropriate medical management and routine observations, some lesions rapidly progress and become life threatening, and it is often unclear when preemptive surgical intervention would be most beneficial. Because AAS progression has been linked to elevated CRP and D dimers, inflammatory activity is thought to play a role in disease progression.[27–29] In recent years, FDG-PET has been sought to help identify patients who are at a heightened risk of disease progression.

Kuehl and colleagues[30] undertook a prospective study of patients with AAS to answer this question. Thirty-three patients with AAS underwent FDG-PET/CT and CT angiography of the aorta. A maximal SUV of 2.5 was defined as the threshold for pathologic uptake, with 11 patients (33%) exhibiting pathologic uptake. Patients were followed up for an average of 224 days and scanned again. Among patients with pathologic uptake, 82% had progression of AAS compared with 45% among those with negative PET results, although on survival analysis, the trend favoring patients with negative PET results was underpowered to achieve significance.

Examining acute aortic dissections (AADs) in particular, Kato and colleagues[31] prospectively followed up 28 patients admitted for AAD and reassessed at 1 and 6 months for an adverse event, defined as death; requirement for surgery; or AAD progression. Patients were scanned once with FDG-PET/CT after admission and were followed up using enhanced CT. Maximum and mean SUVs were significantly greater among patients with adverse events (n = 8) compared with those who were stable ($P<.01$), and mean SUV independently predicted an adverse event (odds ratio, 7.72; 95%

confidence interval, 1.44–41.4; $P = .02$). Similar results have been found in comparison of chronic stable aortic dissections with AAD, with AAD showing significantly greater FDG uptake compared with chronic dissections.[32]

Although there remain limited data for the role of FDG-PET in AAS, these initial studies suggest that FDG-PET/CT may be useful in predicting short-term disease progression with the potential to offer new insights for clinical management.

ROLE OF FDG-PET IN LARGE VESSEL VASCULITIS

Vasculitis is an inflammatory condition of the blood vessels characterized by inflammatory infiltration of the vessel wall.[33] For vasculitis affecting large vessels, imaging has been sought after to provide early noninvasive diagnosis of often-vague non-specific symptoms.[34] In fact, vasculitis represents up to 17% of all cases of fever of unknown origin, a presentation that is a particular challenge to clinicians.[35] In such cases, imaging may not only provide a diagnosis of vasculitis but also identify the extent of vascular inflammation, reveal early vascular complications of disease, and guide biopsy for definitive diagnosis.

Giant Cell Arteritis

The most common large vessel vasculitides include giant cell arteritis (GCA) and Takayasu arteritis (TA). GCA is by far the more common with approximately 20 cases per 100,000 each year.[36] Patients are usually elderly women who present with fever, headache, jaw pain, visual changes, and, occasionally, concurrent polymyalgia rheumatica. GCA affects mostly supra-aortic vessels, especially the superficial temporary artery, but in at least 15% of cases, extracranial arteries are involved, including the aorta and its major branches.[37] Although most current FDG-PET/CT imaging machines do not have the resolution to identify the superficial temporary artery,[38] several studies have looked to

extracranial involvement and found a potential role for FDG-PET in the diagnosis of GCA (**Fig. 2**).

In a recent study by Lehmann and colleagues,[39] the FDG-PET scan results of 20 patients with either GCA or TA were retrospectively reevaluated and compared with 20 controls. FDG uptake was significantly higher among patients with vasculitis ($P = .016$). The study also found that 2 blinded evaluators agreed on the presence of disease 85% of the time and suggested that the method was highly reproducible. A similar study was conducted by Walter and colleagues[40] comparing 26 patients with confirmed GCA or TA with 26 age- and gender-matched controls. The investigators found pathologic FDG uptake in 18 of 26 patients and found that FDG uptake was strongly associated with an elevation of CRP and erythrocyte sedimentation rate (ESR) levels.

FDG-PET assessment of GCA has also helped define the extent of vascular involvement. In an early study by Blockmans and colleagues,[41] the investigators compared FDG uptake in patients with polymyalgia rheumatica (n = 5) and GCA (n = 6) with age-matched controls with other inflammatory conditions (n = 23). The study found that patients with polymyalgia rheumatic and GCA were much more likely to have increased FDG uptake in thoracic vessels ($P<.001$) and upper leg vessels ($P<.05$) compared with controls, suggesting a more extensive distribution of vasculitis than previously suspected. In total, inflammatory involvement of the thoracic vasculature was observed in 4 of 6 patients with GCA and in 4 of 5 patients with polymyalgia, supporting observations that patients with GCA are prone to a greater incidence of AAS, which occur most commonly in the thoracic aorta.[42] Extensive extracranial vascular FDG uptake was observed again in a larger study by the same group. Among 35 patients with GCA, FDG uptake was observed in 83% of patients: 74% in the subclavian arteries, 54% in the aorta, 40% in the carotid arteries, and 37% in the iliac and femoral arteries.[43] Based on these

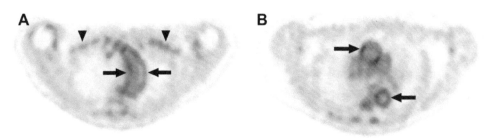

Fig. 2. A 72-year-old woman with a history of breast cancer and GCA. Transverse PET images from FDG-PET/CT examination through levels of aortic arch (*A*) and midascending aorta (*B*) reveal diffusely increased FDG uptake in subclavian arteries (*arrowheads*) and thoracic aorta (*arrows*), in keeping with active GCA.

and other studies, FDG-PET in patients with elevated inflammatory markers is estimated to have a sensitivity of 65% to 92% and a specificity of 80% to 100% for nonspecific vasculitis.[33,39,40,43,44] However, because elevated FDG uptake may be also seen with atherosclerosis, pretest probability and clinical suspicion should drive diagnostic considerations.[37]

When compared with existing imaging technologies, FDG-PET has been found to have several advantages in the diagnosis of GCA. FDG-PET has been shown to have diagnostic parity with duplex sonography, but unlike duplex sonography, FDG-PET is not dependent on operator skill and is able to provide a complete picture of regional vascular inflammation in 1 scan. When FDG-PET was compared with duplex sonography in 22 patients with clinical diagnosis of GCA, FDG-PET showed elevated FDG uptake in anatomic locations in agreement with duplex sonography, except in the temporal arteries (which could not be assessed by FDG-PET).[38] Furthermore, FDG-PET may be more sensitive in detecting extracranial sites of involvement. In a comparison of FDG-PET, MR imaging, and magnetic resonance angiography (MRA) in 15 patients with fever of unknown origin, elevated CRP levels, or elevated ESR levels, FDG-PET detected more involvement of a greater number of vascular sites than MR imaging and MRA.[45] The investigators concluded that FDG-PET was valuable in the primary diagnosis of

aortitis and noted that for a limited number of patients, FDG-PET was also more sensitive for detecting response to immunosuppressive therapy. This latter finding has also been reported in 2 other studies,[46] but despite an observed reduction on follow-up, FDG uptake had no effect on rate of recurrence.[43]

TA

TA is a rare disease characterized by chronic and progressive occlusive vasculitis of the aorta and its branches. In the United Kingdom, the estimated incidence is less than 1 patient per year, with a yearly prevalence of approximately 5 million.[47] In Japan and other Asian countries, the incidence is much higher.[48] TA mostly affects young women and presents a diagnostic challenge until advanced disease when pulseless peripheral arteries become evident. Angiography remains the reference standard diagnosis but is invasive and may not be specific before occlusive disease.[33]

FDG-PET imaging has been proposed as a noninvasive alternative that may have greater sensitivity for detecting early disease (**Fig. 3**). This finding is supported by work from Webb and colleagues[49] who studied 18 patients with suspected TA by angiography, MR imaging, and FDG-PET. Ultimately, 16 of 18 patients met criteria for TA. The investigators concluded that FDG-PET has a sensitivity of 92%, specificity of 100%, negative predictive value of

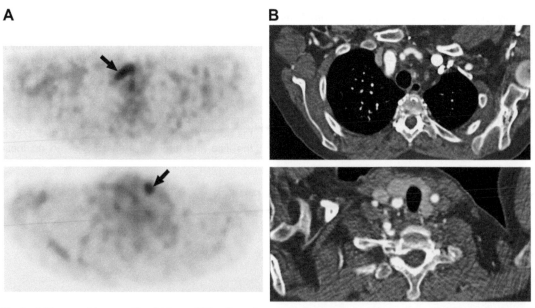

Fig. 3. A 71-year-old man with a history of TA, after prior aortic arch reconstruction, now with left chest and neck pains. Transverse FDG-PET (*A*) and contrast-enhanced CT (*B*) images through proximal and midneck demonstrate increased FDG uptake within left subclavian and left common carotid arteries (*arrows*) along with mild wall thickening on CT, in keeping with active TA.

85%, and positive predictive value of 100%. Similar results were reported by Kobayashi and colleagues[50] in another study comparing 11 patients with active TA and 3 patients with inactive TA with 6 healthy controls using FDG-PET/CT. The highest FDG uptake was seen in active patients, and no significant accumulation was observed in either inactive TA or health controls. The investigators estimated that FDG-PET had a sensitivity of 91% and a specificity of 89%.

As in patients with GCA, FDG-PET may also have a role in monitoring response to therapy. This finding was suggested by a small study by Andrews and colleagues[51] in which the investigators followed 6 confirmed cases of TA. Five patients went into remission, and FDG-PET showed a corresponding decrease in FDG uptake ($P<.04$). In the patient whose TA remained active, FDG uptake remained stable. A similar result was observed by Kobayashi and colleagues.[50] Notably, the FDG-PET results were sensitive to changes in disease activity despite stable inflammatory biomarkers of disease, which correlate with disease severity in only about 50% of all TA cases.[50,52]

ROLE OF FDG-PET IN VASCULAR GRAFT INFECTION

Vascular graft infection is a serious complication that is associated with high morbidity and mortality.[53] However, the onset may be insidious, whereby patients may present with vague symptoms or fever of unknown origin.[54] In acute cases, a rapid and accurate diagnosis is needed to both identify the infection and localize it for surgical planning. Conventional tools for diagnosis include CT and MR imaging, but several studies and case reports support an expanded role for FDG-PET (Fig. 4).

Numerous studies have compared the diagnostic abilities of FDG-PET and reference standard CT. In the first of these, Fukuchi and colleagues[55] studied 33 patients with suspected arterial vascular graft infection. Eleven (33%) patients were ultimately diagnosed with vascular graft infection. When

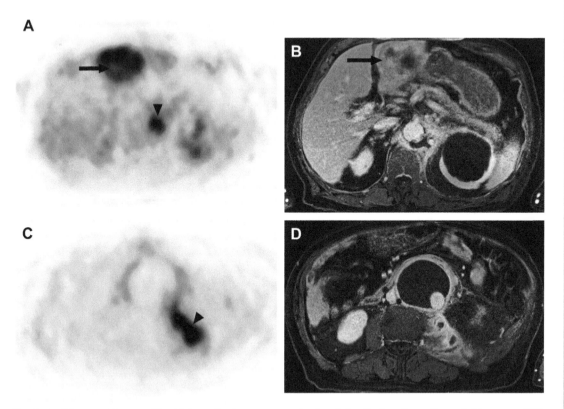

Fig. 4. An 80-year-old man with a history of colon cancer and prior abdominal aortic graft repair. Transverse FDG-PET and delayed postcontrast fat-suppressed T1-weighted MR images at upper abdominal (*A, B*) and midabdominal (*C, D*) levels show asymmetric increased FDG uptake (*arrowheads*) within thickened enhancing soft tissue on MR imaging along superior aspect of graft repair and also increased FDG uptake (*arrowheads*) within the left retroperitoneal enhancing soft tissue and fluid on MR imaging, in keeping with aortic graft infection and retroperitoneal abscess. Also note incidental FDG uptake in the left hepatic lobe abscess (*arrows*).

overall FDG uptake was considered (diffuse and focal), FDG-PET had a greater sensitivity (91%) than CT (64%), but lower specificity (64% vs 86%), resulting in 8 false-positive results. Remarkably, when the investigators altered their criteria for a positive PET result to include only focal FDG uptake in the aorta (defined as dotted nonconsecutive uptake), the specificity increased to 95%, whereas the sensitivity remained constant. The investigators noted that diffuse versus focal uptake strongly differentiated between normal and infected grafts, a finding that suggests a chronic process, such as underlying atherosclerosis, is responsible for diffuse FDG uptake. The investigators concluded that focal FDG uptake assessed by FDG-PET is superior to conventional CT in the diagnosis of graft infections.

This study has since been replicated with similar results. Keidar and colleagues[56] used FDG-PET/CT to assess 39 patients with suspected vascular graft infection. Similar to Fukuchi and colleagues,[55] Keidar and colleagues looked for focal FDG uptake on FDG-PET/CT as evidence of graft infection and found inflammatory foci localized to the vascular graft in 16 patients. Of these, 14 (88%) were ultimately diagnosed with graft infection. FDG-PET/CT had a sensitivity of 93%, specificity of 91%, positive predictive value of 88%, and negative predictive value of 96%, which was highly consistent with the results of Fukuchi and colleagues. More recently, Bruggink and colleagues[57] compared FDG-PET, CT, and FDG-PET/CT in 25 patients with clinically suspected vascular graft infection and compared readings by 2 observers. Similar to previous findings, the investigators report the best results with FDG-PET (sensitivity, 93%; specificity, 70%; positive predictive value, 82%; and negative predictive value, 88%), with fused FDG-PET/CT also showing significant improvement over CT alone. Reproducibility was excellent

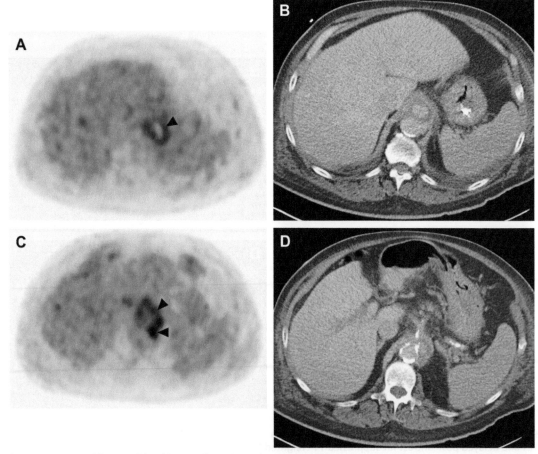

Fig. 5. A 67-year-old man with a history of persistent bacteremia. Transverse FDG-PET and contrast-enhanced CT images at retrocrural (A, B) and celiac arterial (C, D) levels reveal focal asymmetric increased FDG uptake (arrowheads) within the wall of a partially thrombosed saccular abdominal aortic aneurysm seen on CT, in keeping with mycotic aortic aneurysm.

for FDG-PET ($\kappa = 1.00$) but was much lower for CT and FDG-PET/CT (0.63 and 0.66, respectively). Spacek and colleagues[58] prospectively evaluated 76 patients with FDG-PET/CT and found similarly high sensitivity for the detection of vascular graft infections, noting in particular that focal uptake and irregular boundaries were highly specific.

Taken together, these studies strongly advocate for the inclusion of FDG-PET in the diagnostic workup of suspected vascular graft infection. In addition, advances in the FDG-PET and CT fusion should improve the anatomic correlation in combined imaging techniques. In their study, Keidar and colleagues[56] specifically note that FDG-PET/CT provided sufficient anatomic correlation to differentiate between vascular graft infections and neighboring soft tissue infections. The accuracy of FDG-PET/CT to localize the site of graft infection, even in the presence of aortoenteric fistula, has also been corroborated by numerous case reports and case series.[54,59-63] This localization is a crucial parameter for the accurate and rapid diagnosis of conditions that require surgical intervention and allows FDG-PET/CT to play an increasing role in the diagnosis of vascular infections.

NOVEL APPLICATIONS OF FDG-PET IN VASCULAR DISEASE

The rapidly expanding role of FDG-PET has seen novel applications of FDG-PET in numerous areas concerning vascular biology and disease. In some fields, such as chronic periaortitis[64] and vascular gene therapy,[65] the role of FDG-PET is just beginning to be explored. In others, the utility of FDG-PET warrants further consideration. Notable examples include assessment of mycotic aneurysms, fever of unknown origin, and vascular inflammation in novel populations.

Mycotic aneurysm is rare condition but has long posed a diagnostic dilemma with significant consequences in terms of morbidity and mortality. With the decline of valvular heart disease, aortitis has become the most common cause of mycotic aneurysms.[66] In numerous case reports, FDG-PET has aided in the timely diagnosis of mycotic aneurysms (**Fig. 5**) and has been suggested for use in long-term monitoring.[67-70]

There is also a growing interest in the utility of FDG-PET in the evaluation of fever of unknown origin. Although the various causes of fever of unknown origin are numerous, a significant number result from vasculitis and vascular wall infections as discussed earlier. In addition, several studies have supported a broader role for FDG-PET/CT in the diagnostic workup to take advantage of its ability to assess numerous tissues for metabolic and anatomic abnormalities. A study of 48 patients with fever of unknown origin assessed patients with FDG-PET/CT.[71] Nearly two-thirds of all 27 patients had a positive finding, and in 22 patients (46%), FDG-PET/CT identified the underlying disease (most commonly inflammation, infection, or malignancy). The negative predictive value was 100%. These impressive results have been replicated by other studies[72] and suggest that FDG-PET/CT may have a role in the diagnosis of fever of unknown origin.[73]

Finally, FDG-PET has been recently employed to investigate vascular inflammation in novel populations. In a recent work by Mehta and colleagues,[74] the investigators used FDG PET/CT to compare aortic inflammation in 6 patients with psoriasis with 4 age and gender-matched controls. They reported greater aortic inflammation in patients with psoriasis independent of known cardiovascular risk factors, suggesting a site of systemic inflammation that may have important clinical consequences. While such novel applications of FDG-PET technology remain in the realm of research, they help illustrate potential future applications of FDG-PET imaging in the assessment of vascular disease.

SUMMARY

The current clinical experience of FDG-PET in thoracic vascular imaging suggests a growing role for the early detection of vascular disease. For atherosclerosis, there is a growing body of literature supporting its role to both screen for subclinical atherosclerotic disease and monitor the response of vascular inflammation to drug therapy. Determination of the diagnostic performance of FDG-PET compared with existing imaging outputs, such as coronary arterial calcium scores, or clinical outcomes is important for future prospective studies. Although the literature is more limited regarding other applications of FDG-PET for evaluation of thoracic vascular disease, the role of FDG-PET seems to be similar. For conditions that may rapidly progress to highly morbid disease and for which conventional diagnostic guidelines have poor sensitivity, such as large vessel vasculitis, AAS, vascular graft infections, and mycotic aneurysms, FDG-PET seems to be uniquely sensitive to areas of active disease, detecting clinically significant lesions even when conventional diagnostic tests are inconclusive. The benefits of FDG-PET imaging as a diagnostic alternative in these and other vascular conditions will need to be explored further in future research, but existing studies demonstrate great potential for FDG-PET in the evaluation of patients with thoracic vascular disease.

REFERENCES

1. Vallabhajosula S, Fuster V. Atherosclerosis: imaging techniques and the evolving role of nuclear medicine. J Nucl Med 1997;38(11):1788–96.

2. Yun M, Yeh D, Araujo LI, et al. F-18 FDG uptake in the large arteries: a new observation. Clin Nucl Med 2001;26(4):314–9.

3. Xu J, Kochanek KD, Murphy SL, et al. Deaths: final data for 2007. Natl Vital Stat Rep 2010;58(19):1–135.

4. Burke AP, Farb A, Malcom GT, et al. Coronary risk factors and plaque morphology in men with coronary disease who died suddenly. N Engl J Med 1997;336(18):1276–82.

5. Virmani R, Kolodgie FD, Burke AP, et al. Lessons from sudden coronary death: a comprehensive morphological classification scheme for atherosclerotic lesions. Arterioscler Thromb Vasc Biol 2000;20(5): 1262–75.

6. Rudd JH, Warburton EA, Fryer TD, et al. Imaging atherosclerotic plaque inflammation with [18F]-fluorodeoxyglucose positron emission tomography. Circulation 2002;105(23):2708–11.

7. Ogawa M, Ishino S, Mukai T, et al. 18F-FDG accumulation in atherosclerotic plaques: immunohistochemical and PET imaging study. J Nucl Med 2004;45(7): 1245–50.

8. Tawakol A, Migrino RQ, Bashian GG, et al. In vivo 18F-fluorodeoxyglucose positron emission tomography imaging provides a noninvasive measure of carotid plaque inflammation in patients. J Am Coll Cardiol 2006;48(9):1818–24.

9. Worthley SG, Zhang ZY, Machac J, et al. In vivo noninvasive serial monitoring of FDG-PET progression and regression in a rabbit model of atherosclerosis. Int J Cardiovasc Imaging 2009;25(3):251–7.

10. Aziz K, Berger K, Claycombe K, et al. Noninvasive detection and localization of vulnerable plaque and arterial thrombosis with computed tomography angiography/positron emission tomography. Circulation 2008;117(16):2061–70.

11. Tahara N, Kai H, Nakaura H, et al. The prevalence of inflammation in carotid atherosclerosis: analysis with fluorodeoxyglucose-positron emission tomography. Eur Heart J 2007;28(18):2243–8.

12. Arauz A, Hoyos L, Zenteno M, et al. Carotid plaque inflammation detected by 18F-fluorodeoxyglucose-positron emission tomography: pilot study. Clin Neurol Neurosurg 2007;109(5):409–12.

13. Rudd JHF, Myers KS, Bansilal S, et al. 18Fluorodeoxyglucose positron emission tomography imaging of atherosclerotic plaque inflammation is highly reproducible: implications for atherosclerosis therapy trials. J Am Coll Cardiol 2007;50(9):892–6.

14. Rudd JH, Myers KS, Bansilal S, et al. Atherosclerosis inflammation imaging with 18F-FDG PET: carotid, iliac, and femoral uptake reproducibility, quantification methods, and recommendations. J Nucl Med 2008; 49(6):871–8.

15. Bural GG, Torigian DA, Chamroonrat W, et al. FDG-PET is an effective imaging modality to detect and quantify age-related atherosclerosis in large arteries. Eur J Nucl Med Mol Imaging 2008;35(3):562–9.

16. Bural GG, Torigian DA, Botvinick E, et al. A pilot study of changes in (18)F-FDG uptake, calcification and global metabolic activity of the aorta with aging. Hell J Nucl Med 2009;12(2):123–8.

17. Wassélius J, Larsson S, Jacobsson H. FDG-accumulating atherosclerotic plaques identified with 18F-FDG-PET/CT in 141 patients. Mol Imaging Biol 2009;11(6):455–9.

18. Tahara N, Kai H, Yamagishi S, et al. Vascular inflammation evaluated by [18F]-fluorodeoxyglucose positron emission tomography is associated with the metabolic syndrome. J Am Coll Cardiol 2007;49(14): 1533–9.

19. Paulmier B, Duet M, Khayat R, et al. Arterial wall uptake of fluorodeoxyglucose on PET imaging in stable cancer disease patients indicates higher risk for cardiovascular events. J Nucl Cardiol 2008; 15(2):209–17.

20. Rominger A, Saam T, Wolpers S, et al. 18F-FDG PET/CT identifies patients at risk for future vascular events in an otherwise asymptomatic cohort with neoplastic disease. J Nucl Med 2009;50(10): 1611–20.

21. Rudd JHF, Narula J, Strauss HW, et al. Imaging atherosclerotic plaque inflammation by fluorodeoxyglucose with positron emission tomography: ready for prime time? J Am Coll Cardiol 2010;55(23): 2527–35.

22. Ogawa M, Magata Y, Kato T, et al. Application of 18F-FDG PET for monitoring the therapeutic effect of antiinflammatory drugs on stabilization of vulnerable atherosclerotic plaques. J Nucl Med 2006; 47(11):1845–50.

23. Tahara N, Kai H, Ishibashi M, et al. Simvastatin attenuates plaque inflammation: evaluation by fluorodeoxyglucose positron emission tomography. J Am Coll Cardiol 2006;48(9):1825–31.

24. Corti R, Fayad ZA, Fuster V, et al. Effects of lipid-lowering by simvastatin on human atherosclerotic lesions: a longitudinal study by high-resolution, noninvasive magnetic resonance imaging. Circulation 2001;104(3):249–52.

25. Corti R, Fuster V, Fayad ZA, et al. Lipid lowering by simvastatin induces regression of human atherosclerotic lesions: two years' follow-up by high-resolution noninvasive magnetic resonance imaging. Circulation 2002;106(23):2884–7.

26. Lee SJ, On YK, Lee EJ, et al. Reversal of vascular 18F-FDG uptake with plasma high-density lipoprotein elevation by atherogenic risk reduction. J Nucl Med 2008;49(8):1277–82.

27. Golledge J, Muller R, Clancy P, et al. Evaluation of the diagnostic and prognostic value of plasma D-dimer for abdominal aortic aneurysm. Eur Heart J 2011;32(3):354–64.

28. Ohlmann P, Faure A, Morel O, et al. Diagnostic and prognostic value of circulating D-dimers in patients with acute aortic dissection. Crit Care Med 2006; 34(5):1358–64.

29. Schillinger M, Domanovits H, Bayegan K, et al. C-reactive protein and mortality in patients with acute aortic disease. Intensive Care Med 2002; 28(6):740–5.

30. Kuehl H, Eggebrecht H, Boes T, et al. Detection of inflammation in patients with acute aortic syndrome: comparison of FDG-PET/CT imaging and serological markers of inflammation. Heart 2008;94(11): 1472–7.

31. Kato K, Nishio A, Kato N, et al. Uptake of 18F-FDG in acute aortic dissection: a determinant of unfavorable outcome. J Nucl Med 2010;51(5):674–81.

32. Reeps C, Pelisek J, Bundschuh RA, et al. Imaging of acute and chronic aortic dissection by 18F-FDG PET/CT. J Nucl Med 2010;51(5):686–91.

33. Zerizer I, Tan K, Khan S, et al. Role of FDG-PET and PET/CT in the diagnosis and management of vasculitis. Eur J Radiol 2010;73(3):504–9.

34. Zeidler M, Hughes T, Zeman A. Confused by arteritis. Lancet 2000;355(9201):374.

35. Vanderschueren S, Knockaert D, Adriaenssens T, et al. From prolonged febrile illness to fever of unknown origin: the challenge continues. Arch Intern Med 2003;163(9):1033–41.

36. Salvarani C, Cantini F, Hunder GG. Polymyalgia rheumatica and giant-cell arteritis. Lancet 2008; 372(9634):234–45.

37. Belhocine T, Blockmans D, Hustinx R, et al. Imaging of large vessel vasculitis with 18FDG PET: illusion or reality? A critical review of the literature data. Eur J Nucl Med Mol Imaging 2003;30(9):1305–13.

38. Brodmann M, Lipp RW, Passath A, et al. The role of 2-18F-fluoro-2-deoxy-D-glucose positron emission tomography in the diagnosis of giant cell arteritis of the temporal arteries. Rheumatology (Oxford) 2004;43(2):241–2.

39. Lehmann P, Buchtala S, Achajew N, et al. 18F-FDG PET as a diagnostic procedure in large vessel vasculitis—a controlled, blinded re-examination of routine PET scans. Clin Rheumatol 2011;30(1):37–42.

40. Walter MA, Melzer RA, Schindler C, et al. The value of [18F]FDG-PET in the diagnosis of large-vessel vasculitis and the assessment of activity and extent of disease. Eur J Nucl Med Mol Imaging 2005;32(6): 674–81.

41. Blockmans D, Maes A, Stroobants S, et al. New arguments for a vasculitic nature of polymyalgia rheumatica using positron emission tomography. Rheumatology (Oxford) 1999;38(5):444–7.

42. Eberhardt RT, Dhadly M. Giant cell arteritis: diagnosis, management, and cardiovascular implications. Cardiol Rev 2007;15(2):55–61.

43. Blockmans D, de Ceuninck L, Vanderschueren S, et al. Repetitive 18F-fluorodeoxyglucose positron emission tomography in giant cell arteritis: a prospective study of 35 patients. Arthritis Rheum 2006;55(1): 131–7.

44. Bleeker-Rovers CP, Bredie SJ, van der Meer JW, et al. F-18-fluorodeoxyglucose positron emission tomography in diagnosis and follow-up of patients with different types of vasculitis. Neth J Med 2003;61(10):323–9.

45. Meller J, Strutz F, Siefker U, et al. Early diagnosis and follow-up of aortitis with [(18)F]FDG PET and MRI. Eur J Nucl Med Mol Imaging 2003;30(5): 730–6.

46. de Leeuw K, Bijl M, Jager PL. Additional value of positron emission tomography in diagnosis and follow-up of patients with large vessel vasculitides. Clin Exp Rheumatol 2004;22(6 Suppl 36):S21–6.

47. Watts R, Al-Taiar A, Mooney J, et al. The epidemiology of Takayasu arteritis in the UK. Rheumatology (Oxford) 2009;48(8):1008–11.

48. Toshihiko N. Current status of large and small vessel vasculitis in Japan. Int J Cardiol 1996;54(Suppl):S91–8.

49. Webb M, Chambers A, AL-Nahhas A, et al. The role of 18F-FDG PET in characterising disease activity in Takayasu arteritis. Eur J Nucl Med Mol Imaging 2004;31(5):627–34.

50. Kobayashi Y, Ishii K, Oda K, et al. Aortic wall inflammation due to Takayasu arteritis imaged with 18F-FDG PET coregistered with enhanced CT. J Nucl Med 2005;46(6):917–22.

51. Andrews J, Al-Nahhas A, Pennell DJ, et al. Non-invasive imaging in the diagnosis and management of Takayasu's arteritis. Ann Rheum Dis 2004;63(8): 995–1000.

52. Kerr G. Takayasu's arteritis. Curr Opin Rheumatol 1994;6(1):32–8.

53. van der Vaart MG, Meerwaldt R, Slart RH, et al. Application of PET/SPECT imaging in vascular disease. Eur J Vasc Endovasc Surg 2008;35(5):507–13.

54. van Assen S, Houwerzijl EJ, van den Dungen JJ, et al. Vascular graft infection due to chronic Q fever diagnosed with fusion positron emission tomography/computed tomography. J Vasc Surg 2007; 46(2):372.

55. Fukuchi K, Ishida Y, Higashi M, et al. Detection of aortic graft infection by fluorodeoxyglucose positron emission tomography: comparison with computed tomographic findings. J Vasc Surg 2005;42(5): 919–25.

56. Keidar Z, Engel A, Hoffman A, et al. Prosthetic vascular graft infection: the role of 18F-FDG PET/CT. J Nucl Med 2007;48(8):1230–6.

57. Bruggink JL, Glaudemans AW, Saleem BR, et al. Accuracy of FDG-PET-CT in the diagnostic work-up

of vascular prosthetic graft infection. Eur J Vasc Endovasc Surg 2010;40(3):348–54.

58. Spacek M, Belohlavek O, Votrubova J, et al. Diagnostics of "non-acute" vascular prosthesis infection using 18F-FDG PET/CT: our experience with 96 prostheses. Eur J Nucl Med Mol Imaging 2009;36(5): 850–8.

59. Tegler G, Sorensen J, Bjorck M, et al. Detection of aortic graft infection by 18-fluorodeoxyglucose positron emission tomography combined with computed tomography. J Vasc Surg 2007;45(4):828–30.

60. Lauwers P, Van den Broeck S, Carp L, et al. The use of positron emission tomography with (18)F-fluorodeoxyglucose for the diagnosis of vascular graft infection. Angiology 2007;58(6):717–24.

61. Wasikova S, Staffa R, Kriz Z, et al. Treatment of vascular prosthesis infection and aorto-enteric fistula as a late complication after reconstructive surgery of the abdominal aorta—a case report. Rozhl Chir 2007; 86(10):522–4 [in Czech].

62. Krupnick AS, Lombardi JV, Engels FH, et al. 18-fluorodeoxyglucose positron emission tomography as a novel imaging tool for the diagnosis of aortoenteric fistula and aortic graft infection—a case report. Vasc Endovascular Surg 2003;37(5):363–6.

63. Basu S, Chryssikos T, Moghadam-Kia S, et al. Positron emission tomography as a diagnostic tool in infection: present role and future possibilities. Semin Nucl Med 2009;39(1):36–51.

64. Blockmans D, Van Moer E, Dehem J, et al. Positron emission tomography can reveal abdominal periaortitis. Clin Nucl Med 2002;27(3):211–2.

65. Manninen HI, Yang X. Imaging after vascular gene therapy. Eur J Radiol 2005;56(2):165–70.

66. Brown SL, Busuttil RW, Baker JD, et al. Bacteriologic and surgical determinants of survival in patients with mycotic aneurysms. J Vasc Surg 1984;1(4):541–7.

67. Spacek M, Stadler P, Belohlavek O, et al. Contribution to FDG-PET/CT diagnostics and post-operative monitoring of patients with mycotic aneurysm of the thoracic aorta. Acta Chir Belg 2010;110(1): 106–8.

68. Bonekamp D, Smith JD, Aygun N. Avid FDG uptake in a rapidly enlarging common carotid artery mycotic aneurysm, mimicking lymphadenopathy. Emerg Radiol 2009;16(5):383–6.

69. Davison JM, Montilla-Soler JL, Broussard E, et al. F-18 FDG PET-CT imaging of a mycotic aneurysm. Clin Nucl Med 2005;30(7):483–7.

70. Helleman JN, Hendriks JM, Deblier I, et al. Mycotic aneurysm of the descending thoracic aorta. Review and case report. Acta Chir Belg 2007;107(5): 544–7.

71. Keidar Z, Gurman-Balbir A, Gaitini D, et al. Fever of unknown origin: the role of 18F-FDG PET/CT. J Nucl Med 2008;49(12):1980–5.

72. Jaruskova M, Belohlavek O. Role of FDG-PET and PET/CT in the diagnosis of prolonged febrile states. Eur J Nucl Med Mol Imaging 2006;33(8):913–8.

73. Meller J, Sahlmann CO, Scheel AK. 18F-FDG PET and PET/CT in fever of unknown origin. J Nucl Med 2007;48(1):35–45.

74. Mehta NN, Yu Y, Saboury B, et al. Systemic and vascular inflammation in patients with moderate to severe psoriasis as measured by [18F]-fluorodeoxyglucose positron emission tomography-computer tomography (FDG-PET/CT). Arch Derm 2011. [Epub ahead of print].

Review of Physiologic and Pathophysiologic Sources of Fluorodeoxyglucose Uptake in the Chest Wall on PET

Marc Hickeson, MD, FRCP*, Gad Abikhzer, MD

KEYWORDS

- Chest wall • FDG • PET/CT • Physiologic • Benign
- Malignant

The chest wall can be defined as the osseous and soft tissue structures that form the outer framework of the thorax and move during breathing. The topics covered in this article include physiologic uptake of fluorodeoxyglucose (FDG), benign diseases of the chest wall, and malignant tumors of the chest wall.

PHYSIOLOGIC ACTIVITY
Intense Exercise

In general, skeletal muscles show low FDG activity at rest. FDG-PET commonly shows physiologic muscle uptake caused by excessive muscle activity during the uptake phase or within a few days preceding the study, which can be seen in various muscle groups including the chest wall.[1] The pattern can be observed after recent intense physical exercises or muscle tension. It is usually, but not always, relatively symmetric and diffuse in various muscle groups (**Fig. 1**).

Inadequate Fasting and Recent Insulin Administration

Increased serum insulin levels either from exogenous administration or endogenous secretion of insulin associated with insufficient fasting may result in a hyperinsulinemic state and affect the diagnostic quality of FDG-PET imaging. It is typically associated with diffuse muscular and myocardial uptake. Diffusely decreased hepatic uptake may also be shown.[2] A minimum fast of 4 to 6 hours is recommended in both the Society of Nuclear Medicine and European Association of Nuclear Medicine guidelines before FDG-PET (**Fig. 2**).[3,4]

Physiologic Brown Fat Uptake

The distribution of hypermetabolism caused by brown adipose tissue was previously considered to be related to muscular uptake on dedicated PET scanners. The precise anatomic localization of the hypermetabolism achievable on PET/computed tomography (CT) showed that this uptake corresponds to fatty tissue. Brown adipose tissue is a thermogenesis organ with the main function of generating heat.[2] Unlike white adipose tissue, it is associated with high cellularity, rich vascularization, and innervation, and contains considerably more mitochondria than white fat.

Brown adipose tissue was originally described as hypermetabolism corresponding to adipose

The investigators have nothing to disclose.
Division of Nuclear Medicine, McGill University Health Centre, Royal Victoria Hospital, 687 Pine Avenue West, M2.11, Montreal, Quebec H3A 1A1, Canada
* Corresponding author.
E-mail address: marc.hickeson@muhc.mcgill.ca

PET Clin 6 (2011) 339–364
doi:10.1016/j.cpet.2011.04.004
1556-8598/11/$ – see front matter © 2011 Elsevier Inc. All rights reserved.

pet.theclinics.com

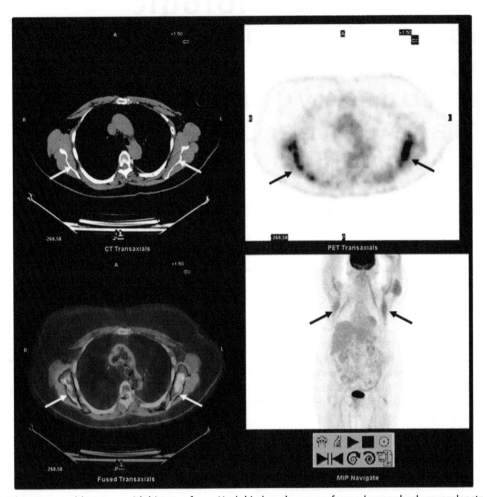

Fig. 1. This 73-year-old woman with history of non-Hodgkin lymphoma performed upper body muscular strength training exercise in a fitness gymnasium the evening before the FDG-PET/CT study. Imaging shows hypermetabolism in the musculature of the shoulder girdle bilaterally (*arrows*) and bilateral proximal upper limbs.

tissue in bilateral supraclavicular regions on PET/CT imaging.[5] It can also be shown in the posterior cervical region, suprasternal notch, bilateral upper axillae, mediastinum, bilateral paravertebral regions, cardiac apex, and bilateral pararenal spaces.[6] The distribution is usually relatively symmetric but may be asymmetric, particularly in a patient with altered innervation of brown adipose tissue from surgical interruption of sympathetic neurons.[2] Brown adipose tissue is most commonly seen on FDG-PET/CT imaging in young patients, patients with low body-mass index, and in women.[7,8]

The appearance of physiologic brown fat uptake can generally be easily recognized by the distribution of intense hypermetabolism corresponding to adipose tissue. However, it may pose a challenge with the presence of known space-occupying lesions surrounded by this physiologic uptake. Several approaches, both pharmacologic and nonpharmacologic, are available to suppress this physiologic brown fat uptake. These approaches are summarized in **Box 1 (Box 1; Fig. 3)**.[5,9–13]

Bone Marrow Hyperplasia

A mild to moderate degree of FDG activity is normally shown on PET/CT. Bone marrow hyperplasia refers to increased bone marrow cellularity and can be attributed to decreased peripheral blood cell counts or induction by pharmacologic agents. Bone marrow hyperplasia is commonly shown in patients with malignancies who have been treated with chemotherapy and bone marrow stimulating agents (granulocyte colony-stimulating factor). There are also multiple other causes such as anemia,[14] leukemia,[15] and treatment with erythropoietin.[16] PET imaging generally shows diffuse hypermetabolism within the imaged

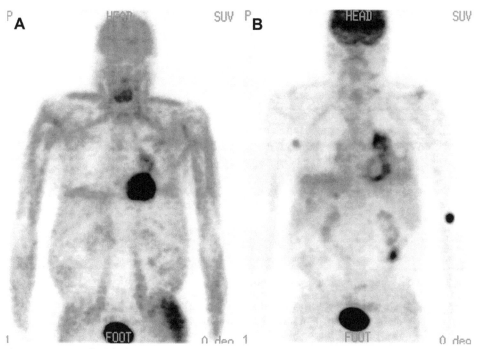

Fig. 2. First FDG-PET study (*A*) the patient had breakfast immediately before traveling for 2 hours before the FDG-PET study. The serum glucose was 10.0 mmol/L at the time of FDG injection. The study was nondiagnostic, with extensive hypermetabolism in the cardiac and skeletal muscle. Repeat FDG-PET study performed 5 days later (*B*) the serum glucose was 5.5 mmol before FDG injection and the patient adequately fasted before the study. Imaging shows focal hypermetabolic lesions that were not clearly evident on the first study, including in the right axillary, porta hepatic, and subhepatic regions.

bone marrow and less intensely increased uptake in the spleen.[17,18] This pattern of diffuse hypermetabolism in the skeleton and the spleen should be recognized as being most likely caused by bone marrow hyperplasia and should not be mistaken for diffuse metastatic disease. This finding can be confirmed by the absence of diffuse

hypermetabolism in the skeleton on a baseline pretreatment study (**Fig. 4**).

Chronic Obstructive Pulmonary Disease

Chronic obstructive pulmonary disease (COPD) is a major health problem, and is an important cause of mortality in many countries. COPD is a phenotypically heterogeneous chronic condition of the lung and airways that is characterized by airflow obstruction, and is composed of variable amounts of alveolar lung tissue destruction (emphysema) and airway disease (chronic bronchitis, asthma). COPD causes resistance to airflow that is not completely reversible, which reduces the ability of the airways to remain open during expiration. This airway narrowing is related to loss of elastic recoil of the lung in emphysema caused by decreased radial traction on airways. This situation results in increased workload of the respiratory muscles in patients with COPD compared with the healthy population. Patients with COPD use their intercostal and abdominal muscles extensively during expiration to overcome the increased resistance to airflow in airways and loss of lung elasticity.

Box 1
Methods to reduce FDG uptake in brown adipose tissue

- Nonpharmacologic

  - Avoid cold exposure[5]
  - Warm ambient temperature[9]
  - Warm clothing at the time of the study[9]
  - Cover patient with warm blanket[9]
  - Low-carbohydrate and high-fat diet[10]
  - Avoid cigarettes and nicotine[11]
  - Avoid adrenergic agents[11]

- Pharmacologic

  - Benzodiazepines[12]
  - Fentanyl[12]
  - Propanolol[13]
  - Reserpine[13]

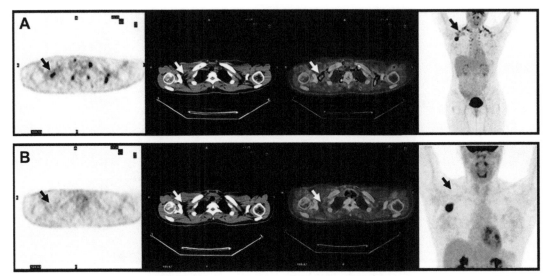

Fig. 3. This 31-year-old woman presented with a known biopsy-proven adenocarcinoma in the apex of the right axilla. (*A*) An FDG-PET/CT was subsequently performed to evaluate for any other sites of disease and showed extensive FDG uptake in brown adipose tissue in the neck, bilateral axillae (*arrow*), superior mediastinum, and bilateral paraspinal regions. (*B*) The patient returned 2 days later for repeat FDG-PET/CT imaging after the intravenous administration of 5 mg of diazepam, which showed resolution of this brown adipose tissue uptake (*arrow*) and persistent hypermetabolic lesion in the right axilla without evidence of metabolically active disease elsewhere.

As a result of the increased workload of the expiratory muscles, COPD is associated with extensive and relatively symmetric areas of excessive metabolic activity on FDG-PET in the thoracic and abdominal expiratory musculature, including the intercostal, subscapular, rectus abdominis, and abdominal oblique muscles.[19,20] Other findings commonly observed with COPD are increased lung volume, diffusely diminished FDG activity in the lungs, increased anteroposterior thoracic diameter, flattening of the diaphragm, and prominent right ventricular FDG uptake (**Figs. 5–7**).[21–23]

BENIGN DISEASES OF THE CHEST WALL
Benign Tumors of the Chest Wall

Benign tumors are seen on FDG-PET mostly as incidental findings in patients being evaluated for other neoplastic diseases. The role of FDG-PET in these lesions is not clearly defined. In general, benign tumors with intense FDG uptake are usually characterized as histiocytic or giant cell-containing lesions, fibrous dysplasia, schwannoma,[24] or elastofibroma dorsi.[25] Other benign tumors generally show low uptake of FDG.[26] These are briefly summarized in **Tables 1** and **2** (**Figs. 8** and **9**; **Tables 1** and 2).[24–34]

Previous Surgery of the Chest Wall

A history of recent surgery is a common occurrence in patients undergoing an FDG-PET study. The recognition of this cause for benign FDG uptake is important for the appropriate management of these patients. Postsurgical FDG uptake at the surgical site is mainly diffuse, corresponds

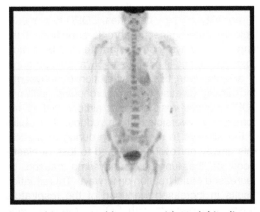

Fig. 4. This 29-year-old woman with Hodgkin disease underwent a PET/CT study after the second cycle of chemotherapy. FDG-PET imaging shows diffuse hypermetabolism within the axial and proximal appendicular skeleton caused by bone marrow stimulation from granulocyte colony-stimulating factor.

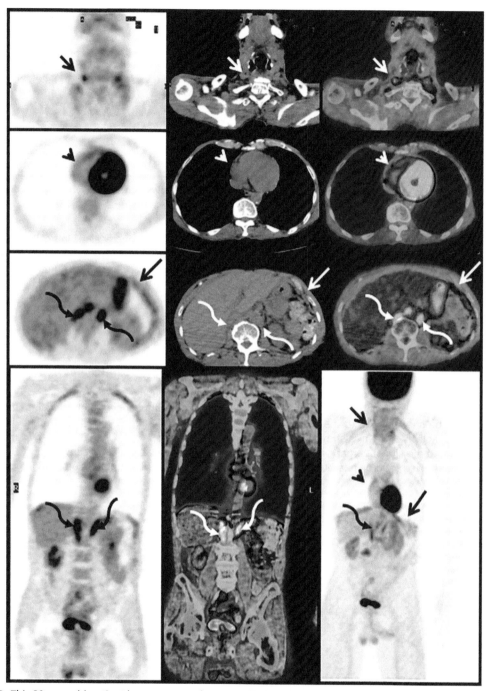

Fig. 5. This 80-year-old patient has severe emphysema. PET/CT imaging showed hypermetabolism of the scalene muscles (*small arrow*), diaphragmatic muscles (*large arrow*), diaphragmatic crura (*curved arrow*), and prominent right ventricle uptake (*arrow head*). Increased lung volume is also evident on the coronal and maximal intensity projection images.

to the site of surgery, decreases in intensity with time, and is often not associated with any distinct space-occupying lesion on the corresponding CT images. This benign pattern of FDG uptake should not be mistaken for recurrent neoplastic disease, which is expected to show focal FDG uptake and increase in intensity and/or size with time (**Fig. 10**).[35]

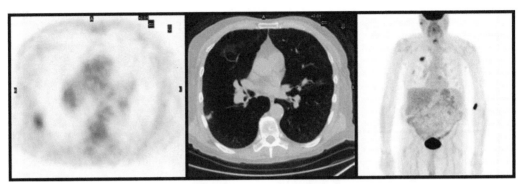

Fig. 6. The FDG-PET/CT study of this 72-year-old man with emphysema shows increased anteroposterior diameter of the thoracic cavity.

Infections of the Chest Wall

Imaging with FDG-PET has been shown to have a promising role for the evaluation of bone and soft tissue infection.[36–40] The increased uptake of FDG in infection can be attributed to the increased expression of glucose transporters in activated inflammatory cells.[41] In the chest wall, FDG uptake may be seen in sites of cellulitis and osteomyelitis as well as in areas of normal postoperative change, which could pose a challenge when evaluating patients for infection or local recurrence of tumor. The presence of infection in the postoperative site can be suspected with the presence of intense FDG activity with a distribution that is noncongruent to the site of surgery, the presence of fat-stranding, fluid, and/or gas bubbles on CT imaging, and by increasing intensity of FDG uptake on follow-up FDG-PET imaging. To differentiate a fracture related to trauma or surgery from infection, the period of FDG-PET after the fracture may be of value. Zhuang and colleagues[42] reported that FDG uptake in fracture should normalize within 3 months unless complicated by infection or malignancy (**Figs. 11–13**).

Radiation Sequelae in the Chest Wall

Radiation sequelae are commonly encountered in patients with cancer after radiation therapy. Radiation is recognized as a potent inducer of inflammation.[43,44] On FDG-PET/CT imaging, radiation sequelae generally show mildly to moderately increased FDG uptake corresponding to the

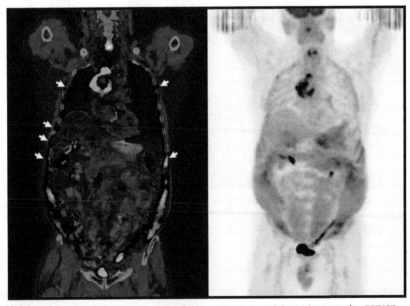

Fig. 7. Increased FDG uptake in the intercostals muscle uptake (*arrows*) is evident on the PET/CT study of this 75-year-old patient with emphysema. (*Courtesy of* Dr Chris Rush, Department of Nuclear Medicine, Jewish General Hospital, Montreal, Quebec, Canada.)

Table 1
Appearance of benign chest wall tumors on FDG-PET

Usually Low FDG Uptake	Variable FDG Uptake	Usually High FDG Uptake
Cavernous hemangioma	Fibrous dysplasia	Aneurysmal bone cyst
Osteochondroma	Schwannoma	Giant cell tumor
Ossifying fibromyxoid tumor	Elastofibroma dorsi	Eosinophilic granuloma
Lipoma		Paraganglioma
Neurofibroma		Chondromyxoid fibroma
Desmoid tumor		

Data from Refs. [24–30]

sites of radiation therapy, which gradually decreases in intensity. The duration of this hypermetabolism attributed to radiation has yet to be established. Generally, FDG uptake seen 6 months after completion of radiation therapy should have normalized and any focal FDG uptake should be considered as tumor recurrence.[45]

MALIGNANT TUMORS OF THE CHEST WALL

The chest wall consists of muscles, bone, cartilage, fat, fibrous connective tissue, nerves, breast tissue, and blood and lymphatic vessels.[46] Tumors may arise from any of these tissues and produce chest wall masses, which are typical clinical presentations of malignant tumors of the chest wall. Chest wall pain is the most common presenting symptom and, unlike with benign chest wall tumors, occurs in most patients. Malignant tumors of the chest wall can be classified as skeletal or extraskeletal in origin and as primary or metastatic in nature.

Primary Osseous Tumors

Chondrosarcoma

Chondrosarcomas are malignant bone tumors that produce chondroid matrix.[47] They are the most common chest wall primary osseous neoplasms, accounting for approximately 20% of all primary chest wall malignancies. Two peak periods of prevalence have been identified, with the first peak at less than 20 years of age and the second at greater than 50 years of age. This malignancy most commonly arises along the costochondral junctions of the first 5 ribs but may also originate from any of the bones of the chest wall. Most of these neoplasms are primary lesions. However, approximately 10% arise from preexisting benign tumors such as enchondromas and osteochondromas. Prognosis is variable and is highly dependent on the histologic grade. Approximately 90% are of low-grade histology, which are slow growing, have low propensity to metastasize,

and are considered to be poorly responsive to chemotherapy and radiation therapy. Approximately 10% are of high-grade histology,[48] which have high metastatic potential, poor prognosis, but a higher rate of response to chemotherapy and radiation therapy.

On FDG-PET imaging, low-grade chondrosarcomas show low uptake of FDG generally with a maximum standardized uptake value (SUV) of less than 5.0. On the other hand, a chondrosarcoma showing intense FDG activity with a maximum SUV of greater than 5.0 is typically associated with high-grade histology.[49] The lesion typically appears as a mass with irregular contour associated with bone destruction and multiple foci of calcification on the corresponding CT images (**Figs. 14** and **15**).

Osteosarcoma

Osteosarcomas are mesenchymal malignancies that produce osteoid matrix or immature bone. They most commonly originate in the metaphyses of long bones and rarely occur in the thorax. The ribs, scapulae, and clavicles are the most frequent sites of chest wall osteosarcomas, although they may occur in any bone. The usual clinical presentation of chest wall osteosarcomas is typically a painful mass. This neoplasm is associated with a frequent local recurrence rate, high propensity to metastasize to the regional lymph nodes, and a worse prognosis compared with osteosarcomas originating from the appendicular skeleton. There is a bimodal age distribution, with peaks in adolescence and in adults older than 60 years.[50] Unlike those in children, osteosarcomas in older adults are secondary to preexisting bone disease such as Paget disease, fibrous dysplasia, multiple chondromas, or to previous radiation or chemotherapy in more than 50% of cases.[51]

On FDG-PET imaging, osteosarcomas usually show intense uptake. They are also associated with markedly heterogeneous FDG activity with areas of high metabolic activity most often in the peripheral regions of the tumor mass. Large

Table 2
Clinical findings and appearance of CT for benign chest wall tumors

Benign Tumor	Age	Prevalence	Findings on Nonenhanced CT
Superficial Soft Tissue Lesions			
Cavernous hemangioma	Infancy or early adulthood	Uncommon	Cutaneous mass with ill-defined contours
Lipoma	Adulthood	Common	Soft tissue lesion with fat attenuation, well-defined contours, and internal homogeneity most frequent in the obese
Spindle cell lipoma	Adulthood	Uncommon	Soft tissue lesion in neck or shoulder region with well-defined contours and internal heterogeneity most frequent in men
Deep Soft Tissue Lesions			
Desmoid tumor	Adolescence to early adulthood	Common	Noncalcified nonneoplastic fibrous mass with infiltrating or nodular pattern
Elastofibroma dorsi	Middle to late adulthood	Rare	Soft tissue mass, often bilateral, usually in the deep dorsal region between the thoracic wall and the lower third of the scapula, often containing fat
Ganglioneuroma	Early adulthood	Uncommon	Soft tissue lesion located in paravertebral region with well-defined contour and whorled appearance
Neurofibroma	Early adulthood	Uncommon	Associated with type 1 neurofibromatosis, well-defined soft tissue lesion with plexiform contour, osseous scalloping and calcification
Paraganglioma	Adolescence to early adulthood	Rare	Soft tissue lesion with well-defined contours in midthorax; often associated with additional adrenal or extrathoracic paraganglionic tumors
Schwannoma	Adulthood	Common	Encapsulated, typically slow-growing soft tissue lesion with osseous scalloping; large lesions with cystic, necrotic, fatty, or calcific changes
Bone Lesions			
Aneurysmal bone cyst	Early adulthood	Uncommon	Expansile osteolytic bone lesion with blood-filled cyst associated with cortical thinning
Chondromyxoid fibroma	Early adulthood	Rare	Expansile bone lesion with sclerotic band located in rib, spine, or scapula
Fibrous dysplasia	Adolescence to early adulthood	Uncommon	Fusiform-shaped, usually monostotic osteolytic bone lesion with mild osseous expansion, ground glass matrix, fracture, or deformity
Giant cell tumor	Early to middle adulthood	Common	Eccentric osteolytic bone lesion with cortical thinning located in subchondral regions of flat or tubular bones

(continued on next page)

Table 2
(continued)

Benign Tumor	Age	Prevalence	Findings on Nonenhanced CT
Ossifying fibromyxoid tumor	Adulthood	Rare	Bone lesion with sclerotic band and osteolytic change and confluent contours
Osteochondroma	Adulthood	Common	Bone lesion with eccentric growth pattern and cartilaginous cap at costochondral junction associated with fracture or deformity

Data from Refs. [31–34]

lesions commonly show large areas of low uptake of FDG as a result of necrosis. The maximum SUV within the lesion correlates well with the histologic grade.[49,52] The site of highest FDG uptake can be used to indicate the biopsy site of the tumor. The corresponding CT images show calcification within the lesion, with the areas of mineralization typically greater at the center than in the periphery (**Fig. 16**).

Ewing sarcoma

Ewing sarcoma is an uncommon malignancy of mesenchymal origin with the highest incidence between the ages of 10 and 20 years. Ewing sarcomas express one of several different reciprocal translocations, with 85% to 90% of cases associated with translocations between chromosomes 11 and 22-t(11;22)(q24;q12). It is a highly aggressive malignancy with high propensity to metastasize, with the most common sites being the lungs, followed by the bone marrow and bone.[53] The most common presenting symptom is localized pain or swelling of a few weeks' or months' duration.[54] Constitutional signs and symptoms such as fever, weight loss, fatigue and anemia are present in approximately 10% to 20% of cases at initial presentation and are often associated with advanced disease.

On baseline FDG-PET imaging, Ewing sarcoma generally appears as an intensely hypermetabolic lesion and is usually diaphyseal or metaphyseal in location with or without adjacent soft tissue involvement. It can arise from any bone[55] but the most common sites in the chest wall are the spine and ribs. The corresponding CT images typically show a predominantly osteolytic ill-defined lesion with a heterogeneous appearance attributed by extensive cystic degeneration that may or may not be associated with calcification (**Fig. 17**).[56]

Hematologic Malignancies

Lymphomas

Primary malignant lymphomas of the chest wall are uncommon, with few cases arising from the pleura, the rib, or the sternum having been reported.[57–61] The most common histology is diffuse large B-cell lymphoma.[62] They usually appear intensely hypermetabolic on FDG-PET imaging. They may be associated with a soft tissue mass or, if involving the bone, a pure osteolytic or mixed osteolytic-osteosclerotic pattern on corresponding CT imaging (**Fig. 18**).[63]

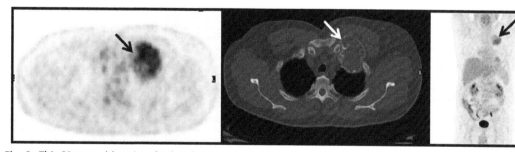

Fig. 8. This 60-year-old patient had undergone a PET/CT study, which shows an FDG-avid eccentric expansile left chest wall mass (*arrow*) involving the first rib with a maximum SUV of 5.4 with no other hypermetabolic lesions elsewhere. This finding corresponds to an expansile lytic lesion with sclerotic margins (*arrow*) on the CT images. The final diagnosis of a chondromyxoid fibroma was established after subsequent excisional biopsy.

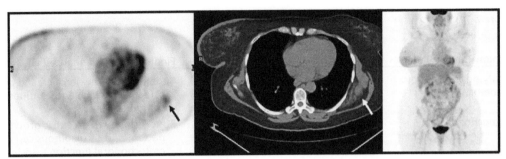

Fig. 9. The FDG-PET/CT of this 57-year-old woman with previous breast cancer shows mild hypermetabolism (*arrow*), which corresponds to the poorly defined soft tissue changes containing linear low-attenuation streaks from fat in the subscapular region on the left side of the chest wall (*arrow*). The location, low uptake of FDG, and appearance on CT imaging are characteristic for elastofibroma dorsi.

Solitary plasmacytoma and multiple myeloma

Solitary plasmacytoma and multiple myeloma are characterized by the neoplastic proliferation of a single clone of plasma cells producing a monoclonal immunoglobulin.[64] Multiple myelomas are the most common primary bone malignancies. Solitary plasmacytomas present as a solitary lesion, most commonly in the skeleton and rarely outside the skeleton. They have a peak incidence at the age of approximately 50 years. On the other hand, multiple myeloma presents as multiple lesions and is diagnosed later in life with a median age of approximately 66 years at diagnosis.[65] The diagnostic criteria for solitary plasmacytoma and multiple myeloma are summarized in **Box 2**.[66,67] Solitary plasmacytomas may progress to multiple myeloma.

On FDG-PET imaging, previously untreated solitary plasmacytomas appear as hypermetabolic lesions corresponding to a multicystic expansile or purely osteolytic lesion without expansion. Extraosseous plasmacytoma presents as a hypermetabolic soft tissue mass. Previously untreated multiple myeloma most commonly appears as either multifocal or diffuse bone marrow hypermetabolism.[68]

The corresponding CT images show osteolytic lesions at the sites of the hypermetabolic lesions. Sclerosis may appear at the sites of the lesions after pathologic fracture, chemotherapy, or radiotherapy. Untreated lesions not associated with fractures may rarely appear as sclerotic lesions (see **Box 2**).[33]

Primary Soft Tissue Tumors

Soft tissue sarcomas

Sarcomas are a heterogeneous group of malignant neoplasms of mesenchymal origin involving the bone and soft tissues. The most common histologic origins of soft tissue sarcomas are liposarcomas, malignant fibrous histiosarcomas, leiomyosarcomas, and synovial sarcomas in adults. In children, rhabdomyosarcomas account for approximately 70% of childhood soft tissue sarcomas. In the chest wall, liposarcoma is the most common type of soft tissue sarcoma, followed by malignant fibrous histiocytoma (MFH), malignant peripheral nerve sheath tumor, dermatomyosarcoma protuberans, and leiomyosarcoma.[33] All of these tumors are discussed in the next sections.

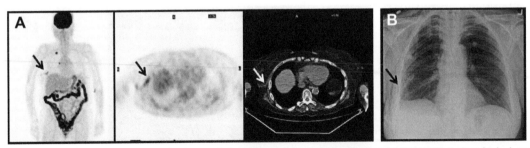

Fig. 10. (*A*) This 72-year-old patient had recently had a chest tube removed before FDG-PET/CT study, which shows mild linear hypermetabolism at the level of the right fifth intercostal space (*arrows*). (*B*) The recent CT scan of the chest and chest radiograph performed 2 weeks before the PET/CT show evidence of the chest tube in place (*arrows*).

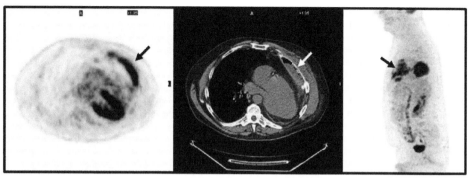

Fig. 11. This 65-year-old man had previously undergone a left pneumonectomy, en bloc chest wall resection, and chest wall reconstruction with Gore-Tex synthetic prosthetic mesh for locally extensive lung cancer. He developed a chest wall abscess overlying the prosthetic mesh in the left anterior chest wall. The FDG-PET/CT study shows extensive hypermetabolism at the site of the infection (*arrows*). The patient subsequently underwent abscess drainage, removal of the infected mesh, and redo thoracotomy.

Liposarcoma

Liposarcoma is a neoplastic disease of adipose tissues. It is most prevalent during adulthood, with a peak age incidence between the ages of 40 and 60 years. There are several histologic variants of liposarcomas. The most common histologies are well-differentiated liposarcomas followed by dedifferentiated liposarcomas. Myxoid, round-cell, and pleomorphic variants also exist but are more uncommon. Approximately 10% of all liposarcomas originate from the chest wall. Morphologically, well-differentiated liposarcomas have similar characteristics as mature adipose tissue, whereas dedifferentiated liposarcomas are more cellular and have similar characteristics to other solid neoplasms.

On FDG-PET imaging, well-differentiated liposarcomas appear as mildly hypermetabolic large

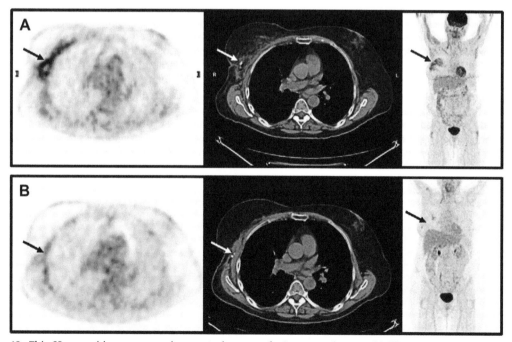

Fig. 12. This 63-year-old woman was known to have a soft tissue purulent methicillin-resistant *Staphylococcus aureus* infection deep to the right breast. The initial FDG-PET/CT study (*A*) showed extensive soft tissue hypermetabolism (*arrow*) on PET images corresponding to fat-stranding and gas bubbles (*arrow*) on CT images. This hypermetabolism was subsequently debrided. The patient improved clinically and the follow-up FDG-PET/CT study (*B*) showed marked regression of the hypermetabolism.

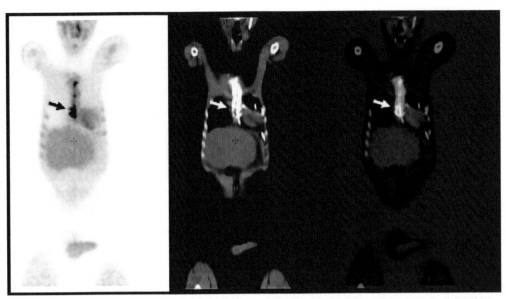

Fig. 13. This 16-year-old boy developed a sternal osteomyelitis after a Fontan procedure. The FDG-PET/CT study showed heterogeneous hypermetabolism at the site of the sternotomy, which is most intense inferiorly (*arrow*). The patient improved clinically after debridement and treatment with antibiotics. (*Courtesy of* Dr Sophie Turpin, Department of Nuclear Medicine, Sainte-Justine Hospital, Montreal, Quebec, Canada.)

masses. On the corresponding CT images, these liposarcomas have slightly higher attenuation than that of normal adipose tissue because these tumors consist of both adipose and soft tissues. These lesions usually have heterogeneous appearance because of their variable cellularity.[33] Regions of calcification and ossification are sometimes present and suggest a myxoid subtype. Dedifferentiated subtypes typically appear intensely hypermetabolic on FDG-PET and have the appearance and attenuation of soft tissue masses on CT imaging.

Well-differentiated liposarcomas are low-grade malignancies, whereas dedifferentiated liposarcomas are high-grade malignancies. Dedifferentiated liposarcomas are associated with high local recurrence rates, propensity to metastasize, and a 6-fold increase in mortality compared with well-differentiated liposarcomas.[69,70] It is believed that dedifferentiated liposarcomas arise from well-differentiated liposarcomas, and well-differentiated liposarcomas may recur as dedifferentiated liposarcomas. Liposarcomas are in general very large at the time of diagnosis. Thus, liposarcomas can contain varying regions of necrotic tissue, dedifferentiated tissue, and other tissue components such that tissue sampling errors can result in errors at histopathologic diagnosis. Brenner and colleagues[71] reported that the maximum SUV was a stronger predictor of

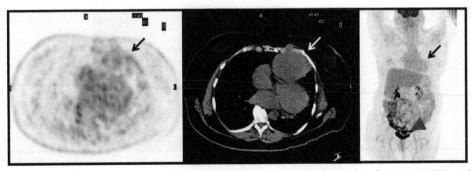

Fig. 14. This 60-year-old woman is known to have endometrial carcinoma (*arrowhead*). FDG-PET/CT imaging also shows a soft tissue mass (*arrows*) involving the left anterior rib cage and anterior mediastinum associated with low uptake of FDG, with maximum SUV of 3.0. The final diagnosis of low-grade chondrosarcoma was subsequently established after en bloc resection of that mass.

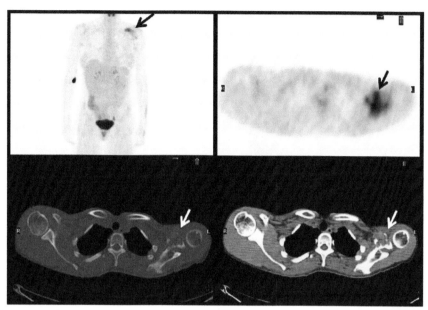

Fig. 15. This 35-year-old woman has a large osteochondroma with secondary malignant transformation into a high-grade chondrosarcoma emanating from the glenoid process of the left scapula. The FDG-PET/CT study showed a lobulated hypermetabolic lesion (with maximum SUV 5.7) associated with multifocal osseous destruction, a soft tissue component, and multiple foci of calcification (*arrows*).

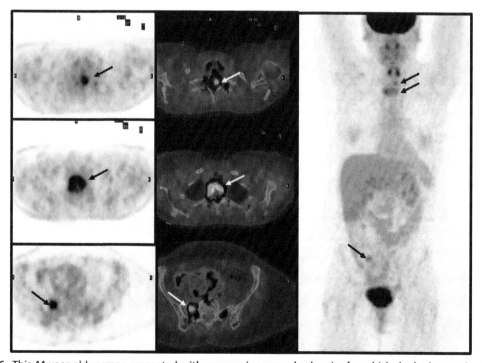

Fig. 16. This 44-year-old woman presented with progressive upper back pain, for which she had extensive investigations including an FDG-PET/CT study. This study showed multiple hypermetabolic lesions, including the entire T2 vertebral body (*arrows*) extending into the right paravertebral space (maximum SUV 6.4). This lesion corresponds to extensive sclerosis visualized on the CT images. Additional lesions (*arrows*) were shown in the left posterior aspect of the T1 vertebral body (maximal SUV 5.6) and the right upper aspect of the sacrum (SUV 7.1), both of which are not clearly visualized on the CT images. The final diagnosis of metastatic high-grade osteosarcoma was established with the biopsies of the lesions in T2 and in the sacrum.

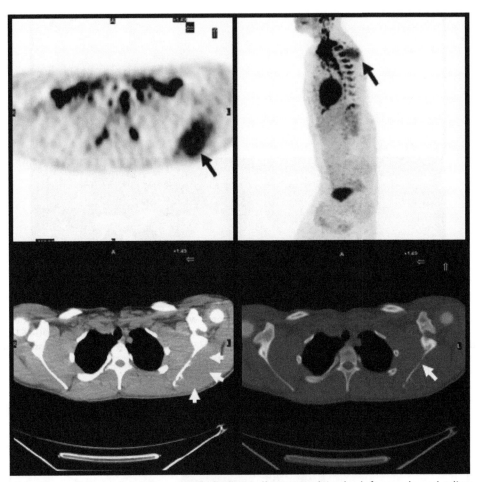

Fig. 17. This 18-year-old man has a hypermetabolic lesion (*long arrow*) in the left scapula and adjacent soft tissues posteriorly with a maximal SUV of 7.5 on FDG-PET imaging. This finding corresponds to a permeative destructive lesion (*medium arrow*) extending into the adjacent soft tissues posteriorly (*short arrows*) on the CT images. The diagnosis of Ewing sarcoma was established by biopsy. Extensive hypermetabolism caused by brown adipose tissue is also noted.

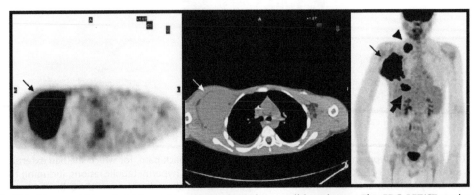

Fig. 18. This 12-year-old boy has biopsy-proven anaplastic large cell lymphoma. The FDG-PET/CT study showed intensely hypermetabolic lesions in the right axilla (*thin arrow*) with a maximum SUV of 22, the right supraclavicular region (*arrow head*) with a maximum SUV of 18, and the right fifth intercostal space and sixth rib anteriorly with a maximum SUV of 16 (*thick arrow*).

> **Box 2**
> **Diagnostic criteria for solitary plasmacytoma and multiple myeloma**
>
> - Solitary plasmacytoma
>   - All 4 criteria must be met:
>   - biopsy-proven bone or soft tissue lesion with evidence of plasma cells
>   - normal bone marrow with no evidence of clonal plasma cells
>   - normal skeletal survey on magnetic resonance (MR) imaging of spine and pelvis (except for the primary solitary lesion)
>   - absence of end-organ damage such as calcium level increase, renal insufficiency, anemia, and bone abnormality (CRAB) lesions that can be attributed to lympho-plasma cell proliferative disorder
> - Multiple myeloma
>   - All 3 criteria must be met:
>   - presence of a serum or urinary monoclonal protein
>   - presence of clonal plasma cells in the bone marrow or a plasmacytoma
>   - presence of end-organ damage thought to be related to the plasma cell dyscrasia, such as:
>   - increased calcium concentration
>   - lytic bone lesions
>   - anemia, or
>   - renal failure

disease-specific survival than the histologic grade of liposarcomas.

MFH

MFH, the most common soft tissue sarcoma in late adult life, rarely occurs in the chest well. MFH is of uncertain cellular origin and may arise in soft tissue or bone. There has been evidence that MFH has no evidence of clear-cut histiocytic differentiation and represents a sarcomatous disease that has undergone the final common pathway of dedifferentiation in tumors.[72] For these reasons, MFH has been formally declassified and renamed as undifferentiated pleomorphic sarcoma not otherwise specified by the World Health Organization in 2002.[73]

MFH has a broad range of histologic appearance, with 4 main subtypes: storiform-pleomorphic, myxoid, giant cell, and inflammatory.[72] Of these subtypes, the most common are storiform-pleomorphic and myxoid, accounting for approximately 70% and 20%, respectively, of MFHs.

On FDG-PET imaging, MFH typically appears as an intensely hypermetabolic mass corresponding to a heterogeneous lesion with no calcification on CT imaging.[49] The myxoid variant of MFH is associated with at least 50% of myxoid areas and, as a result of its relatively low cellularity, a lower intensity of FDG uptake than other histologic variants of MFH. The myxoid MFH also appears as having low attenuation in the myxoid components compared with the more cellular regions on CT imaging (**Fig. 19**).[33]

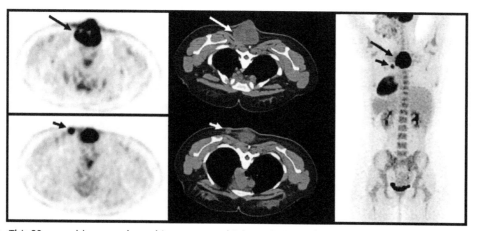

Fig. 19. This 29-year-old woman has a biopsy-proven high-grade MFH ulcerating in the subcutaneous tissues of the upper back. On FDG-PET/CT imaging, this lesion (*large arrows*) appears intensely hypermetabolic with a maximum SUV of 24.9 and is associated with a nonmetabolic center caused by necrosis. A second satellite subcutaneous lesion (*small arrows*) is shown in the left upper thorax with a maximum SUV of 10.9.

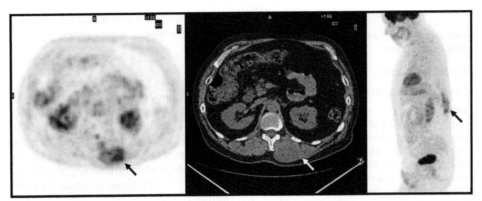

Fig. 20. This 70-year-old man presented with a biopsy-proven high-grade leiomyosarcoma in the midback. PET/CT imaging showed a hypermetabolic and heterogeneous mass (*arrow*) in the left paraspinal musculature at the levels of T12 to L2. The maximal SUV was 6.0.

Leiomyosarcoma

Leiomyosarcoma is a malignant neoplastic disease derived from smooth muscle cells. It accounts for approximately 5% to 10% of all soft tissue sarcomas[74] and most commonly occurs during adulthood, with a peak age incidence of approximately 60 years. It can occur at any site of the body, even in the skeleton, but most commonly originates in the gastrointestinal tract, uterus, and uncommonly in the chest wall.

On FDG-PET imaging, a previously untreated leiomyosarcoma typically appears as a hypermetabolic lesion with a high degree of correlation of intensity of FDG activity and lesion grade.[49,75] The corresponding CT images most commonly show a large mass that frequently includes areas of necrosis or cystic changes and displacement or distortion of vessels and absence of calcification (**Fig. 20**).[33]

Synovial sarcoma

Synovial sarcoma accounts for between 5% and 10% of all soft tissue sarcomas and most commonly occurs near joint capsules, bursae, and tendon sheaths, and is rare in the chest wall.

It can occur at any age but occurs predominantly in adolescents and young adults, with a median age of 34 years at diagnosis.[76]

On FDG-PET imaging, synovial sarcoma usually appears as a hypermetabolic lesion but occasionally has low uptake of FDG. The corresponding CT images typically show a soft tissue mass associated with slightly higher attenuation than that of muscles, and may show infiltration of adjacent structures and cortical bone erosion or invasion.[33] Intratumoral calcifications are present in 20% to 30% of cases.[77]

Synovial sarcoma is generally considered and treated as a high-grade sarcoma.[78] Nevertheless, it has a varied biologic aggressiveness with the disease-specific survival probability negatively influenced by the primary tumor size (larger than 5 cm), patient age (older than 25 years), and histologic evidence of poorly differentiated tumor.[78] Pretherapy FDG-PET imaging has prognostic implications because a high maximum SUV is associated with a decreased disease-free survival and high risk for local recurrences and metastatic disease compared with a low maximum SUV (**Fig. 21**).[79]

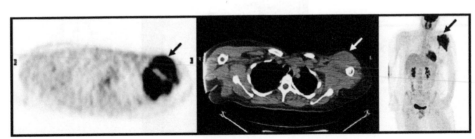

Fig. 21. This 25-year-old woman has a large soft tissue mass in the left shoulder, left humerus, and left lateral chest wall. The FDG-PET/CT shows intense and heterogeneous hypermetabolism at the site of the mass (*arrows*) with a maximum SUV of 15.2. The diagnosis of monophasic synovial sarcoma was established by ultrasound-guided biopsy.

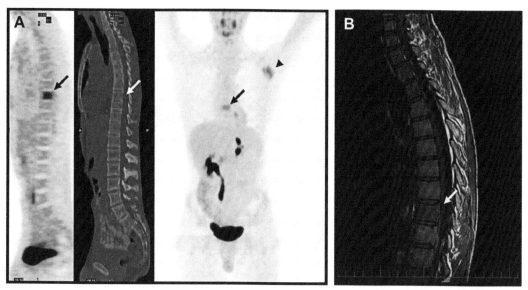

Fig. 22. This 18-year-old man is known to have rhabdomyosarcoma in the left hand. The FDG-PET/CT study (*A*) showed a hypermetabolic lesion in the left axilla (*arrowhead*) with a maximum SUV of 5.6, corresponding to a soft tissue mass and a hypermetabolic lesion in the T8 vertebral body (*arrows*) with a maximum SUV of 4.6. The T1-weighted images of a subsequent MR image (*B*) of the thoracic spine subsequently supported the diagnosis of metastatic disease to the T8 vertebral body.

Rhabdomyosarcoma

Rhabdomyosarcoma is a high-grade mesenchymal neoplasm with skeletal muscle differentiation. It is usually diagnosed in patients younger than 45 years and accounts for approximately 50% of soft tissue sarcomas in childhood. It most commonly occurs in the abdomen, head, or neck. Chest wall involvement is relatively uncommon.[33] Metastatic disease is present in approximately 15% of children with rhabdomyosarcoma at the time of initial diagnosis.[80] Approximately half of these cases of metastatic disease

occur at only 1 site, most commonly the lung (36%), bone marrow (22%), or bone (7%).[81] Thus, accurate staging is particularly important in patients with newly diagnosed rhabdomyosarcoma for selection of appropriate therapy.

FDG-PET CT imaging typically shows a noncalcified soft tissue mass associated with intense hypermetabolism (**Fig. 22**).[33,49]

Malignant peripheral nerve sheath tumor

Malignant peripheral nerve sheath tumor is generally a highly aggressive malignant neoplasm of the

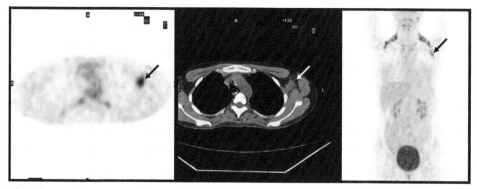

Fig. 23. This 25-year-old woman with neurofibromatosis type 1 has a growing soft tissue mass in the left brachial plexus. On FDG-PET/CT imaging, this mass (*arrows*) appears hypermetabolic, with a maximum SUV of 5.1, corresponding to a heterogeneous soft tissue lesion. This mass turned out to be a high-grade malignant peripheral nerve sheath tumor on subsequent excisional biopsy. Physiologic brown adipose tissue uptake in the neck bilaterally is also shown.

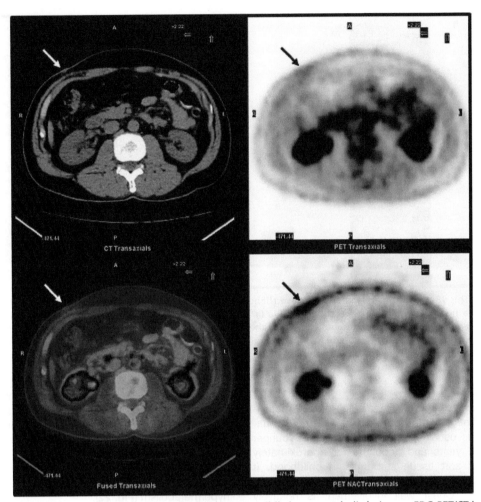

Fig. 24. This 56-year-old woman has a small subcutaneous mildly hypermetabolic lesion on FDG-PET/CT imaging in the right thoracoabdominal junction corresponding to a 1.5-cm nodule on CT imaging (*arrows*). The maximum SUV is 1.9. The diagnosis was a low-grade DFSP on subsequent excisional biopsy.

peripheral nerve. It accounts for approximately 10% of all soft tissue sarcomas and can present as a rapidly growing mass. It most commonly occurs in the deep soft tissue close to a nerve trunk, and the most common sites are the sciatic nerve, brachial plexus, and sacral plexus.[82] It usually occurs during adulthood, with a mean age at diagnosis of 42 years, and an association

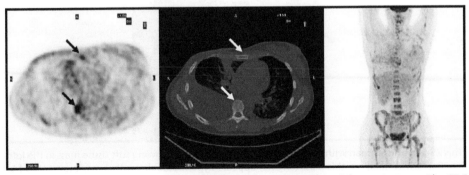

Fig. 25. This 35-year-old woman has a history of breast cancer status after right mastectomy. The FDG-PET/CT study shows innumerable hypermetabolic lesions scattered throughout the skeleton, including these visualized in the sternum (*arrow*) and T7 vertebral body (*arrows*).

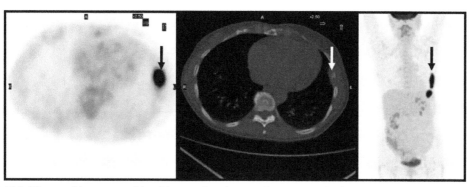

Fig. 26. This 59-year-old woman with a history of endometrial carcinoma had undergone an FDG PET/CT study, which showed 2 hypermetabolic foci in the left sixth rib (*arrows*) with maximum SUV of 16.2 and 15.3, corresponding to bone destruction on the CT images. The diagnosis of metastases from endometrial carcinoma was histologically confirmed after partial resection of that rib.

with type I neurofibromatosis is present in approximately 50% of patients.[83]

FDG-PET imaging typically shows a heterogeneously and intensely hypermetabolic large mass. This finding corresponds on CT imaging to a large noncalcified heterogeneous mass, occasionally accompanied by bone destruction (**Fig. 23**).[33]

Dermatofibrosarcoma protuberans

Dermatofibrosarcoma protuberans (DFSP) is a low-grade to intermediate-grade soft tissue neoplasm arising from the dermal layer of the skin that accounts for approximately 1% of all soft tissue sarcomas. The most commonly involved regions are the trunk (almost 50%), followed by the lower limbs, upper limbs, and less commonly the head and neck.[84] Although it rarely metastasizes, it is associated with a high local recurrence rate. The disease-specific survival probability of patients with DFSP is generally excellent except when there is fibrosarcomatous transformation. The prognosis is usually poor in this small subset of patients.[85]

On FDG-PET imaging, DFSP is associated with focal hypermetabolism in a subcutaneous lesion.[86] This finding corresponds to a nodular subcutaneous lesion with attenuation that is equal

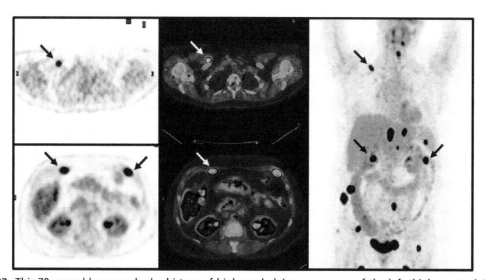

Fig. 27. This 70-year-old woman had a history of high-grade leiomyosarcoma of the left thigh resected 1 year before this FDG-PET/CT study. This study showed numerous soft tissue hypermetabolic lesions in the skeletal muscles, including the superior aspects of the transversus abdominis muscles (*arrow*) and in the right pectoralis major muscle (*arrow*). One of the lesions was subsequently biopsied to establish the diagnosis of metastatic high-grade leiomyosarcoma.

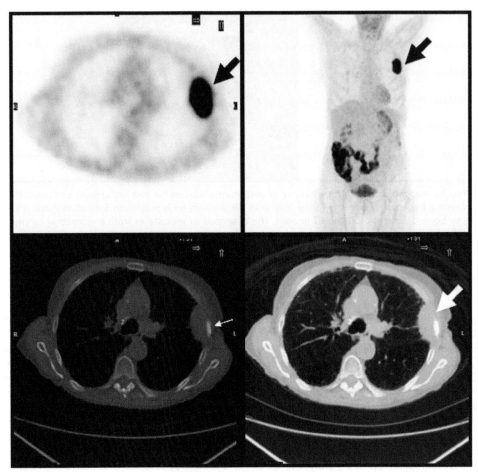

Fig. 28. This 75-year-old woman with bronchogenic carcinoma had undergone an FDG-PET/CT study, which showed an intensely hypermetabolic lesion (*large arrows*) with a maximum SUV of 28.1 in the left upper lobe. This lesion is associated with invasion of the left fourth rib laterally as evidenced by the sclerotic changes in that rib as seen on CT images (*small arrow*). There was no evidence of metabolically active neoplastic lesions elsewhere on that study. The presence of chest wall invasion was subsequently confirmed intraoperatively.

Table 3
Appearance of primary malignant chest wall tumors on FDG-PET

Usually Low FDG Uptake	Variable FDG Uptake	Usually High FDG Uptake
Liposarcoma (unless high grade)	Plasmacytoma	Osteosarcoma
DFSP	Multiple myeloma	Ewing sarcoma
Chondrosarcoma (unless high grade)		Lymphoma
		MFH
		Rhabdomyosarcoma
		Neuroblastoma
		Synovial sarcoma
		Leiomyosarcoma

Data from Basu S, Nair N, Banavali S. Uptake characteristics of fluorodeoxyglucose (FDG) in deep fibromatosis and abdominal desmoids: potential clinical role of FDG-PET in the management. Br J Radiol 2007;80(957):750–6; and Charest M, Hickeson M, Lisbona R, et al. FDG PET/CT imaging in primary osseous and soft tissue sarcomas: a retrospective review of 212 cases. Eur J Nucl Med Mol Imaging 2009;36(12):1944–51.

to or slightly higher than that of skeletal muscle.[33] The presence of a mildly hypermetabolic lesion corresponding to a well-defined soft tissue lesion without evidence of muscle invasion suggests a low-grade lesion. In contrast, the presence of a large intensely hypermetabolic lesion associated with muscle invasion suggests an aggressive process such as a higher-grade DFSP (**Fig. 24**).

Table 4
Clinical findings and appearance of CT for primary malignant chest wall tumors

Malignant Tumor	Age	Prevalence	Findings on Nonenhanced CT
Soft Tissue Tumors			
DFSP	Adolescence	Uncommon	Well-defined subcutaneous nodule with attenuation slightly higher or similar to muscle
Leiomyosarcoma	Late adulthood	Uncommon	Large mass with low-attenuation regions
Liposarcoma	Middle adulthood	Common	Soft tissue mass that may have visible fat attenuation
MFH	Late adulthood	Uncommon	Heterogeneous, ill-defined lesion with no calcification
Malignant peripheral nerve sheath tumor	Adulthood	Uncommon	Large noncalcified heterogeneous mass, associated with neurofibromatosis type I
Neuroblastoma	Childhood	Rare	Ill-defined mass with low-attenuation regions and spotty calcifications
Rhabdomyosarcoma	Adolescence to early adulthood	Rare	Noncalcified soft tissue mass
Synovial sarcoma	Adolescence to early adulthood	Rare	Soft tissue mass, slightly higher attenuation than muscle; may show calcifications
Hematologic Malignancies			
Lymphoma	Any age	Uncommon	Soft tissue mass
Multiple myeloma	Late adulthood	Common	Osteolytic or multicystic bone lesion with or without expansion; uncommonly, soft tissue mass with no calcification
Plasmacytoma	Middle to late adulthood	Common	Osteolytic or multicystic bone lesion with or without expansion; uncommonly, soft tissue mass with no calcification
Primary Osseous Tumors			
Chondrosarcoma	Early or middle adulthood	Common	Lesion with chondroid calcifications
Ewing sarcoma	Adolescence	Uncommon	Osteolytic ill-defined heterogeneous mass with or without extension into adjacent soft tissues
Osteosarcoma	Bimodal peak: adolescence and late adulthood	Rare	Mass containing ossifications

Other Soft Tissue Neoplasms

Neuroblastoma/ganglioneuroma

Neuroblastoma is the most common extracranial solid neoplastic disease in childhood[87] and constitutes approximately 97% of neuroblastic tumors. It is primarily a disease of infants and young children and rarely occurs after the age of 10 years. It has a broad spectrum of behavior, which can range from spontaneous regression, maturation into a benign ganglioneuroma, or aggressive features associated with disseminated metastatic disease leading to demise. In children, neuroblastoma accounts for approximately 6% of childhood cancers.[87] Neuroblastoma consists primarily of immature neuroblasts, whereas ganglioneuroma consists of a variable component of mature glial and ganglion cells.[88] Thoracic neuroblastomas and ganglioneuroblastomas most commonly originate in the extraadrenal sympathetic ganglia of the chest wall.

On FDG-PET, previously untreated neuroblastoma typically avidly accumulates FDG[89] corresponding to an ill-defined mass on the CT images. Spotty calcifications and low attenuation regions of necrosis in neuroblastoma are frequently evident on the CT images.[88]

Metastatic Disease and Direct Chest Wall Extension of Malignancy

The most common cause of malignant disease in the chest wall is metastatic disease. Metastases often appear as multiple lesions but may appear as a solitary lesion. When multiple, metastases typically have a random distribution. Within the chest wall, metastases most commonly occur in the bone marrow of the osseous structures: spine, ribs, sternum, scapulae, and ribs. Although virtually any malignancy can metastasize to bone marrow, the most common primary cancers resulting in metastatic disease to these sites arise from the breast, prostate, lung, and kidney in adults.[90] However, metastatic disease can also occur in the soft tissues of the chest wall (Figs. 25–27).

Chest wall invasion can occur in lung cancer,[91] malignant pleural mesothelioma,[92] mediastinal neoplasms,[93,94] sarcomas,[95] and breast cancer.[95] However, the most common primary neoplasm to invade the chest wall is locally advanced lung cancer.[96] When chest wall invasion from lung cancer is present, the lesion is staged as at least T3. On FDG-PET imaging, chest wall invasion by lung cancer typically appears as a hypermetabolic lung mass extending into the chest wall.[97] On CT imaging, signs of chest wall invasion include osseous destruction, pleural thickening, loss of the extrapleural fat plane, an obtuse angle between the mass and chest wall, and greater than $3(f \times 1)$cm of contact between a lung mass and the chest wall. Of all of these criteria, the only reliable sign of chest wall invasion is evidence of definite bone destruction.[98] The accurate determination of chest wall invasion is often not established until the time of surgery.[99] MR imaging may be useful as an adjunct for more definitive evaluation of chest wall invasion (Fig. 28; Tables 3 and 4).[34,49]

SUMMARY

Benign and malignant diseases of the chest wall are of diverse origin. The patient's age, clinical presentation, and imaging appearance of the lesions on PET/CT (as well as on other imaging studies such as plain film radiography, CT, or MR imaging) are valuable for the differential diagnosis of the disease process. Physiologic uptake in the chest wall is commonly shown on PET/CT. The typical appearance of this physiologic uptake should be recognized to avoid misinterpretation of the PET/CT study.

ACKNOWLEDGMENTS

The authors acknowledge and greatly appreciate William Makis for the preparation of the teaching file from McGill University Health Center, from which some of the cases were used for this article.

REFERENCES

1. Jackson RS, Schlarman TC, Hubble WL, et al. Prevalence and patterns of physiologic muscle uptake detected with whole-body 18F-FDG PET. J Nucl Med Technol 2006;34(1):29–33.
2. Cohade C. Altered biodistribution on FDG-PET with emphasis on brown fat and insulin effect. Semin Nucl Med 2010;40(4):283–93.
3. Delbeke D, Coleman RE, Guiberteau MJ, et al. Procedure guideline for tumor imaging with 18F-FDG PET/CT 1.0. J Nucl Med 2006;47(5):885–95.
4. Boellaard R, O'Doherty MJ, Weber WA, et al. FDG PET and PET/CT: EANM procedure guidelines for tumour PET imaging: version 1.0. Eur J Nucl Med Mol Imaging 2010;37(1):181–200.
5. Cohade C, Osman M, Pannu HK, et al. Uptake in supraclavicular area fat ("USA-Fat"): description on 18F-FDG PET/CT. J Nucl Med 2003;44(2):170–6.
6. Hany TF, Gharehpapagh E, Kamel EM, et al. Brown adipose tissue: a factor to consider in symmetrical tracer uptake in the neck and upper chest region. Eur J Nucl Med Mol Imaging 2002;29(10):1393–8.

7. Cypess AM, Lehman S, Williams G, et al. Identification and importance of brown adipose tissue in adult humans. N Engl J Med 2009;360(15):1509–17.

8. van Marken Lichtenbelt WD, Vanhommerig JW, Smulders NM, et al. Cold-activated brown adipose tissue in healthy men. N Engl J Med 2009;360(15): 1500–8.

9. Garcia CA, Van Nostrand D, Atkins F, et al. Reduction of brown fat 2-deoxy-2-[F-18]fluoro-D-glucose uptake by controlling environmental temperature prior to positron emission tomography scan. Mol Imaging Biol 2006;8(1):24–9.

10. Williams G, Kolodny GM. Method for decreasing uptake of 18F-FDG by hypermetabolic brown adipose tissue on PET. AJR Am J Roentgenol 2008;190(5):1406–9.

11. Baba S, Tatsumi M, Ishimori T, et al. Effect of nicotine and ephedrine on the accumulation of 18F-FDG in brown adipose tissue. J Nucl Med 2007; 48(6):981–6.

12. Gelfand MJ, O'Hara SM, Curtwright LA, et al. Premedication to block [(18)F]FDG uptake in the brown adipose tissue of pediatric and adolescent patients. Pediatr Radiol 2005;35(10):984–90.

13. Tatsumi M, Engles JM, Ishimori T, et al. Intense (18) F-FDG uptake in brown fat can be reduced pharmacologically. J Nucl Med 2004;45(7):1189–93.

14. Shammas A, Lim R, Charron M. Pediatric FDG PET/CT: physiologic uptake, normal variants, and benign conditions. Radiographics 2009;29(5):1467–86.

15. Takalkar A, Yu JQ, Kumar R, et al. Diffuse bone marrow accumulation of FDG in a patient with chronic myeloid leukemia mimics hematopoietic cytokine-mediated FDG uptake on positron emission tomography. Clin Nucl Med 2004;29(10):637–9.

16. Blodgett TM, Ames JT, Torok FS, et al. Diffuse bone marrow uptake on whole-body F-18 fluorodeoxyglucose positron emission tomography in a patient taking recombinant erythropoietin. Clin Nucl Med 2004;29(3):161–3.

17. Sugawara Y, Fisher SJ, Zasadny KR, et al. Preclinical and clinical studies of bone marrow uptake of fluorine-1-fluorodeoxyglucose with or without granulocyte colony-stimulating factor during chemotherapy. J Clin Oncol 1998;16(1):173–80.

18. Sugawara Y, Zasadny KR, Kison PV, et al. Splenic fluorodeoxyglucose uptake increased by granulocyte colony-stimulating factor therapy: PET imaging results. J Nucl Med 1999;40(9):1456–62.

19. Aydin A, Hickeson M, Yu JQ, et al. Demonstration of excessive metabolic activity of thoracic and abdominal muscles on FDG-PET in patients with chronic obstructive pulmonary disease. Clin Nucl Med 2005;30(3):159–64.

20. Alavi A, Gupta N, Alberini JL, et al. Positron emission tomography imaging in nonmalignant thoracic disorders. Semin Nucl Med 2002;32(4):293–321.

21. Arakawa H, Kurihara Y, Nakajima Y, et al. Computed tomography measurements of overinflation in chronic obstructive pulmonary disease: evaluation of various radiographic signs. J Thorac Imaging 1998;13(3):188–92.

22. Rothpearl A, Varma AO, Goodman K. Radiographic measures of hyperinflation in clinical emphysema. Discrimination of patients from controls and relationship to physiologic and mechanical lung function. Chest 1988;94(5):907–13.

23. Basu S, Alzeair S, Li G, et al. Etiopathologies associated with intercostal muscle hypermetabolism and prominent right ventricle visualization on 2-deoxy-2 [F-18]fluoro-D-glucose-positron emission tomography: significance of an incidental finding and in the setting of a known pulmonary disease. Mol Imaging Biol 2007;9(6):333–9.

24. Beaulieu S, Rubin B, Djang D, et al. Positron emission tomography of schwannomas: emphasizing its potential in preoperative planning. AJR Am J Roentgenol 2004;182(4):971–4.

25. Onishi Y, Kitajima K, Senda M, et al. FDG-PET/CT imaging of elastofibroma dorsi. Skeletal Radiol 2011;40(7):849–53.

26. Aoki J, Watanabe H, Shinozaki T, et al. FDG PET of primary benign and malignant bone tumors: standardized uptake value in 52 lesions. Radiology 2001;219(3):774–7.

27. Taieb D, Sebag F, Barlier A, et al. 18F-FDG avidity of pheochromocytomas and paragangliomas: a new molecular imaging signature? J Nucl Med 2009; 50(5):711–7.

28. Cardona S, Schwarzbach M, Hinz U, et al. Evaluation of F18-deoxyglucose positron emission tomography (FDG-PET) to assess the nature of neurogenic tumours. Eur J Surg Oncol 2003;29(6):536–41.

29. Fisher MJ, Basu S, Dombi E, et al. The role of [18F]-fluorodeoxyglucose positron emission tomography in predicting plexiform neurofibroma progression. J Neurooncol 2008;87(2):165–71.

30. Hamada K, Tomita Y, Qiu Y, et al. (18)F-FDG PET analysis of schwannoma: increase of SUVmax in the delayed scan is correlated with elevated VEGF/VPF expression in the tumors. Skeletal Radiol 2009;38(3):261–6.

31. Tateishi U, Gladish GW, Kusumoto M, et al. Chest wall tumors: radiologic findings and pathologic correlation: part 1. Benign tumors. Radiographics 2003;23(6):1477–90.

32. Brandser EA, Goree JC, El-Khoury GY. Elastofibroma dorsi: prevalence in an elderly patient population as revealed by CT. AJR Am J Roentgenol 1998; 171(4):977–80.

33. Tateishi U, Gladish GW, Kusumoto M, et al. Chest wall tumors: radiologic findings and pathologic correlation: part 2. Malignant tumors. Radiographics 2003;23(6):1491–508.

34. Basu S, Nair N, Banavali S. Uptake characteristics of fluorodeoxyglucose (FDG) in deep fibromatosis and abdominal desmoids: potential clinical role of FDG-PET in the management. Br J Radiol 2007;80(957): 750–6.

35. Gorenberg M, Bar-Shalom R, Israel O. Patterns of FDG uptake in post-thoracotomy surgical scars in patients with lung cancer. Br J Radiol 2008; 81(970):821–5.

36. Robiller FC, Stumpe KD, Kossmann T, et al. Chronic osteomyelitis of the femur: value of PET imaging. Eur Radiol 2000;10(5):855–8.

37. De Winter F, Vogelaers D, Gemmel F, et al. Promising role of 18-F-fluoro-D-deoxyglucose positron emission tomography in clinical infectious diseases. Eur J Clin Microbiol Infect Dis 2002;21(4):247–57.

38. Kalicke T, Schmitz A, Risse JH, et al. Fluorine-18 fluorodeoxyglucose PET in infectious bone diseases: results of histologically confirmed cases. Eur J Nucl Med 2000;27(5):524–8.

39. Zhuang H, Alavi A. 18-fluorodeoxyglucose positron emission tomographic imaging in the detection and monitoring of infection and inflammation. Semin Nucl Med 2002;32(1):47–59.

40. Zhuang H, Duarte PS, Pourdehand M, et al. Exclusion of chronic osteomyelitis with F-18 fluorodeoxyglucose positron emission tomographic imaging. Clin Nucl Med 2000;25(4):281–4.

41. Love C, Tomas MB, Tronco GG, et al. FDG PET of infection and inflammation. Radiographics 2005; 25(5):1357–68.

42. Zhuang H, Sam JW, Chacko TK, et al. Rapid normalization of osseous FDG uptake following traumatic or surgical fractures. Eur J Nucl Med Mol Imaging 2003;30(8):1096–103.

43. Johnston CJ, Williams JP, Elder A, et al. Inflammatory cell recruitment following thoracic irradiation. Exp Lung Res 2004;30(5):369–82.

44. Van der Meeren A, Monti P, Lebaron-Jacobs L, et al. Characterization of the acute inflammatory response after irradiation in mice and its regulation by interleukin 4 (Il4). Radiat Res 2001;155(6):858–65.

45. Kazama T, Faria SC, Varavithya V, et al. FDG PET in the evaluation of treatment for lymphoma: clinical usefulness and pitfalls. Radiographics 2005;25(1):191–207.

46. Jeung MY, Gangi A, Gasser B, et al. Imaging of chest wall disorders. Radiographics 1999;19(3):617–37.

47. Murphey MD, Walker EA, Wilson AJ, et al. From the archives of the AFIP: imaging of primary chondrosarcoma: radiologic-pathologic correlation. Radiographics 2003;23(5):1245–78.

48. Frassica FJ, Unni KK, Beabout JW, et al. Dedifferentiated chondrosarcoma. A report of the clinicopathological features and treatment of seventy-eight cases. J Bone Joint Surg Am 1986;68(8):1197–205.

49. Charest M, Hickeson M, Lisbona R, et al. FDG PET/CT imaging in primary osseous and soft tissue sarcomas: a retrospective review of 212 cases. Eur J Nucl Med Mol Imaging 2009;36(12): 1944–51.

50. Mirabello L, Troisi RJ, Savage SA. Osteosarcoma incidence and survival rates from 1973 to 2004: data from the Surveillance, Epidemiology, and End Results Program. Cancer 2009;115(7):1531–43.

51. Huvos AG. Osteogenic sarcoma of bones and soft tissues in older persons. A clinicopathologic analysis of 117 patients older than 60 years. Cancer 1986;57(7):1442–9.

52. Folpe AL, Lyles RH, Sprouse JT, et al. (F-18) fluorodeoxyglucose positron emission tomography as a predictor of pathologic grade and other prognostic variables in bone and soft tissue sarcoma. Clin Cancer Res 2000;6(4):1279–87.

53. Meyers PA, Gorlick R. Osteosarcoma. Pediatr Clin North Am 1997;44(4):973–89.

54. Widhe B, Widhe T. Initial symptoms and clinical features in osteosarcoma and Ewing sarcoma. J Bone Joint Surg Am 2000;82(5):667–74.

55. Grier HE. The Ewing family of tumors. Ewing's sarcoma and primitive neuroectodermal tumors. Pediatr Clin North Am 1997;44(4):991–1004.

56. Winer-Muram HT, Kauffman WM, Gronemeyer SA, et al. Primitive neuroectodermal tumors of the chest wall (Askin tumors): CT and MR findings. AJR Am J Roentgenol 1993;161(2):265–8.

57. Tori M, Fujii Y, Minami M, et al. Hodgkin's disease of the chest wall: report of a case. Surg Today 1998; 28(8):853–6.

58. Hirai S, Hamanaka Y, Mitsui N, et al. Primary malignant lymphoma arising in the pleura without preceding long-standing pyothorax. Ann Thorac Cardiovasc Surg 2004;10(5):297–300.

59. Lones MA, Sanger W, Perkins SL, et al. Anaplastic large cell lymphoma arising in bone: report of a case of the monomorphic variant with the t(2;5)(p23;q35) translocation. Arch Pathol Lab Med 2000;124(9):1339–43.

60. Faries PL, D'Ayala M, Santos GH. Primary immunoblastic B-cell lymphoma of the sternum. J Thorac Cardiovasc Surg 1997;114(4):684–5.

61. Hsu PK, Hsu HS, Li AF, et al. Non-Hodgkin's lymphoma presenting as a large chest wall mass. Ann Thorac Surg 2006;81(4):1214–8.

62. Clayton F, Butler JJ, Ayala AG, et al. Non-Hodgkin's lymphoma in bone. Pathologic and radiologic features with clinical correlates. Cancer 1987; 60(10):2494–501.

63. Mengiardi B, Honegger H, Hodler J, et al. Primary lymphoma of bone: MRI and CT characteristics during and after successful treatment. AJR Am J Roentgenol 2005;184(1):185–92.

64. Smith A, Wisloff F, Samson D. Guidelines on the diagnosis and management of multiple myeloma 2005. Br J Haematol 2006;132(4):410–51.

65. Kyle RA, Gertz MA, Witzig TE, et al. Review of 1027 patients with newly diagnosed multiple myeloma. Mayo Clin Proc 2003;78(1):21–33.

66. Group IMW. Criteria for the classification of monoclonal gammopathies, multiple myeloma and related disorders: a report of the International Myeloma Working Group. Br J Haematol 2003; 121(5):749–57.

67. Kyle RA, Rajkumar SV. Criteria for diagnosis, staging, risk stratification and response assessment of multiple myeloma. Leukemia 2009;23(1):3–9.

68. Durie BG, Waxman AD, D'Agnolo A, et al. Whole-body (18)F-FDG PET identifies high-risk myeloma. J Nucl Med 2002;43(11):1457–63.

69. Lahat G, Anaya DA, Wang X, et al. Resectable well-differentiated versus dedifferentiated liposarcomas: two different diseases possibly requiring different treatment approaches. Ann Surg Oncol 2008;15(6): 1585–93.

70. Singer S, Antonescu CR, Riedel E, et al. Histologic subtype and margin of resection predict pattern of recurrence and survival for retroperitoneal liposarcoma. Ann Surg 2003;238(3):358–70 [discussion: 370–1].

71. Brenner W, Eary JF, Hwang W, et al. Risk assessment in liposarcoma patients based on FDG PET imaging. Eur J Nucl Med Mol Imaging 2006;33(11): 1290–5.

72. Hollowood K, Fletcher CD. Malignant fibrous histiocytoma: morphologic pattern or pathologic entity? Semin Diagn Pathol 1995;12(3):210–20.

73. Murphey MD. World Health Organization classification of bone and soft tissue tumors: modifications and implications for radiologists. Semin Musculoskelet Radiol 2007;11(3):201–14.

74. Gustafson P, Willen H, Baldetorp B, et al. Soft tissue leiomyosarcoma. A population-based epidemiologic and prognostic study of 48 patients, including cellular DNA content. Cancer 1992;70(1):114–9.

75. Punt SE, Eary JF, O'Sullivan J, et al. Fluorodeoxyglucose positron emission tomography in leiomyosarcoma: imaging characteristics. Nucl Med Commun 2009;30(7):546–9.

76. Sultan I, Rodriguez-Galindo C, Saab R, et al. Comparing children and adults with synovial sarcoma in the Surveillance, Epidemiology, and End Results program, 1983 to 2005: an analysis of 1268 patients. Cancer 2009;115(15):3537–47.

77. Sanchez Reyes JM, Alcaraz Mexia M, Quinones Tapia D, et al. Extensively calcified synovial sarcoma. Skeletal Radiol 1997;26(11):671–3.

78. Bergh P, Meis-Kindblom JM, Gherlinzoni F, et al. Synovial sarcoma: identification of low and high risk groups. Cancer 1999;85(12):2596–607.

79. Lisle JW, Eary JF, O'Sullivan J, et al. Risk assessment based on FDG-PET imaging in patients with synovial sarcoma. Clin Orthop Relat Res 2009; 467(6):1605–11.

80. Crist W, Gehan EA, Ragab AH, et al. The third intergroup rhabdomyosarcoma study. J Clin Oncol 1995; 13(3):610–30.

81. Raney RB Jr, Tefft M, Maurer HM, et al. Disease patterns and survival rate in children with metastatic soft-tissue sarcoma. A report from the Intergroup Rhabdomyosarcoma Study (IRS)-I. Cancer 1988; 62(7):1257–66.

82. Hrehorovich PA, Franke HR, Maximin S, et al. Malignant peripheral nerve sheath tumor. Radiographics 2003;23(3):790–4.

83. Sordillo PP, Helson L, Hajdu SI, et al. Malignant schwannoma–clinical characteristics, survival, and response to therapy. Cancer 1981;47(10):2503–9.

84. Bowne WB, Antonescu CR, Leung DH, et al. Dermatofibrosarcoma protuberans: a clinicopathologic analysis of patients treated and followed at a single institution. Cancer 2000;88(12):2711–20.

85. Abbott JJ, Oliveira AM, Nascimento AG. The prognostic significance of fibrosarcomatous transformation in dermatofibrosarcoma protuberans. Am J Surg Pathol 2006;30(4):436–43.

86. Basu S, Baghel NS. Recurrence of dermatofibrosarcoma protuberans in post-surgical scar detected by 18F-FDG-PET imaging. Hell J Nucl Med 2009;12(1):68.

87. Grovas A, Fremgen A, Rauck A, et al. The national cancer data base report on patterns of childhood cancers in the United States. Cancer 1997;80(12):2321–32.

88. Lonergan GJ, Schwab CM, Suarez ES, et al. Neuroblastoma, ganglioneuroblastoma, and ganglioneuroma: radiologic-pathologic correlation. Radiographics 2002;22(4):911–34.

89. Shulkin BL, Hutchinson RJ, Castle VP, et al. Neuroblastoma: positron emission tomography with 2-[fluorine-18]-fluoro-2-deoxy-D-glucose compared with metaiodobenzylguanidine scintigraphy. Radiology 1996;199(3):743–50.

90. Cooke KS, Kirpekar M, Abiri MM, et al. US case of the day. Skeletal metastasis from poorly differentiated carcinoma of unknown origin. Radiographics 1997;17(2):542–4.

91. Bandi V, Lunn W, Ernst A, et al. Ultrasound vs. CT in detecting chest wall invasion by tumor: a prospective study. Chest 2008;133(4):881–6.

92. Spitilli MG, Treglia G, Calcagni ML, et al. Malignant pleural mesothelioma: utility of 18 F-FDG PET. Ann Ital Chir 2007;78(5):393–6.

93. Makis W, Hickeson M, Derbekyan V. Myeloid sarcoma presenting as an anterior mediastinal mass invading the pericardium: serial imaging with F-18 FDG PET/CT. Clin Nucl Med 2010;35(9):706–9.

94. Gross JL, Rosalino UA, Younes RN, et al. Characteristics associated with complete surgical resection of primary malignant mediastinal tumors. J Bras Pneumol 2009;35(9):832–8.

95. Novoa N, Benito P, Jimenez MF, et al. Reconstruction of chest wall defects after resection of large

neoplasms: ten-year experience. Interact Cardiovasc Thorac Surg 2005;4(3):250–5.

96. O'Sullivan P, O'Dwyer H, Flint J, et al. Malignant chest wall neoplasms of bone and cartilage: a pictorial review of CT and MR findings. Br J Radiol 2007; 80(956):678–84.

97. Plathow C, Aschoff P, Lichy MP, et al. Positron emission tomography/computed tomography and whole-body magnetic resonance imaging in staging of advanced nonsmall cell lung cancer–initial results. Invest Radiol 2008;43(5):290–7.

98. Quint LE. Staging non-small cell lung cancer. Cancer Imaging 2007;7:148–59.

99. Rohren EM, Lowe VJ. Update in PET imaging of non-small cell lung cancer. Semin Nucl Med 2004;34(2): 134–53.

PET Assessment of Brown Fat

Maarten L. Donswijk, MD[a],*,
Henny S. Broekhuizen-de Gast, MD[a],
Drew A. Torigian, MD, MA[b], Abass Alavi, MD[b],
Thomas C. Kwee, MD, PhD[a], Marnix G.E.H. Lam, MD, PhD[a]

KEYWORDS

- Brown fat • Brown adipose tissue • Fluorodeoxyglucose
- Positron emission tomography

Brown fat or brown adipose tissue (BAT) is an organ specific to mammals. The brown adipocyte is discerned from the white by having numerous fat vacuoles and a much higher number of iron-containing mitochondria creating the brown color.[1] Brown fat is richly innervated by sympathetic nerves and is characterized by its unique protein, uncoupling protein-1 (UCP1) or thermogenin, which is essential for the function of brown fat: to convert food into heat.[2,3] UCP1 uncouples mitochondrial respiration from adenosine triphosphate (ATP) synthesis, thereby stimulating heat production at the expense of energy in the form of ATP ("nonshivering" thermogenesis). Brown fat plays a crucial function in maintaining normal body temperature in small rodents and in newborn infants.[4]

In human autopsy series from several decades ago, it was shown that brown fat was distributed widely across the body in the first decade, but disappeared from most areas with increased age only to persist around the kidneys, adrenal glands, aorta, and in the neck and mediastinum.[5] Until the advent of hybrid PET/computed tomography (CT) imaging, brown fat was not thought to be metabolically significant. Then, in several studies, it was suggested that in some patients and under certain circumstances, brown fat was present and metabolically active.[6–8] In more recent studies, hypermetabolic areas in healthy volunteers or

patients suspected to be brown fat were confirmed to be brown fat at histopathological analysis.[9–12] Moreover, it was shown that brown fat hypermetabolism is not a rare phenomenon, but can be induced in a substantial number of younger adult subjects and even in some older subjects as well. These findings have incited further research into the determinants of the presence and metabolic activity of brown fat, and the relation between brown fat metabolism, energy expenditure, and obesity.[13–15]

BROWN FAT AND CLINICAL PET IMAGING

Physiologic uptake of [^{18}F]fluorodeoxyglucose (FDG) in normal structures may mimic pathologic processes. In oncology, FDG-PET is widely used to stage patients at initial disease presentation, and to assess for tumor recurrence and the effects of therapy. Incorrect interpretation obviously can have serious consequences. **Fig. 1** is a representation of interference of brown fat uptake with image interpretation in an oncologic patient. Since the time when clinical FDG-PET was first implemented, increased symmetric FDG uptake in the cervical and thoracic spinal region has been frequently encountered, although earlier it was generally regarded as muscular uptake. It was argued that increased FDG uptake would generally correspond

The authors have nothing to disclose.
[a] Department of Radiology and Nuclear Medicine, University Medical Center Utrecht, Heidelberglaan 100, 3584 CX Utrecht, The Netherlands
[b] Department of Radiology, Hospital of the University of Pennsylvania, University of Pennsylvania School of Medicine, 3400 Spruce Street, Philadelphia, PA 19104, USA
* Corresponding author.
E-mail address: M.L.Donswijk@umcutrecht.nl

PET Clin 6 (2011) 365–375
doi:10.1016/j.cpet.2011.04.005
1556-8598/11/$ – see front matter © 2011 Elsevier Inc. All rights reserved.

pet.theclinics.com

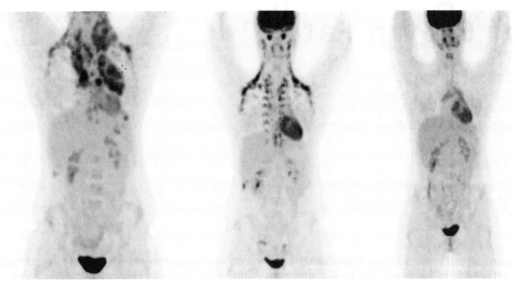

Fig. 1. Coronal maximum intensity projection (MIP) images of 3 total-body FDG-PET scans in an 18-year old woman with Hodgkin lymphoma. Left image shows extensive pathologic uptake in cervical and mediastinal lymph nodes, as well as in brown fat in supraclavicular areas. Four of 5 subsequent follow-up PET scans showed marked brown fat activation, with the fifth shown in the middle image. Based on pattern, uptake was regarded as brown fat activation except in right flank, which was due to traumatic rib lesion. Image on right shows last follow-up scan 6 months later after administration of 80 mg propranolol orally 2 hours before FDG injection. No brown fat activation is seen on the last scan, contrary to earlier scans. Moreover, no residual or recurrent lymphoma is seen.

well to origins and insertions of the neck and back muscles, and it was observed that diazepam, a muscle-relaxant, seemed to reduce FDG uptake.[16] However, as the spatial resolution of PET imaging improved over time and hybrid PET/CT technology was introduced, new opportunities to reevaluate these assumed explanations for physiologic FDG uptake were made available. Hany and colleagues[6] first proposed brown fat as a potential source of physiologic FDG uptake, followed by others.[7,8] Since then, much research has been conducted to assess which factors influence brown fat activation.

TYPICAL SITES OF APPEARANCE

From autopsy studies, it is known that brown fat is present not only in infants but also in adults.[5] The distribution pattern of brown fat was found to be quite similar in adults and infants. However, the chance of finding brown fat depots in adults at typical sites as seen in children decreased with age. Typical sites where depots of brown fat can be found in both children and adults are: the neck, around the carotids and cervical muscles; the supraclavicular areas (hence the old, somewhat limited phrase "uptake in supraclavicular area [USA]" fat); the paravertebral region; the mediastinum; around the abdominal aorta; and in the perinephric region.[5,7]

These findings correspond well with areas of brown fat uptake as visualized with FDG-PET.[6–8,17,18]

Hany and colleagues[6] described two patterns of FDG uptake in brown fat. An extensive pattern showed FDG uptake in the lower cervical spine, the shoulder region, and the upper thoracic spine in the costovertebral region, with activity comparable to brain activity. A less extensive pattern involved only intermediate FDG uptake in the lower cervical spine and shoulder region or in the shoulder region alone. Patients with the extensive patterns were all female and tended to be leaner in comparison with patients with the less extensive pattern. Kim and colleagues[17] studied FDG uptake patterns in 4 different areas in which brown fat activity frequently is seen, and found FDG uptake in brown fat in 42 of 1495 studies (2.8%). All mediastinal uptake coexisted with supraclavicular uptake, all suprarenal uptake coexisted with paravertebral uptake, and nearly all paravertebral uptake (93%) coexisted with supraclavicular uptake. Supraclavicular uptake was seen in 40 of 42 studies (95%) and coexisted with paravertebral uptake in 68%, mediastinal uptake in 58%, and suprarenal uptake in 28% of studies. However, Truong and colleagues[19] described brown fat uptake isolated to the mediastinum in 5 of 15 patients with brown fat uptake in a cohort of 845 oncologic patients. Brown fat uptake is symmetric, but asymmetric uptake is rarely seen in patients with a unilateral sympathetic nerve lesion, which prevents ipsilateral brown fat from being activated.[20,21]

Fig. 2 shows a typical brown fat distribution as can be visualized with FDG-PET.

INCIDENCE AND DETERMINANTS OF FDG UPTAKE IN BROWN FAT

Initial hybrid PET/CT studies in mixed patient populations reported FDG uptake in supposed brown fat areas with an incidence ranging from 2.5% to 6.7%.[6–8] A later study reported a 45% incidence of FDG uptake in a middle-aged female population and with repeated scanning.[22] Other studies specifically designed to visualize activated brown fat in young healthy adults reported incidences of FDG uptake of greater than 90% in histologically confirmed brown tissue.[9,10] Virtanen and colleagues[9] studied 5 healthy male volunteers who underwent two FDG-PET/CT studies, one of which was performed during cold exposure and the other during warm conditions. Cold exposure consisted of

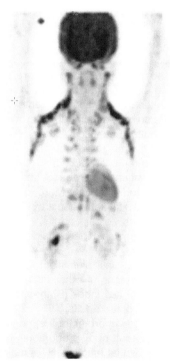

Fig. 2. Coronal MIP image of total-body FDG-PET scan in a 14-year-old girl. This follow-up PET scan was made after treatment for dysgerminoma. Prior imaging showed para-aortic lymph node metastases at level of kidneys. CT scan (not shown) performed at the same time as the current PET scan showed no residual disease. A typical brown fat FDG uptake pattern in supraclavicular and paravertebral areas is seen, as well as some uptake in the superior abdominal para-aortic region.

spending 2 hours in a room with an ambient temperature of 17°C to 19°C while wearing light clothing before scanning and placing the subject's feet intermittently in iced water during scanning. During cold exposure, high FDG uptake was seen in the supraclavicular area in all 5 subjects, whereas this was not seen in any of the subjects during warm conditions. In 3 of 5 subjects, biopsies were taken from the supraclavicular area, which showed morphologic features of brown adipocytes that expressed UCP1. Van Marken Lichtenbelt and colleagues[10] studied 24 young (aged 20–32 years) healthy male volunteers. Wearing clothing with standardized intermediate isolation properties, these volunteers were exposed to an ambient temperature of 16°C for 2 hours before PET/CT scanning. In 23 of 24 subjects, high FDG uptake was seen in supraclavicular fat tissue as assessed by the coregistered CT images, which was considered to be brown fat. Rescanning of 3 subjects under thermoneutral (22°C) conditions showed resolution of detectable uptake in brown fat. Biopsies obtained from the supraclavicular region during surgery in a patient with multinodular goiter showed brown fat tissue and revealed the presence of UCP1.

The findings of Virtanen and van Marken Lichtenbelt groups suggest that brown fat is present and can be activated in nearly all, at least young and healthy, humans. Moreover, these findings and the wide range of reported incidences in other studies indicate that brown fat activity is greatly influenced by patient-related and environmental factors before or during FDG-PET scanning. Several studies have assessed these factors, and are discussed in the following sections. Numerous studies have assessed the influence of multiple factors not only on the incidence, but on the degree of brown fat activity as well.[9–11,15,23–26] Although measurements of brown fat activity have been well performed and delicately elaborated, these data are not discussed separately. Factors influencing the degree of brown fat activity are the same as those influencing the incidence of brown fat activation, as was shown in these studies. It should be kept in mind that brown fat activation is not simply an on-off phenomenon, but is a more gradational process. Regarding this, most of the discussed factors should be regarded as modulators of brown fat activation, not as prerequisites. However, some factors may have a threshold under which no brown fat activation takes place and above which a "dose-dependent" degree of brown fat activity takes place. This situation may especially apply to sympathetic stimulants like cold temperature and exposure to sympathetic activity modulating agents. Furthermore, brown fat activity is related to brown fat volume, and larger amounts of brown fat are able to generate more heat. Barnard and colleagues[27] showed that brown fat activity and volume were increased in rats that were chronically exposed to cold environments. Smaller mammals have a higher surface area to body weight ratio, which causes more heat dissipation and makes them more vulnerable to hypothermia. In smaller mammals, heat generation by brown fat is crucial for thermoregulation. With increasing age and size, relative functional capacity of BAT decreases in larger mammals.[28] From the aforementioned autopsy studies in humans, it was known that infants have a more extensive distribution pattern of brown fat than adults.[5] Infants also possess a greater volume of brown fat tissue relative to total body weight. Enerbäck and colleagues[29] report that whereas brown fat makes up 5% to 10% of the total body weight in mice, the corresponding values in infants and adults are estimated to be 2% to 5% and 0.05% to 0.1%, respectively. The relationship between brown fat activity and volume is supported by the studies of Ouellet and colleagues[15] and Pfannenberg and colleagues,[25] who found a clear overlap between factors that influence brown fat activation and brown fat volume in human adults. Visualization of FDG uptake in brown fat is dependent on spatial resolution and on signal to background ratio (which depends on brown fat volume and degree of activation along with FDG uptake in surrounding tissues). Recognition of brown fat uptake on imaging also depends on the skill and time availability of the interpreting physicians, and on the availability of other imaging modalities for comparison purposes. All these considerations have to be taken into account when assessing studies that report on the incidence of brown fat activation and the factors that influence brown fat activation.

Temperature

In the absence of pathology such as endocrine malignancy, which has been reported to be associated with brown fat activation, exposure to cold temperature is the main stimulus for brown fat activation.[30,31] This is not unexpected, as the function of brown fat is to produce heat to maintain thermoregulation under cold circumstances. Significantly higher incidences of brown fat activation were found during cold seasons or with lower room temperature in multiple retrospective studies.[15,18,23,24,32,33] These factors remained significant in some large multivariate analyses.[15,18,24] The largest study to date comprising 6652 PET/CT scans in 4842 patients had been performed by Ouellet and colleagues.[15] These investigators found a significant inverse relationship between the incidence of brown

fat activation and outdoor temperature on the day of scanning ($P<.0001$), despite patients having stayed for 60 minutes in a 24°C room between FDG injection and PET scanning. Cohade and colleagues[32] found the strongest correlation between low environmental temperature and brown fat activation after a prolonged period of cold weather. However, Kim and colleagues[33] suggest that brown fat activation is merely an acute response to cold weather. The findings of Ouellet and colleagues[15] seem to favor the latter idea, because although during the cold season (winter) a higher incidence of brown fat activation was seen ($P = .04$), the already described inverse relationship with temperature on the day of scanning was stronger. Finally, a few studies, including the aforementioned studies of Virtanen and colleagues and van Marken Lichtenbelt and colleagues, implemented induction of brown fat activation by acute exposure of subjects to cold conditions.[9–11,26] An interesting finding, reported by several different studies, was that brown fat activation was associated more with photoperiod (day length) than with environmental temperature.[15,23] With a shorter day, the incidence of brown fat activation was found to be higher, although this was not confirmed in a multivariate analysis.

Age

Age is the most studied patient-related factor influencing brown fat activation. As in smaller mammals, thermoregulation in infants and children relies more on heat generation by brown fat than it does in adults, because of their relatively high body surface area to weight ratio. Although no direct measurements of brown fat activity in infants are available, the abundance of brown fat in infants supports this view. Moreover, higher incidences of brown fat activation are seen in children. Compared with older adults, young adults consistently show a higher incidence of brown fat activation as well.[8,11,12,15,18,19,24,25,32–36] This observation remains significant in multivariate analyses, regardless of other influencing factors such as body mass index (BMI), which tends to be higher in older adults.[12,15,18,24,25] Although brown fat is less important for thermogenesis after attainment of adult body proportions, the findings show that brown fat functionality is maintained for several decades of human life but eventually decreases with increasing age.

Gender

Significantly higher female to male incidence ratios of brown fat activation are described, ranging from 1.5:1 to 6.7:1.[8,12,18,19,23–25,32,33,36] Some studies reported an age by gender interaction, albeit with conflicting directions of this interaction.[15,25] However, in multivariate analysis most studies found gender to be an independent factor affecting brown fat activation.[12,15,18,24,25] An explanation for this observation may be found in the sexual dimorphism that has been reported in animal studies. It was shown that testosterone decreases brown fat activity.[37] Regarding female sex hormones, ambivalent results have been reported. Bartness and Wade[38] report that estrogen increases brown fat activity, while Abelenda and colleagues[39] found that 17β-estradiol and progesterone inhibit brown fat activation. Whether independent or by interaction with sex hormones, another mechanism might involve gender-dependent differences in temperature threshold for brown fat activation. Under thermoneutral circumstances (22°C), female rats possess greater amounts of active brown fat tissue in relation to their body weight.[37] However, when both sexes were exposed to cold temperatures (4°C), this difference disappeared. If interest, Saito and colleagues[11] noted no difference in brown fat activity between male and female human subjects after exposure to cold (in a 19°C room) while wearing light clothing and intermittently placing their legs on an ice block.

Body Mass Index

The BMI measures a person's weight (kg) in relation to the square of height (m). A high BMI reflects a high body mass compared with length. Subjects with a lower BMI therefore have a higher surface area to body weight ratio. BMI has been found to be inversely correlated with brown fat activation.[10–12,15,18,22,24,25,35] In most prospective or multivariate analyses, this correlation remained significant.[10–12,15,24,25] It is striking that the only subject in 24 volunteers studied by van Marken Lichtenbelt and colleagues[10] that showed no brown fat activation during cold exposure was the one with the highest BMI (38.7 kg/m^2). Low BMI, and thus higher surface area to body weight ratio, causes more heat dissipation, as mentioned earlier. Therefore, it seems plausible that subjects with lower BMI show higher incidences of brown fat activation. This process may even take place under "thermoneutral" temperatures of 22°C, which may actually be too cold for subjects with lower BMI while lying still during FDG-PET preparation and scanning.

Other Determinants

Of the other potentially influential factors regarding brown fat activation, one of the most described is the plasma glucose level. Several studies have found this factor to be inversely correlated with brown fat activity, although none found plasma glucose level to be an independent factor in multivariate analysis.[11,12,14,15,18] Only Ouellet and colleagues[15] found the diabetic state to be associated with lower incidences of brown fat activation ($P = .0003$). These findings would imply that in the absence of diabetes, plasma glucose levels do not influence brown fat activity, whereas insulin resistance may decrease brown fat activity. This finding is supported by the study of Saito and colleagues,[11] who found a significant inverse relation of brown fat activity with plasma insulin levels. These findings have incited the idea that the metabolic syndrome may be related in some way to brown fat activity, which may provide new directions in the study of novel therapeutics against diabetes and obesity.

Hadi and colleagues[30] found higher levels of circulating catecholamines to be related to brown fat activation in groups of patients with and without pheochromocytoma (n = 65 and n = 27, respectively, and $P = .01$). Cypess and colleagues[18] found smoking to be correlated with a lower incidence of brown fat activation ($P = .02$). This result is somewhat paradoxic, as nicotine is known to be a sympathetic stimulant. Both studies did not confirm their findings in multivariate analyses. However, these reports indicate that the sympathetic involvement in brown fat activation in humans corresponds with what is observed in rodents, as discussed later.

STRATEGIES TO REDUCE OR HANDLE BROWN FAT FDG UPTAKE

As mentioned earlier, brown fat uptake on routine clinical FDG-PET scanning is an undesirable phenomenon. In the following sections methods to prevent, diminish, or deal with brown fat uptake on FDG-PET scanning are discussed.

Nonpharmacologic Methods

Preventing exposure to cold temperature
As a major factor, or perhaps even a prerequisite, for brown fat activation, exposure to cold temperature is an obvious factor to avoid. It is easily achieved, does not bring inconvenience for the patient, and avoids the use of medication. Many studies have observed a decrease in or resolution of brown fat FDG uptake during repeat PET scanning under warmer conditions.[10,40,41] Whether a high environmental temperature is able to eliminate brown fat uptake has been prospectively assessed in multiple studies. Christensen and colleagues[40] achieved complete or near-complete resolution in 9 of 10 patients. These investigators concluded that

instructing patients to dress warmly and to avoid exposure to cold during transit to the imaging center, along with covering patients with blankets in a 22°C to 24°C room during the 60 to 90 minutes between radiotracer injection and PET imaging, was sufficient to effectively prevent brown fat uptake. Garcia and colleagues[41] reported similar findings with an additional preinjection phase of up to 2 hours in a room with a temperature of at least 24°C Zukotynski and colleagues[42] eliminated brown fat uptake in 13 of 14 pediatric patients by increasing room temperature from 21°C to 24°C 30 minutes before and 60 minutes after radiotracer injection. These studies suggest that avoidance of cold exposure and an environmental temperature of 24°C at least 30 minutes before injection might be reasonable and sufficient to prevent FDG uptake in brown fat. Larger-scale prospective studies may determine the optimal temperature for this purpose.

Diet

Williams and Kolodny[43] reasoned that as fatty acid loading suppresses glucose metabolism in the myocardium, this mechanism might be applicable to another mitochondria-rich tissue, namely, brown fat. These investigators retrospectively studied 1970 FDG-PET scans obtained during winter months (October 2002 to April 2003), and observed a significantly lower incidence of brown fat uptake in the 741 scans when patients had a high-fat, low-carbohydrate dietary preparation the night before and on the day of scanning compared with 1229 scans when patients were fasted on the day of scanning ($P<.0002$). Furthermore, blood glucose levels were significantly lower in the high-fat dietary preparation group. These data do not provide direct evidence of prevention of brown fat uptake, but suggest an interesting influence of diet on brown fat activation.

Avoidance of sympathetic stimulants

From animal studies, it is known that sympathetic stimulation with nicotine, ephedrine, or ketamine causes brown fat activation.[44,45] However, in these studies caffeine did not have a significant influence on brown fat uptake. As mentioned earlier, higher levels of catecholamines were associated with brown fat uptake in humans as well.[30] These data suggest that patients should avoid the use of sympathetic stimulating substances prior to PET scanning in order to decrease FDG uptake in brown fat.

Pharmacologic Methods

Reducing sympathetic activity

The most effective pharmacologic intervention to reduce brown fat uptake is most likely blockade of sympathetic activity. As brown fat adipocytes are under direct control of sympathetic nerves and circulating catecholamines, blockade of these pathways substantially reduces brown fat activity.[28] Tatsumi and colleagues[44] have prospectively studied the effect of sympathetic blocking agents in rodents. A first group of rodents was treated with ketamine-based anesthesia or with a sympathetic activity stimulating agent, or exposed to cold. Histologic examinations showed that uptake in brown fat increased 14-fold and 4.9-fold, respectively. In contradistinction, FDG uptake in brown fat significantly decreased to 16% and 28% of baseline after injection of high doses of propranolol (a β-blocking agent) and reserpine (a catecholamine blocking agent), respectively. Similarly, PET/CT showed only faint to mild FDG uptake in brown fat in the second group of rodents as opposed to intense uptake in the first group. Some other organs also had a marked decrease in FDG uptake. For instance, myocardial uptake decreased to 30% to 40% of baseline values for both the propranolol group and the reserpine group. Therefore, Tatsumi and colleagues[44] suggested that sympathetic blockade may diminish FDG uptake in pathologic processes as well; this would warrant clinical testing before widespread routine administration of β-blockers could be implemented. However, in their experience, active tumors and inflammation generally show intense FDG uptake regardless of the degree of FDG uptake in brown fat or sympathetic activity. Furthermore, sympathetic blockade for various other indications such as hypertension does not seem to interfere with the interpretation of routine clinical FDG-PET.

Studies in human subjects seem to confirm the effectiveness of reducing sympathetic activity as well.[46] Parysow and colleagues[46] found increased FDG uptake in brown fat in 26 cancer patients, representing 3.2% of the total number of studies performed. Repeated PET scanning after administering a single dose of 20 mg propranolol orally 60 minutes before FDG injection was performed within 2 to 14 days. Mean basal brown fat maximum standardized uptake value (SUV_{max}) was 5.52 ± 2.3, whereas mean SUV_{max} after propranolol was 1.39 ± 0.42 ($P<.0001$). This action reduced brown fat uptake in all patients sufficiently enough to discern brown fat from malignant tissue. Although no immediate administration of propranolol and subsequent rescanning was performed, the investigators stated that scanning conditions on the different occasions were comparable. Similar results in similarly designed studies were reported by Soderlund and colleagues[47] and Agrawal and colleagues,[48] using a single oral dose of 80 mg propranolol 2 hours before and 40 mg propranolol 60 minutes before FDG injection, respectively. Soderlund and colleagues found complete or near-complete resolution of brown fat uptake in all 11 patients, whereas Agrawal and colleagues found resolution in 36 of 40 (90%) patients.[47,48] In their studies, Parysow and colleagues[46] and Soderlund and colleagues[47] addressed the suggestion of Tatsumi and colleagues[44] that sympathetic blockade may obscure pathologic processes. After administration of propranolol, no significant reduction of FDG uptake was found in malignant tissues. Parysow and colleagues reported a basal mean tumor SUV_{max} of 8.07 ± 6.4 and 7.88 ± 5.9 before and after propranolol administration, respectively ($P = .53$). Soderlund and colleagues found a mean tumor SUV_{max} change from 2.4 ± 1.3 to 2.7 ± 1.1 before and after propranolol, respectively. These data imply that a single oral dose of 20 mg propranolol 60 minutes before FDG injection is an effective and safe method to suppress brown fat activation. A representative image of brown fat uptake before and after administering a single dose of 80 mg propranolol is shown in **Fig. 1**.

Sedatives

The use of a single dose of oral diazepam before scanning has been advocated to diminish muscular uptake through its muscle-relaxant effect.[16] In several studies, the effect of benzodiazepines on brown tissue FDG uptake has been investigated.[35,44,49–51] The brown fat adipocyte is known to express benzodiazepine receptors, which appear to be able to downregulate brown fat activity.[52] In addition, the central anxiolytic effect of benzodiazepines may diminish sympathetic nervous system activity. Nonetheless, no significant reduction of brown fat activity has been demonstrated either in rodent studies using high-dose intravenous diazepam or in human subjects receiving moderate doses (up to 10 mg) of oral diazepam.[44,49–51]

Among other drugs, opiates are known to decrease the central temperature threshold for cold-induced responses.[53] Gelfand and colleagues[49] retrospectively assessed the effect of a single dose of intravenous fentanyl (≤ 1 μg/kg, maximum of 50 μg) premedication on the FDG uptake in brown fat tissue. These investigators reviewed 118 PET scans in a pediatric population from 69 patients. A significant reduction of brown fat activity in patients treated with intravenous fentanyl was reported as compared with low-dose oral diazepam or no drugs ($P<.004$). However, Gelfand and colleagues state that compared

with oral β-blockers, the use of fentanyl might be too laborious for practical clinical use because of the requirement for patient monitoring.

Other Solutions

If preventive measurements fail, brown fat uptake may complicate correct interpretation of the PET images. Comparison with CT images can have great additional value and may prevent incorrect interpretation.[6,7,19,22] Correct coregistration of PET and CT images is important, so hybrid PET/CT scanning is preferred.

Kim and colleagues[17] proposed the idea of evaluating patterns of brown fat activation to differentiate between malignant tissue and brown fat uptake when CT coregistration is not available (see section "Typical sites of appearance"). Brown fat uptake in one region would generally be symmetric and accompanied by brown fat uptake in another region. However, Truong and colleagues[19] reported differently, finding brown fat uptake in 15 of 845 oncologic patients. Of these, 5 patients showed focal hypermetabolic brown fat isolated to the mediastinum. Hence, this should be regarded as an unreliable method.

Box 1 gives a summary of information about brown fat.

Box 1
Summary of information about brown fat

1. Brown Fat Sites of Predilection

    a. Supraclavicular area
    b. Mediastinum
    c. Paravertebral area
    d. Perinephric area

2. Brown Fat Activation Stimulating Factors

    a. Cold exposure
    b. Young age
    c. Female gender
    d. Low BMI
    e. Nondiabetic state
    f. Sympathetic stimulants

3. Strategies to Reduce Brown Fat Uptake (in order of effectiveness)

    a. Avoiding cold exposure
    b. Ambient temperature $\geq 24°C$ from 30 minutes before FDG injection
    c. Oral propranolol before FDG injection
    d. Intravenous fentanyl before FDG injection
    e. High-fat, low-carbohydrate diet ≥ 12 hours prior to PET scanning
    f. Avoidance of sympathetic stimulants on day of PET scanning

QUANTIFICATION OF BROWN FAT FDG UPTAKE ON PET IMAGING

An interesting method to differentiate brown fat from malignant tissue was proposed by Alkhawaldeh and Alavi,[54] who studied the degree and pattern of FDG uptake in brown fat on dual time-point FDG-PET imaging in response to many studies, and reported promising results of this technique in differentiating benign from malignant lesions. Dual time-point FDG-PET imaging obtained at 1 and 2 hours after injection of FDG typically shows a decrease in SUV in benign and an increase in SUV in malignant lesions over time. Malignant cells typically express high numbers of glucose transporters on their membranes, as well as high levels of hexokinase and low levels of glucose-6-phosphatase. These findings lead to

an accumulation of FDG within the malignant cell, enhancing the contrast between malignant lesions and the normal surrounding tissues.[55] However, on dual time-point imaging, there was a progressive increase (12%–192%) in SUV_{max} within most (76%) of the hypermetabolic brown fat areas. In some instances, there even was an increase in the number of visualized brown fat areas. Esen and colleagues[56] reported similar results on acquiring images 1 and 2 hours after FDG injection. FDG uptake increased in 80.6% of brown fat areas for an average increase of 69% $\pm$ 25%. Alkhawaldeh and Alavi[54] suggested that the high mitochondrial level in the brown fat adipocyte may account for this phenomenon. Levels of glucose-6-phosphatase and hexokinase, unlike in malignancy, would not be an explanation. From these studies, it appears that this approach

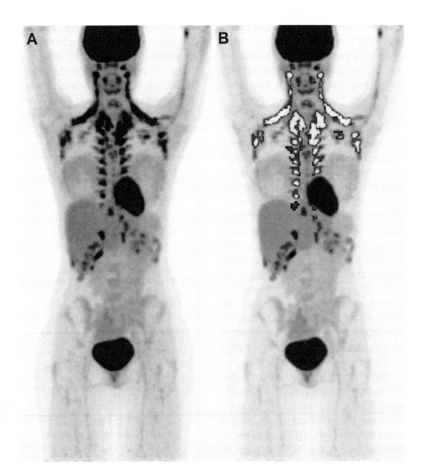

Fig. 3. Coronal MIP PET image without (A) and with (B) computer-assisted color-overlay segmentation from FDG-PET/CT examination of a 23-year-old woman with a history of Hodgkin lymphoma. Note typical symmetric distribution of FDG uptake within brown fat in neck, supraclavicular fossae, and paravertebral locations. Through use of computer-assisted segmentation and quantification (ROVER software, ABX GmbH, Germany) (B), brown fat total metabolically active volume (MAV) (141.57 cc), total mean metabolic volumetric product (MVP_{mean}) (656.72 SUV cc), and total partial volume corrected mean metabolic volumetric product ($cMVP_{mean}$) (1823.33 SUV cc) were calculated.

does not discriminate between FDG uptake in brown fat and malignant lesions. However, Basu and colleagues[57] reported continued FDG accumulation in malignant tissues seen on PET imaging during an extended time course of 8 hours in 3 patients with non–small cell lung carcinoma, whereas surrounding normal tissues showed declining or stable values with time. Studies assessing brown fat uptake over longer time periods may provide insight regarding whether dual time-point FDG-PET imaging with a prolonged interval can differentiate between brown fat and malignant tissue, although this may be impractical to perform in clinical practice because of the prolonged patient wait times.

Technical considerations other than timing of image acquisition also have to be taken into account when quantifying brown fat uptake. Technical factors such as image reconstruction parameters and attenuation correction methods can affect SUV measurements. SUV_{max} increases with the number of iterations of correction. Artifacts due to patient motion and misregistration may also affect SUV. Partial volume effects severely affect the accuracy of SUV measurements, leading to an underestimation of the true values. To overcome this problem, the exact volume of a lesion of interest can be defined by measuring the true lesion size on coregistered CT or from PET images using computer-assisted methods, allowing for assessment of FDG uptake in the true lesion volume. Moreover, multiple volumes of interest can be identified and assessed quantitatively.[58,59] As such, brown fat total metabolically active volume (MAV), total mean metabolic volumetric product ($MVP_{mean} = SUV_{mean} \times MAV$), and total partial volume corrected mean metabolic volumetric product ($cMVP_{mean}$ = partial volume corrected $SUV_{mean} \times MAV$) can be calculated using computer-assisted methods.[59] This approach provides for practical quantitative global assessment of the amount and degree of activity of active brown fat in human subjects. See **Fig. 3** for a representative image. These quantifications may help to further understand brown fat metabolism in pathologic conditions such as obesity and diabetes, and to provide a means for quantitative response assessment. PET/magnetic resonance imaging (MRI) technology may also be useful for localization and quantification of brown fat.[60]

SUMMARY

In recent years there has been a tremendous increase of interest in brown fat. Brown fat is present and metabolically active in adults, and is involved in physiologic and presumably pathologic

processes as well. Sites of predilection for brown fat are the supraclavicular, mediastinal, paravertebral, and perinephric areas. Exposure to cold temperature is more or less a prerequisite for brown fat activation, whereas age, gender, and BMI are the major modulating factors. Brown fat activation can seriously interfere with correct FDG-PET image interpretation if not recognized, although this can be overcome through hybrid PET/CT and PET/MRI technologies. Identification of typical distribution patterns, as well as pharmacologic and non-pharmacologic interventions to reduce brown fat uptake, can also be applied to overcome this problem. Advanced quantitative PET imaging techniques may be used to quantify total brown fat volume and metabolic activity for assessment prior to and following various interventions, and will likely to contribute to further understanding of brown fat.

REFERENCES

1. Enerbäck S. The origins of brown adipose tissue. N Engl J Med 2009;360(19):2021–3.
2. Aquila H, Link TA, Klingenberg M. The uncoupling protein from brown fat mitochondria is related to the mitochondrial ADP/ATP carrier. Analysis of sequence homologies and of folding of the protein in the membrane. EMBO J 1985;4(9):2369–76.
3. Heaton GM, Wagenvoord RJ, Kemp A Jr, et al. Brown-adipose-tissue mitochondria: photoaffinity labelling of the regulatory site of energy dissipation. Eur J Biochem 1978;82(2):515–21.
4. Lean ME. Brown adipose tissue in humans. Proc Nutr Soc 1989;48(2):243–56.
5. Heaton JM. The distribution of brown adipose tissue in the human. J Anat 1972;112(Pt 1):35–9.
6. Hany TF, Gharehpapagh E, Kamel EM, et al. Brown adipose tissue: a factor to consider in symmetrical tracer uptake in the neck and upper chest region. Eur J Nucl Med Mol Imaging 2002;29(10):1393–8.
7. Cohade C, Osman M, Pannu HK, et al. Uptake in supraclavicular area fat ("USA-Fat"): description on ^{18}F-FDG PET/CT. J Nucl Med 2003;44(2):170–6.
8. Yeung HW, Grewal RK, Gonen M, et al. Patterns of (18)F-FDG uptake in adipose tissue and muscle: a potential source of false-positives for PET. J Nucl Med 2003;44(11):1789–96.
9. Virtanen KA, Lidell ME, Orava J, et al. Functional brown adipose tissue in healthy adults. N Engl J Med 2009;360(15):1518–25.
10. van Marken Lichtenbelt WD, Vanhommerig JW, Smulders NM, et al. Cold-activated brown adipose tissue in healthy men. N Engl J Med 2009;360(15):1500–8.
11. Saito M, Okamatsu-Ogura Y, Matsushita M, et al. High incidence of metabolically active brown adipose tissue in healthy adult humans: effects of

cold exposure and adiposity. Diabetes 2009;58(7): 1526–31.

12. Lee P, Greenfield JR, Ho KK, et al. A critical appraisal of the prevalence and metabolic significance of brown adipose tissue in adult humans. Am J Physiol Endocrinol Metab 2010;299(4):E601–6.

13. Ravussin E, Kozak LP. Have we entered the brown adipose tissue renaissance? Obes Rev 2009;10(3): 265–8.

14. Jacene HA, Cohade CC, Zhang Z, et al. The relationship between patients' serum glucose levels and metabolically active brown adipose tissue detected by PET/CT. Mol Imaging Biol 2010. [Epub ahead of print].

15. Ouellet V, Routhier-Labadie A, Bellemare W, et al. Outdoor temperature, age, sex, body mass index, and diabetic status determine the prevalence, mass, and glucose-uptake activity of ^{18}F-FDG-detected BAT in humans. J Clin Endocrinol Metab 2011;96(1):192–9.

16. Barrington SF, Maisey MN. Skeletal muscle uptake of fluorine-18-FDG: effect of oral diazepam. J Nucl Med 1996;37(7):1127–9.

17. Kim S, Krynyckyi BR, Machac J, et al. Concomitant paravertebral FDG uptake helps differentiate supraclavicular and suprarenal brown fat uptake from malignant uptake when CT coregistration is not available. Clin Nucl Med 2006;31(3):127–30.

18. Cypess AM, Lehman S, Williams G, et al. Identification and importance of brown adipose tissue in adult humans. N Engl J Med 2009;360(15):1509–17.

19. Truong MT, Erasmus JJ, Munden RF, et al. Focal FDG uptake in mediastinal brown fat mimicking malignancy: a potential pitfall resolved on PET/CT. AJR Am J Roentgenol 2004;183(4):1127–32.

20. Lebron L, Chou AJ, Carrasquillo JA. Interesting image. Unilateral F-18 FDG uptake in the neck, in patients with sympathetic denervation. Clin Nucl Med 2010;35(11):899–901.

21. Cohade C. Altered biodistribution on FDG-PET with emphasis on brown fat and insulin effect. Semin Nucl Med 2010;40(4):283–93.

22. Rousseau C, Bourbouloux E, Campion L, et al. Brown fat in breast cancer patients: analysis of serial (18)F-FDG PET/CT scans. Eur J Nucl Med Mol Imaging 2006;33(7):785–91.

23. Au-Yong IT, Thorn N, Ganatra R, et al. Brown adipose tissue and seasonal variation in humans. Diabetes 2009;58(11):2583–7.

24. Pace L, Nicolai E, D'Amico D, et al. Determinants of physiologic (18)F-FDG uptake in brown adipose tissue in sequential PET/CT examinations. Mol Imaging Biol 2010. [Epub ahead of print].

25. Pfannenberg C, Werner MK, Ripkens S, et al. Impact of age on the relationships of brown adipose tissue with sex and adiposity in humans. Diabetes 2010; 59(7):1789–93.

26. Yoneshiro T, Aita S, Matsushita M, et al. Brown adipose tissue, whole-body energy expenditure, and thermogenesis in healthy adult men. Obesity (Silver Spring) 2011;19(1):13–6.

27. Barnard T, Skala J, Lindberg O. Changes in interscapular brown adipose tissue of the rat during perinatal and early postnatal development and after cold acclimation. I. Activities of some respiratory enzymes in the tissue. Comp Biochem Physiol 1970;33(3):499–508.

28. Cannon B, Nedergaard J. Brown adipose tissue: function and physiological significance. Physiol Rev 2004;84(1):277–359.

29. Enerbäck S. Human brown adipose tissue. Cell Metab 2010;11(4):248–52.

30. Hadi M, Chen CC, Whatley M, et al. Brown fat imaging with (18)F-6-fluorodopamine PET/CT, (18) F-FDG PET/CT, and (123)I-MIBG SPECT: a study of patients being evaluated for pheochromocytoma. J Nucl Med 2007;48(7):1077–83.

31. Kuji I, Imabayashi E, Minagawa A, et al. Brown adipose tissue demonstrating intense FDG uptake in a patient with mediastinal pheochromocytoma. Ann Nucl Med 2008;22(3):231–5.

32. Cohade C, Mourtzikos KA, Wahl RL. "USA-Fat": prevalence is related to ambient outdoor temperature-evaluation with ^{18}F-FDG PET/CT. J Nucl Med 2003; 44(8):1267–70.

33. Kim S, Krynyckyi BR, Machac J, et al. Temporal relation between temperature change and FDG uptake in brown adipose tissue. Eur J Nucl Med Mol Imaging 2008;35(5):984–9.

34. Bar-Shalom R, Gaitini D, Keidar Z, et al. Non-malignant FDG uptake in infradiaphragmatic adipose tissue: a new site of physiological tracer biodistribution characterised by PET/CT. Eur J Nucl Med Mol Imaging 2004;31(8):1105–13.

35. Dobert N, Menzel C, Hamscho N, et al. Atypical thoracic and supraclavicular FDG-uptake in patients with Hodgkin's and non-Hodgkin's lymphoma. Q J Nucl Med Mol Imaging 2004;48(1):33–8.

36. Wehrli NE, Bural G, Houseni M, et al. Determination of age-related changes in structure and function of skin, adipose tissue, and skeletal muscle with computed tomography, magnetic resonance imaging, and positron emission tomography. Semin Nucl Med 2007;37(3):195–205.

37. Rodriguez-Cuenca S, Pujol E, Justo R, et al. Sex-dependent thermogenesis, differences in mitochondrial morphology and function, and adrenergic response in brown adipose tissue. J Biol Chem 2002;277(45):42958–63.

38. Bartness TJ, Wade GN. Effects of interscapular brown adipose tissue denervation on body weight and energy metabolism in ovariectomized and estradiol-treated rats. Behav Neurosci 1984;98(4): 674–85.

39. Abelenda M, Castro C, Venero C, et al. Reduced oxygen consumption of brown adipocytes isolated from progesterone-treated rats. Can J Physiol Pharmacol 1994;72(10):1226–30.

40. Christensen CR, Clark PB, Morton KA. Reversal of hypermetabolic brown adipose tissue in F-18 FDG PET imaging. Clin Nucl Med 2006;31(4):193–6.

41. Garcia CA, Van ND, Atkins F, et al. Reduction of brown fat 2-deoxy-2-[F-18]fluoro-D-glucose uptake by controlling environmental temperature prior to positron emission tomography scan. Mol Imaging Biol 2006;8(1):24–9.

42. Zukotynski KA, Fahey FH, Laffin S, et al. Seasonal variation in the effect of constant ambient temperature of 24 degrees C in reducing FDG uptake by brown adipose tissue in children. Eur J Nucl Med Mol Imaging 2010;37(10):1854–60.

43. Williams G, Kolodny GM. Method for decreasing uptake of ^{18}F-FDG by hypermetabolic brown adipose tissue on PET. AJR Am J Roentgenol 2008;190(5): 1406–9.

44. Tatsumi M, Engles JM, Ishimori T, et al. Intense (18)F-FDG uptake in brown fat can be reduced pharmacologically. J Nucl Med 2004;45(7):1189–93.

45. Baba S, Tatsumi M, Ishimori T, et al. Effect of nicotine and ephedrine on the accumulation of ^{18}F-FDG in brown adipose tissue. J Nucl Med 2007; 48(6):981–6.

46. Parysow O, Mollerach AM, Jager V, et al. Low-dose oral propranolol could reduce brown adipose tissue F-18 FDG uptake in patients undergoing PET scans. Clin Nucl Med 2007;32(5):351–7.

47. Soderlund V, Larsson SA, Jacobsson H. Reduction of FDG uptake in brown adipose tissue in clinical patients by a single dose of propranolol. Eur J Nucl Med Mol Imaging 2007;34(7):1018–22.

48. Agrawal A, Nair N, Baghel NS. A novel approach for reduction of brown fat uptake on FDG PET. Br J Radiol 2009;82(980):626–31.

49. Gelfand MJ, O'Hara SM, Curtwright LA, et al. Premedication to block [(18)F]FDG uptake in the brown adipose tissue of pediatric and adolescent patients. Pediatr Radiol 2005;35(10):984–90.

50. Sturkenboom MG, Hoekstra OS, Postema EJ, et al. A randomised controlled trial assessing the effect of oral diazepam on ^{18}F-FDG uptake in the neck and upper chest region. Mol Imaging Biol 2009; 11(5):364–8.

51. Aukema TS, Vogel WV, Hoefnagel CA, et al. Prevention of brown adipose tissue activation in ^{18}F-FDG PET/CT of breast cancer patients receiving neoadjuvant systemic therapy. J Nucl Med Technol 2010; 38(1):24–7.

52. Gonzalez SC, Romeo HE, Rosenstein RE, et al. Benzodiazepine binding sites in rat interscapular brown adipose tissue: effect of cold environment, denervation and endocrine ablations. Life Sci 1988;42(4):393–402.

53. Alfonsi P. Postanaesthetic shivering: epidemiology, pathophysiology, and approaches to prevention and management. Drugs 2001;61(15):2193–205.

54. Alkhawaldeh K, Alavi A. Quantitative assessment of FDG uptake in brown fat using standardized uptake value and dual-time-point scanning. Clin Nucl Med 2008;33(10):663–7.

55. Sanz-Viedma S, Torigian DA, Parsons M, et al. Potential clinical utility of dual time point FDG-PET for distinguishing benign from malignant lesions: implications for oncological imaging. Rev Esp Med Nucl 2009;28(3):159–66.

56. Esen AB, Gokaslan D, Guner L, et al. FDG uptake in brown adipose tissue—a brief report on brown fat with FDG uptake mechanisms and quantitative analysis using dual-time-point FDG PET/CT. Rev Esp Med Nucl 2011;30(1):14–8.

57. Basu S, Kung J, Houseni M, et al. Temporal profile of fluorodeoxyglucose uptake in malignant lesions and normal organs over extended time periods in patients with lung carcinoma: implications for its utilization in assessing malignant lesions. Q J Nucl Med Mol Imaging 2009;53(1):9–19.

58. Basu S, Zaidi H, Houseni M, et al. Novel quantitative techniques for assessing regional and global function and structure based on modern imaging modalities: implications for normal variation, aging and diseased states. Semin Nucl Med 2007;37(3):223–39.

59. Torigian DA, Lopez RF, Alapati S, et al. Feasibility and performance of novel software to quantify metabolically active volumes and 3D partial volume corrected SUVs and metabolic volumetric products of spinal bone marrow metastases on FDG-PET/CT. Hell J Nucl Med 2011;14(1):8–14.

60. Hofmann M, Pichler B, Scholkopf B, et al. Towards quantitative PET/MRI: a review of MR-based attenuation correction techniques. Eur J Nucl Med Mol Imaging 2009;36(Suppl 1):S93–104.

Index

Note: Page numbers of article titles are in **boldface** type.

PET Clin 6 (2011) 377–381
doi:10.1016/S1556-8598(11)00088-5
1556-8598/11/$ – see front matter © 2011 Elsevier Inc. All rights reserved.

pet.theclinics.com

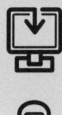

Printed and bound by CPI Group (UK) Ltd, Croydon, CR0 4YY

03/10/2024

01040356-0019